Manual of Traumatic Brain Injury Management

Manual of Traumatic Brain Injury Management

Felise S. Zollman, MD
Co-Project Director
Midwest Regional Traumatic Brain Injury Model System Center

Attending Physician
Brain Injury Medicine and Rehabilitation Program
Rehabilitation Institute of Chicago

Assistant Professor
Departments of Physical Medicine and Rehabilitation & Neurology
Northwestern University Feinberg School of Medicine
Chicago, Illinois

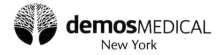

demosMEDICAL
New York

ISBN: 978-1-936287-01-7
eBook ISBN: 978-1-935281-99-3

Acquisitions Editor: Beth Barry
Cover Design: Joe Tenerelli
Compositor: Newgen Imaging
Printer: Hamilton Printing

Visit our website at www.demosmedpub.com

Medicine is an ever-changing science. Research and clinical experience are continually expanding our knowledge, in particular our understanding of proper treatment and drug therapy. The authors, editors, and publisher have made every effort to ensure that all information in this book is in accordance with the state of knowledge at the time of production of the book. Nevertheless, the authors, editors, and publisher are not responsible for errors or omissions or for any consequences from application of the information in this book and make no warranty, express or implied, with respect to the contents of the publication. Every reader should examine carefully the package inserts accompanying each drug and should carefully check whether the dosage schedules mentioned therein or the contraindications stated by the manufacturer differ from the statements made in this book. Such examination is particularly important with drugs that are either rarely used or have been newly released on the market.

Library of Congress Cataloging-in-Publication Data
Manual of traumatic brain injury management / [edited by] Felise S. Zollman.
    p. ; cm.
Includes bibliographical references and index.
ISBN 978-1-936287-01-7
    1. Brain damage—Treatment.   2. Brain damage—Patients—Rehabilitation.
I. Zollman, Felise S. [DNLM: 1. Brain Injuries. WL 354]
RC387.5.M35 2011
617.4981044—dc22   2010054444

Made in the United States of America
12 13 14 15   5 4 3

Contents

Part 5   Traumatic Brain Injury–Related Medical Complications

PART 6 Special Considerations and Traumatic Brain Injury Resources

Preface

The occurrence—and varied manifestations—of traumatic brain injury (TBI) has garnered a great deal of attention in recent years. From sports concussion to severe injuries resulting from motor vehicle collisions or falls to brain injury in the military, issues facing providers caring for those with TBI are wide-ranging and complex. The *Manual of Traumatic Brain Injury Management* has been developed to address the varied needs of clinicians who work with individuals who have sustained a traumatic brain injury. What makes this book unique is that, as a pocket guide, it is designed to provide relevant clinical information in a succinct, readily accessible format. For readers who wish to understand a particular subject in more depth, each chapter concludes with a short list of web-based resources, seminal journal articles, and pertinent textbooks for further exploration.

This book is organized into six parts. Part 1 provides an introduction to core concepts in TBI. Part 2 addresses the epidemiology of TBI as well as injury prevention. Part 3 covers the spectrum of issues pertaining to mild traumatic brain injury (MTBI), including sports concussion, long term sequelae of MTBI, post-concussion disorder, and the co-occurrence of MTBI and post-traumatic stress disorder. Part 4 focuses on moderate to severe TBI, including the spectrum of acute care issues, from pre-hospital care to neurosurgical and intensive care unit management to the transition to the next level of care (e.g., inpatient rehabilitation) and the role of members of the rehabilitation team in caring for those with TBI. Management of the cognitive, behavioral and affective manifestations of TBI is addressed, as is prognosis after TBI and community reintegration. Part 5 discusses TBI-related medical complications, such as postraumatic seizures, endocrine dysfunction, and spasticity. Finally, Part 6 addresses special considerations in TBI management, including TBI in the military, pediatric TBI and TBI in the older adult, use of complementary and alternative medicine modalities in TBI, and recommended additional resources for TBI survivors and their providers. The final chapter offers a unique perspective: living with TBI from a survivor's point of view.

This manual is intended to be relevant to a broad audience, including neurologists, physiatrists, primary care physicians, and physicians-in-training, who will find the practical, medical management focus to be easy to access and implement. Other healthcare providers, from therapists and nurses to social workers and case managers, will find the succinct discussion of various aspects of multidisciplinary care, community resource information, neuropsychiatric, legal and ethical aspects of TBI care to be particularly valuable.

It is my hope that the *Manual of Traumatic Brain Injury Management* will serve as a concise, easy-to-access resource that provides readers with "just enough" information to suit their particular needs. For the user who desires quick access to core concepts, the text will serve as a comprehensive stand-alone resource. If more in-depth understanding of a topic is desired, the "Additional Reading" section at the end of each chapter will provide pointed expert recommendations for further exploration. Ultimately, this pocket guide can serve as both a self-contained resource and as a portal to a comprehensive exploration of the many facets of management of traumatic brain injury.

Felise S. Zollman, MD

Contributors

Bamidele Adeyemo
Clinical Fellow
Department of Physical Medicine
and Rehabilitation
Harvard Medical School
Boston, Massachusetts

Amar Agha, MD, FRCPI
Academic Department of
Neuroendocrinology
Beaumont Hospital and the Royal
College of Surgeons in Ireland
Medical School
Dublin, Ireland

David N. Alexander, MD
Medical Director
Department of Neurology
Neurological Rehabilitation and
Research Unit
University of California
Los Angeles, California

William B. Barr, PhD
Associate Professor
Department of Neurology and
Psychiatry
New York University School of
Medicine
New York, New York

Sarice L. Bassin, MD
Assistant Professor of Neurology,
Neurological Surgery, and
Anesthesiology
Department of Neurology
Northwestern University Feinberg
School of Medicine
Chicago, Illinois

Sheital Bavishi, DO
TBI Fellow
RICVAMC
Department of Physical Medicine
and Rehabilitation
Virginia Commonwealth University
Richmond, Virginia

Lucy-Ann Behan, MB, MRCPI
Academic Department of
Neuroendocrinology
Beaumont Hospital and the Royal
College of Surgeons in Ireland
Medical School
Dublin, Ireland

Debra E. Berens, PhD
Rehabilitation Consultant/
Life Care Planner
Private Practice
Atlanta, Georgia

Ann S. Bines, RN, MS, CCRN
Nurse Manager
Brain Injury Medicine and
Rehabilitation Program
Rehabilitation Institute of Chicago
Chicago, Illinois

Rebecca Brashler, MSW, LCSW
Director
Care Management and Family
Support Services
Rehabilitation Institute of
Chicago
Assistant Professor
Department of Physical Medicine
and Rehabilitation
Northwestern University Feinberg
School of Medicine
Chicago, Illinois

Allen W. Brown, MD
Director, Brain Rehabilitation
    Services
Department of Physical Medicine
    and Rehabilitation
Associate Professor
College of Medicine
Mayo Clinic
Rochester, Minnesota

John J. Bruns, MD[†]
Clinical Assistant Professor
Department of Emergency
    Medicine
Mount Sinai School of Medicine
New York, New York

Catherine Burress, DPT
Doctor of Physical Therapy
Physical Therapist
Brain Injury Medicine and
    Rehabilitation Program
Rehabilitation Institute of Chicago
Chicago, Illinois

Stephen V. Cantrill, MD, FACEP
Emergency Physician
Department of Emergency
    Medicine
Denver Health Medical Center
Denver, Colorado;
Associate Professor
Department of Emergency
    Medicine
University of Colorado School of
    Medicine
Aurora, Colorado

Robert C. Cantu, MD, MA,
    FACS, FACSM
Clinical Professor
Department of Neurosurgery
Boston University School of
    Medicine
Boston, Massachusetts

Michael D. Carter, JD
Attorney
Horwitz, Horwitz and Associates
Chicago, Illinois

Lawrence S. Chin, MD, FACS
Professor and Chairman
Department of Neurosurgery
Boston University School of
    Medicine
Boston, Massachusetts

David Cifu, MD
The Herman J Flax, MD Professor
    and Chairman
Department of Physical Medicine
    and Rehabilitation
Virginia Commonwealth
    University School of Medicine
Richmond, Virginia
National Director
Physical Medicine and
    Rehabilitation Program Office
Veterans Administration Central
    Office
Washington, DC

Sara Cohen, MD
Attending Physician
Braintree Rehabilitation Hospital
Braintree, Massachusetts

Aaron M. Cook, PharmD, BCPS
Pharmacy Specialist
Department of Neurosurgery/
    Critical Care
Assistant Adjunct Professor,
    Pharmacy
UKHealthCare
Department of Pharmacy
    Practice and Science
College of Pharmacy
University of Kentucky
Lexington, Kentucky

[†] Deceased.

John D. Corrigan, PhD
Professor
Department of Physical Medicine
  and Rehabilitation
Ohio State University
Columbus, Ohio

Marie Crandall, MD, MPH
Associate Professor
Department of Surgery
Northwestern University
Chicago, Illinois

Nora Cullen, MD, MSc, FRCPC
Physiatrist
Department of
  NeuroRehabilitation
Toronto Rehabilitation Institute
Assistant Professor
Faculty of Medicine
Toronto, Ontario, Canada

Cherina Cyborski, MD
Attending Physician
Department of Brain Injury
  Medicine and Rehabilitation
Rehabilitation Institute of Chicago
Instructor
Department of Physical Medicine
  and Rehabilitation
Feinberg School of Medicine,
  Northwestern University
Chicago, Illinois

Kristen Dams-O'Connor, PhD
Instructor
Department of Rehabilitation
  Medicine
Mount Sinai School of Medicine
New York, New York

Deirdre R. Dawson, PhD
Associate Professor
Department of Occupational
  Science and Occupational
  Therapy and Graduate
Department of Rehabilitation
  Sciences
University of Toronto
Senior Scientist
Kunin-Lunenfeld Applied
  Research Unit, Baycrest Centre
Toronto, Ontario Canada

Kemesha Delisser, MD
Resident Physician
Department of Rehabilitation
  Medicine
The Mount Sinai Hospital
New York, New York

Ramon Diaz-Arrastia, MD, PhD
Professor
Department of Neurology
University of Texas Southwestern
  Medical School
Dallas, Texas

Ana Durand-Sanchez, MD
Traumatic Brain Injury/Polytrauma
  Fellow, Staff Physician
Physical Medicine and
  Rehabilitation
Michael E. DeBakey VAMC
Brain Injury Fellow
Department of Physical Medicine
  and Rehabilitation
University of Texas Health
  Science Center
Houston, Texas

Elie P. Elovic, MD
Professor
Department of Physical Medicine
  and Rehabilitation
University of Utah
Salt Lake City, Utah

Jennifer Field
J Field Foundation
Whitestone, Virginia

Cynthia D. Fields, MD
Department of Psychiatry
Johns Hopkins University School
of Medicine
Baltimore, Maryland

**Simon Fleminger, MB Bchir,
FRCP, FRCPsych, PhD**
Consultant Neuropsychiatrist
Lishman Brain Injury Unit
Maudsley Hospital
South London and Maudsley NHS
Foundation Trust
London, UK

Louis M. French, PhD
Chief, TBI Service
Department of Orthopaedics and
Rehabilitation
Walter Reed National Military
Medical Center
Assistant Professor
Department of Neurology
Uniformed Services University of
the Health Sciences
Bethesda, Maryland

Christopher Giza, MD
Associate Professor In-Residence
Department of Pediatric
Neurology and Neurosurgery
David Geffen School of Medicine
at UCLA
Mattel Children's Hospital–UCLA
Los Angeles, California

Gary Goldberg, MD
Medical Director, Polytrauma
Network Site and Transitional
Rehabilitation Program
Department of Physical Medicine
and Rehabilitation
Hunter Holmes McGuire Veterans
Administration Medical Center;
Professor
Department of Physical Medicine
and Rehabilitation
Medical College of Virginia/VCU
Health System
Richmond, Virginia

**Diana S. Goldstein, PhD,
ABPP/CN**
Director of Neuropsychology
Michigan Avenue
Neuropsychologists;
Adjunct Faculty
Department of Psychiatry
University of Chicago Pritzker
School of Medicine
Chicago, Illinois

Matthew Goodwin, MD
Attending Physician
Physical Rehabilitation
John L. McClellan Memorial
Veterans Hospital
Little Rock, Arkansas

Wayne A. Gordon, PhD
Professor
Department of Rehabilitation
Medicine
Mount Sinai Medical Center
New York, New York

Michael M. Green, DO
Resident
Department of Physical Medicine
and Rehabilitation
Baylor College of Medicine
and University of Texas
HSC Physical Medicine and
Rehabilitation Alliance
Houston, Texas

Brian Greenwald, MD
Medical Director of Brain Injury
Rehabilitation
Rehabilitation Medicine
Mount Sinai Medical School
New York, New York

Puneet K. Gupta, MD, MSE
Assistant Professor
Department of Neurology and
  Neurotherapeutics
University of Texas Southwestern
  Medical Center
Dallas, Texas

Clare L. Hammell, MB, ChB,
  FRCA
Specialist Registrar
Department of Anaesthesia and
  Critical Care
University Hospital Aintree
Liverpool, UK

Flora Hammond, MD
Covalt Professor of Physical
  Medicine and Rehabilitation
  Chair
Indiana University
Chief of Medical Affairs
Department of Physical Medicine
  and Rehabilitation
Rehabilitation Hospital of Indiana
Indianapolis, Indiana

Robert E. Hanlon, PhD, ABPP
Associate Professor of Psychiatry
  and Neurology
Department of Psychiatry and
  Behavioral Sciences
Northwestern University Feinberg
  School of Medicine
Clinical Neuropsychologist
Neuropsychological Associates of
  Chicago
Chicago, Illinois

Michael Henrie, DO
Visiting Instructor
Department of Physical Medicine
  and Rehabilitation
University of Utah
Salt Lake City, Utah

Pei-Te Hsu, MD
Department of Veterans
  Affairs, Boston
  Healthcare System
Harvard Medical School
Boston, Massachusetts

Hillary R. Irons, MD, PhD
Resident Physician
Department of Emergency
  Medicine
Michigan State University,
  Emergency Medicine
  Residency Program
  (EM-Lansing)
Lansing, Michigan

Grant L. Iverson, PhD
Professor
Department of Psychiatry
University of British Columbia
Vancouver, British Columbia,
  Canada
Researcher
Defense and Veterans Brain
  Injury Center
Washington, DC

Mayur Jayarao, MD
Department of Neurosurgery
Boston Medical Center
Boston, Massachusetts

Ricardo E. Jorge, MD
Associate Professor
Department of Psychiatry
University of Iowa
Iowa City, Iowa

Nathan E. Kegel, PhD
Post Doctoral Fellow
Department of Sports Medicine
University of Pittsburgh Medical
  Center
Pittsburgh, Pennsylvania

Sunil Kothari, MD
Assistant Professor
Department of Rehabilitation
  Medicine
Baylor College of Medicine
Houston, Texas

Richard Kunz, MD
Assistant Clinical Professor
Department of Physical Medicine
  and Rehabilitation
Virginia Commonwealth
  University School of Medicine
Richmond, Virginia

Rael T. Lange, PhD
Research Director/Senior Scientist
Department of Neurology
Defense and Veterans Brain
  Injury Center, Walter Reed
  Army Medical Center
Washington, DC
Clinical Assistant Professor
Department of Psychiatry
University of British Columbia
Vancouver, British Columbia,
  Canada

Michelle C. LaPlaca, PhD
Associate Professor
Wallace H. Coulter Department of
  Biomedical Engineering
Georgia Institute of Technology/
  Emory University
Atlanta, Georgia

Eric B. Larson, PhD
Psychologist
Brain Injury Medicine and
  Rehabilitation Program
Rehabilitation Institute of Chicago
Assistant Professor
Department of Physical Medicine
  and Rehabilitation
Feinberg School of Medicine
Northwestern University
Chicago, Illinois

Henry Lew, MD, PhD
Professor
Department of Physical Medicine
  and Rehabilitation
Virginia Commonwealth
  University School of Medicine
National Consultant
Defense and Veterans Brain
  Injury Center (DVBIC)
Richmond, Virginia

Jeffrey David Lewine, PhD
Professor of Translational
  Neuroscience
Magnetoencephalography Section
MIND Research Network
Albuquerque, New Mexico

Lisa A. Lombard, MD
Assistant Professor, Medical
  Director
Department of Physical Medicine
  and Rehabilitation
Indiana University/Rehabilitation
  Hospital of Indiana
Indianapolis, Indiana

David F. Long, MD
Medical Director, Brain Injury
  Program
Bryn Mawr Rehabilitation
  Hospital
Malvern, Pennsylvania

Mark R. Lovell, PhD
Department of Sports Medicine
University of Pittsburgh Medical
  Center
Pittsburgh, Pennsylvania

John Lowry, DO
Clinical Fellow, Spinal Cord Injury
  Medicine
Department of Physical Medicine
  and Rehabilitation
Harvard Medical School
Boston, Massachusetts

James F. Malec, PhD, ABPP-Cn, Rp
Research Director
Department of Research
Rehabilitation Hospital of Indiana
Professor
Department of Physical Medicine
and Rehabilitation
Indiana University School of
Medicine
Indianapolis, Indiana

Michael McCrea, PhD, ABPP
Executive Director
Neuroscience and Research Institute
ProHealth Care
Waukesha, Wisconsin

Shane D. McNamee, MD
Chief
Department of Physical Medicine
and Rehabilitation
Hunter Holmes McGuire Veterans
Administration Hospital
Assistant Professor
Department of Physical Medicine
and Rehabilitation
Virginia Commonwealth University
Richmond, Virginia

Anne M. Moessner, RN, MSN, CNS
Brain Injury Clinical Nurse
Specialist
Department of Physical Medicine
and Rehabilitation
Mayo Clinic
Rochester, Minnesota

Debjani Mukherjee, PhD
Director
Donnelley Ethics Program
Rehabilitation Institute of Chicago
Assistant Professor
Departments of Physical Medicine
and Rehabilitation & Medical
Humanities and Bioethics

Northwestern University Feinberg
School of Medicine
Chicago, Illinois

Phalgun Nori, MD
Traumatic Brain Injury Fellow
Department of Physical Medicine
and Rehabilitation
JFK Johnson Rehabilitation
Institute
Edison, New Jersey

Kara Kozub O'Dell, MA, CCC-SLP
Allied Health Manager
Brain Injury Medicine and
Rehabilitation Program
The Rehabilitation Institute of
Chicago
Chicago, Illinois

David O. Okonkwo, MD, PhD
Department of Neurological
Surgery
University of Pittsburgh Medical
Center
Pittsburgh, Pennsylvania

Kristine O'Phelan, MD
Assistant Professor, Director of
Neurocritical Care
Department of Neurology
University of Miami, Miller School
of Medicine
Miami, Florida

William V. Padula, OD
Director
Vision Rehabilitation Services
Rehabilitation Center
New Haven, Connecticut
Padula Institute of Vision
Rehabilitation
Guilford Medical Center
Guilford, Connecticut

Ajit B. Pai, MD
Medical Director, Polytrauma
  Rehabilitation Center
Department of PM&R Service
Hunter Holmes McGuire VAMC
Assistant Professor
Department of PM&R
Virginia Commonwealth University
Richmond, Virginia

David M. Panczykowski, MD
University of Pittsburgh Medical
  Center
Pittsburgh, Pennsylvania

Matthew R. Powell, PhD, ABPP
Head of Traumatic Brain Injury
  Clinic
Neuroscience Center
ProHealth Care and Waukesha
  Memorial Hospital
Waukesha, Wisconsin

Jeffrey Radecki, MD
Assistant Professor, Assistant
  Attending Physiatrist
Department of Rehabilitation
  Medicine
NewYork-Presbyterian Hospital,
  Weill Cornell Medical Center
New York, New York

Vani Rao, MBBS, MD
Associate Professor
Department of Psychiatry and
  Behavioral Sciences
Johns Hopkins University
Baltimore, Maryland

Joshua M. Rosenow, MD
Director of Functional
  Neurosurgery/Associate
  Professor of Neurosurgery
Department of Neurosurgery
Northwestern University Feinberg
  School of Medicine
Chicago, Illinois

Angelle M. Sander, PhD
Department of Physical
  Medicine & Rehabilitation
Baylor College of Medicine
Brain Injury Research Center
TIRR Memorial Hermann
Houston, Texas

Daniel Shrey, MD
Fellow Physician
Department of Pediatric
  Neurology
University of California, Los
  Angeles
Los Angeles, California

Brian Steinmetz, DO
Physiatrist
Department of Orthopedics
The Maryland Spine Center
Baltimore, Maryland

Christina Taggart, BA, MA
Research Associate
Department of Research
Toronto Rehabilitation Institute
Toronto, Canada

Pamela Sherron Targett, Med
Collateral Faculty
School of Education
Virginia Commonwealth University
Richmond, Virginia

Gentian Toshkezi, MD
Fellow
Department of Neurosurgery
Boston Medical Center
Boston, Massachusetts

Theodore Tsaousides, PhD
Assistant Professor
Department of Rehabilitation
  Medicine
Mount Sinai School
  of Medicine
New York, New York

William C. Walker, MD
Ernst and Helga Prosser Professor
Department of Physical Medicine
and Rehabilitation
School of Medicine
Virginia Commonwealth University
Site Director and Principal
Investigator
Defense and Veterans Brain
Injury Center
Richmond, Virginia

Erica Wang, MD
Brain Injury Medicine and
Rehabilitation Fellow
Rehabilitation Institute of Chicago
Chicago, Illinois

Roger O. Weed, PhD
Professor
Counseling and Psychological
Services Department
Georgia State University
Atlanta, Georgia

Paul Wehman, PhD
Professor
Physical Medicine and
Rehabilitation
School of Education
Virginia Commonwealth
University
Richmond, Virginia

Cindy Zadikoff, MD, MSc
Assistant Professor,
Department of Neurology
Northwestern University
Chicago, Illinois

Ross Zafonte, DO
Earl P and Ida S. Charlton
Professor and Chair
Department of Physical Medicine
and Rehabilitation

Harvard Medical School
Vice President Medical Affairs,
Research and Education
Spaulding Rehabilitation Network
Chief Physical Medicine and
Rehabilitation
Massachusetts General Hospital
Department of Physical Medicine
and Rehabilitation
Spaulding Rehabilitation
Hospital
Boston, Massachusetts

Donna Zahara, MS
Corporate Director
RIC Academy, Internal Staff
Development
Rehabilitation Institute
of Chicago
Chicago, Illinois

Nathan D. Zasler, MD
CEO and Medical Director
Tree of Life Service, Inc
Concussion Care Center of
Virginia, Ltd.
Richmond, Virginia

Felise S. Zollman, MD
Co-Project Director
Midwest Regional Traumatic
Brain Injury Model System
Center
Attending Physician
Brain Injury Medicine and
Rehabilitation Program
Rehabilitation Institute
of Chicago
Assistant Professor
Departments of Physical
Medicine and Rehabilitation &
Neurology
Northwestern University Feinberg
School of Medicine
Chicago, Illinois

PART 1

Core Concepts

1

Traumatic Brain Injury
Definitions and Nomenclature

Kristine O'Phelan

Traumatic brain injury (TBI) has a broad spectrum of severity, pathology, physiology, and sequela. This chapter will present pertinent definitions, nomenclature, and concepts relevant to the discussion of TBI.

PRIMARY VERSUS SECONDARY INJURY

The distinction is somewhat arbitrary and the specific combination and magnitude of secondary injury is to a great extent determined by the nature of the primary injury.

- **Primary injury**—the physiological or anatomical insult, often but not exclusively the result of direct trauma to head. The primary injury may be associated with structural changes resulting from mechanical forces initially applied during injury. These forces may cause tissue distortion, shearing, and vascular injury as well as destabilization of cell membranes and frank membrane destruction.
- **Secondary injury**—systemic or local changes, which increase tissue damage. Many secondary insults result directly from the primary injury and some are caused by discreet systemic or local phenomena. Secondary injury mechanisms include generation of free radicals, excitotoxicity, disturbance of ionic homeostasis, disruption of the blood-brain barrier, generation of nitric oxide, lipid peroxidation, mitochondrial dysfunction and energy failure, inflammation, secondary hemorrhage, axonal disruption, apoptotic cell death, and ischemia. Ischemia may be due to microvascular changes, or systemic hypotension or hypoxia or elevated intracranial pressure.

CLASSIFICATION OF TBI BY MECHANISM

- **Closed/blunt force**—injury caused by direct force to head, acceleration/deceleration, or rotational forces. Common causes include falls, assault, and motor vehicle collisions.

3

- **Blast injury**—injury caused by overpressure waves generated from high grade explosives. A large amount of thermal, mechanical, and electromagnetic energy is transferred to the brain. Energy can come directly through the cranium or be transmitted indirectly through oscillating pressures in fluid-filled large blood vessels. This may cause damage to the blood-brain barrier or gray-white matter junction, and can cause cerebral edema, axonal injury, apoptosis, and tissue degeneration.
- **Penetrating injury**—injury induced by an object that penetrates the cranial vault. Common causes include gunshot wounds, shrapnel, and knife wounds.

CLINICAL CLASSIFICATION OF TBI

It incorporates the Glasgow Coma Scale (GCS) [1] (Table 1.1). Clinical classification is important because it often guides treatment decisions.

- **Mild TBI (MTBI)**—GCS 13 to 15, the majority of patients with cranial trauma fall in this group. Patients are awake, may be confused but can communicate and follow commands.
- **Moderate TBI**—GCS 9 to 12, these patients are generally drowsy to obtunded but not comatose. They can open their eyes and localize painful stimuli. They are at high risk of clinical deterioration and must be monitored carefully.
- **Severe TBI**—GCS 3 to 8, these patients are comatose, they do not follow commands and may exhibit decerebrate or decorticate posturing. They have significant structural and metabolic brain dysfunction and are at high risk of secondary brain injury and deterioration.

STRUCTURALLY BASED DESCRIPTIONS OF TBI

- **Epidural hematoma (EDH)** (Figure 1.1)—an extradural collection of blood. It is often associated with a skull fracture and has an arterial

Table 1.1 Glasgow Coma Scale

Eye Opening	Best Verbal Response	Best Motor Response
Spontaneous 4	Oriented 5	Obeys commands 6
To speech 3	Confused conversation 4	Localizes pain 5
To pain 2	Inappropriate words 3	Withdrawal 4
None 1	Incomprehensible sounds 2	Abnormal flexion (decorticate) 3
	None 1	Extension (decerebrate) 2
		None 1

origin. Margins of the hematoma do not cross the skull suture lines and often appear convex on imaging studies. If an EDH is evacuated in a timely fashion to reverse mass effect or if the hematoma is small in size, patient outcomes are usually good.

- **Subdural hematoma (SDH)** (Figure 1.2)—a collection of blood in the subdural space. SDHs may be chronic or acute and are caused by venous bleeding from cortical bridging veins. Bleeding may extend over the entire hemisphere. Acute SDHs are significantly associated with seizures. Acute SDHs are also associated with significant alteration

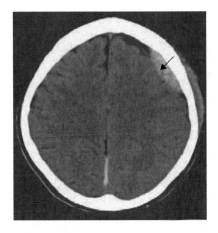

Figure 1.1 Epidural hematoma.

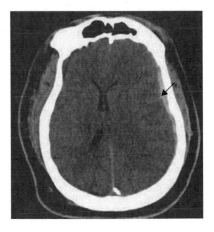

Figure 1.2 Subdural hematoma.

of cerebral blood flow and metabolism of the underlying hemisphere and generally have a worse outcome than EDHs.

- **Traumatic axonal injury** (TAI, also referred to as diffuse axonal injury, or DAI)—injury to axonal connections triggered by inertial forces, predominantly acceleration-deceleration, with subsequent structural and metabolic consequences of mechanical deformation.
- **Traumatic subarachnoid hemorrhage (TSAH or SAH)** (Figure 1.3)— hemorrhage in the subarachnoid space that is not associated with significant mass effect. It often accompanies other types of traumatic hemorrhage. The presence of TSAH has been associated with an increased risk of an unfavorable 6-month outcome in patients with moderate to severe TBI [2].
- **Intraventricular hemorrhage (IVH)**—bleeding into the ventricular system after trauma. It may be associated with acute hydrocephalous and is a risk factor for development of delayed hydrocephalous. IVH is typically seen in conjunction with TSAH.
- **Contusion** (Figure 1.4)—parenchymal hemorrhage, typically in frontal or temporal lobes. Contusions may be "coup" or "contre coup."
  - **Coup injury**—results from direct transmission of force to brain tissue underlying the region of impact.
  - **Contre coup injury**—results from the indirect forces acting in a region contralateral to the region of impact.
- **Skull fractures**—Skull fractures may occur after trauma because of blunt or penetrating injury. They may involve the convexity or the skull base and may be open or closed depending on the presence of an overlying scalp laceration. Large depressed skull fractures may need to be surgically elevated. Depressed skull fractures are associated with an increased risk of seizures [3].

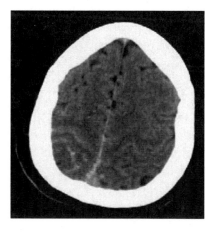

Figure 1.3 Traumatic subarachnoid hemorrhage.

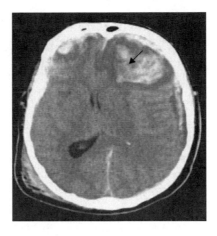

Figure 1.4 Cerebral contusion.

Table 1.2 AAN Practice Parameter Grading System for Concussion

Grade 1
Transient Confusion; no loss of consciousness; symptoms resolve in <15 minutes
Grade 2
Transient confusion; no loss of consciousness; concussion symptoms last >15 minutes
Grade 3
Any loss of consciousness either brief (seconds) or prolonged (minutes)

From Ref. [4].

CONCUSSION

It is altered mental state occurring after trauma, which may or may not include loss of consciousness. Symptoms reflect a functional disturbance rather than structural injury. The American Academy of Neurology (AAN) concussion grading scale [4] (Table 1.2) has been widely used to describe the severity of concussion.

POSTTRAUMATIC AMNESIA

Posttraumatic amnesia (PTA) is the impaired recall of events surrounding the injury. Retrograde PTA involves impaired recollection of events immediately preceding the injury and anterograde PTA is a deficit in forming new memories after the injury [5].

Table 1.3 Symptoms of Postconcussive Disorder

Depression, dizziness, drowsiness
Excess sleep Fatigue Feel "in a fog"
Feel "slowed down," headache irritability
Memory problems, nausea, nervousness
Numbness/tingling, poor balance, poor concentration
Ringing in ears, sadness, sensitivity to light
Sensitivity to noise, trouble falling asleep, vomiting

From Ref. [5].

POSTCONCUSSION DISORDER

Also known as postconcussion syndrome, this term refers to postconcussive symptoms that persist for 3 or more months post injury. Symptoms are quite variable and are not unique to this diagnosis [6].

SECOND IMPACT SYNDROME

A second MTBI occurring while an individual remains symptomatic from the first MTBI may cause the "second impact syndrome." This rare phenomenon involves acute cerebrovascular congestion and loss of cerebrovascular autoregulation resulting in malignant brain swelling, which is life threatening [7].

RECOVERY AND SEQUELAE

- **Diaschisis**—dysfunction in an area of brain that is remote from an area with structural damage but is connected to the damaged area via neuronal pathways.
- **Neuroprotection**—therapies or management strategies that prevent or limit secondary injury leading to improved survival of neurons, microglia, or the supporting microvasculature.
- **Neuroplasticity**—changes in brain structure (neuronal and glial connectivity) and function due to experience. This is a major mechanism for recovery of function after traumatic injury.
- **Gliosis**—formation of a dense network of glial cells in areas of brain injury that do not contribute to functional recovery. This can occur after trauma, stroke, or demyelination.
- **Atrophy**—loss of neurons and glia and their connections. This can occur after TBI and is usually related to the severity of the initial injury.

ADDITIONAL READING

Electronic Reference

Brain Trauma Foundation Web site. http://www.braintrauma.org

Textbooks/Chapters

Reilly P, Bullock MR. *Head Injury: Pathophysiology and Management*. 2nd ed. London: Hodder Arnold; 2005.

Journal Articles

Aarabi B, Simard JM. Traumatic brain injury. *Curr Opin Crit Care*. 2009;15:548–553.

Bouma GJ, Muizelaar JP, Choi SC, Newlon PG, Young HF. Cerebral circulation and metabolism after severe traumatic brain injury: the elusive role of ischemia. *J Neurosurg*. 1991;75(5):685–693.

Buki A, Povlishock JT. All roads lead to disconnection?—traumatic axonal injury revisited. *Acta Neurochirugica*. 2006;148:181–194.

Cernak I, Noble-Haeusslein LJ. Traumatic brain injury: an overview of pathobiology with emphasis on military populations. *J Cereb Blood Flow Metab*. 2010; 30(2):255–266.

Garga N, Lowenstein DH. Posttraumatic epilepsy: a major problem in desperate need of major advances. *Epilepsy Currents*. 2006;6(1):1–5.

Verweij BH, Amelink GJ, Muizelaar JP. Current concepts of cerebral oxygen transport and energy metabolism after severe traumatic brain injury. *Prog Brain Res*. 2007; 161:111–124.

REFERENCES

1. Teasdale G, Jennett B. Assessment of coma and impaired consciousness. A practical scale. *Lancet*. 1974;2:81–84.
2. Steyerberg EW, Mushkudiani N, Perel P, et al. Predicting outcome after traumatic brain injury: development and international validation of prognostic scores based on admission characteristics. *PLoS Med*. 2008;5(8):e165; discussion e165.
3. Temkin NR. Antiepileptogenesis and seizure prevention trials with antiepileptic drugs: meta-analysis of controlled trials. *Epilepsia*. 2001;42(4):515–524.
4. Practice Parameter: The management of concussion in sports (summary statement). *Neurology*. 1997;48:581–585.
5. Cantu RC. Posttraumatic Retrograde and Anterograde Amnesia: Pathophysiology and Implications in Grading and Safe Return to Play. *J Athl Train*. 2001;36(3):244–248.
6. McCrory P, Johnston K, Meeuwisse W, et al. Summary and agreement statement of the 2nd International conference on concussion in Sport, Prague 2004. *Br J Sports Med*. 2005;(39):196–204.
7. Kelly JP, and Rosenberg JH. Diagnosis and management of concussion in sports. *Neurology* 1997;48:575–580.

2

Essential Concepts in Traumatic Brain Injury Neuropathology
Primary Injury, Secondary Injury, and Neuroplasticity

Michelle C. LaPlaca and Hillary R. Irons

GENERAL PRINCIPLES

Traumatic brain injury (TBI) occurs as a continuum of events, from the primary injury to secondary consequences (or secondary injury), to repair.

- *Primary injury/insult*: immediate (milliseconds to seconds) result of the associated traumatic event
- *Secondary injury*: (seconds to minutes to weeks) the cascade of changing events on a cellular, tissue (micro), and systemic (macro) level, which result in additional morbidity and mortality following the primary injury
- *Plasticity*: the brain's ability to reorganize itself by forming new neural connections during development and after injury or disease (weeks to years)

BIOMECHANICS AND PRIMARY INJURY

Traumatic insults: motor vehicle accidents, falls, blows to the head, and so on. Head can hit surface *or* object can hit head. Brain injury is initiated when the insult is severe enough to cause high tissue strain, which leads to either micro- or macrodamage [1].

Role of head acceleration (velocity/time) and impact force (load): Higher acceleration = more injury. Angular acceleration is worse than linear. Higher force = more injury.

Suprathreshold force strains or damages tissue: Strain can be tensile (stretch), compression, and/or shear (Note: brain is especially vulnerable to shear strain).

More force + softer tissue = more strain: for example, for the same force, soft neural tissue deforms more than skull. As a result, the brain can be more damaged than exterior body surface/skull.

Primary insults are heterogeneous and depend on the following:

- **Mechanics of the occurrence** (i.e., multiple insults (polytrauma), level of force, distribution of force, tissue properties, and duration of the insult)
- **State of the individual** (i.e., age, weight, genetic makeup, underlying health conditions, nutritional status, medications, and substance abuse)

Primary insults include structural failure of the tissue surrounding the brain (e.g., muscle and other soft connective tissue injury, osseous fractures from simple to shatter to penetrating), of vascular structures (resulting in bleeding), and of the brain itself. Structural failure of the brain includes microtears, macrotears, compression, tension, and/or shearing within and between brain regions. Insults to the neural tissue may manifest in neuronal damage, axonal stretching and tearing, interruption in normal neuronal synaptic transmission, and glial damage.

SECONDARY INJURY

Injury mechanisms for TBI pathologies are poorly understood because of the following:

- Heterogeneous conditions of injury and individual response
- Complexity of interactions among cellular signaling pathways
- Constantly changing cellular activities and systemic adaptations

Cellular responses can broadly be classified as: *hyperactivity* and *hypoactivity*.

Overall response is the sum of cellular responses and organic, systemic-level responses.

Hyperactivity During Secondary Injury

- Disruption of ion homeostasis (Ca^{2+}/Na^+ influx) [2]
- Excitatory amino acid release (e.g., glutamate); overactivation of glutamate receptors (ionotropic, metabotropic) [3]
- Hyperexcitability, electrophysiological dysfunction [4]
- Hypermetabolism—increased use of ATPase membrane pumps, mitochondrial overload, an increase in CO_2 (hypercapnia), H^+ [5]

- Acute inflammatory response (release of histamines, arachidonic acid, bradykinin, and nitric oxide), activation of astrocytes, microglia, and macrophages (increase in proinflammatory cytokines) [6]
- Increase in hydroxyl radicals, leading to more reactive oxygen species (ROS; e.g., superoxide ions, hydrogen peroxide, and more hydroxyls), causing lipid peroxidation and compounding degradative processes [7]
- Aberrant cell signaling (abnormal activation of G-proteins, second messengers, ion channels, kinases, faulty gene and protein regulation) [8]
- Activation of enzymes that damage proteins such as cytoskeletal structures (e.g., calpain, caspase), lipases (e.g., phospholipase A_2) that damage membranes, and endonucleases that damage nucleic acids [9]

Hypoactivity During Secondary Injury

- Reduced excitability, loss of normal synaptic transmission
- Diminished glucose substrates and oxygen, leading to reduced cellular respiration and less ATP production, acidosis [10]
- Loss of blood vessel wall permeability and blood-brain barrier (BBB) disruption [11,12]
- Cytoskeletal damage affecting axonal transport, second messenger pathways [13]
- Myelin degradation, white matter/axonal damage (axons, oligodendrocytes) [14]
- Membrane damage reduces ability to restore selective membrane transport and stability of the plasma membrane phospholipids [15]
- Aberrant cell signaling [8]
- Altered gene expression [16]
- The aforementioned events are coupled to the corresponding physiological factors such as a metabolic state, reduction in efficient perfusion and therefore low oxygenation, possible anemia, and poor fluid balance among the intravascular, interstitial, and intracellular spaces.

Hyper- and Hypoactivity Often Lead to Cellular Dysfunction and Eventual Cell Death

- Apoptosis: unscheduled "programmed" cell death; portions of cell death pathways are activated by the insult [17]
- Necrosis: traditionally distinct from apoptosis; likely one of many death pathways or features are end-stage; enzymatically driven; exacerbated by inflammation
- Autophagy: self destruction through phagocytic processes [18]

Cerebral Edema and the Monro-Kellie Hypothesis: *Osmolality Rules!*

- The cranium maintains a balance of brain volume (1400 mL), cerebrospinal fluid (CSF, 150 mL), and blood (150 mL).
- Brain edema can occur when osmolality changes, resulting in excess volume in any of these compartments.
- The body tries to maintain a constant osmolality; that is the primary cause of fluid movement from one compartment to another.
- Underlying causes are increased intravascular hydrostatic pressure (vasogenic edema), increased interstitial fluid pressure due to blood pressure and protein leakage or abnormal oncotic pressures (interstitial edema), and cellular swelling due to ionic imbalance and osmosis (cytotoxic edema).

Mitigating Secondary Injury

- *Systems management* of normotension and adequate oxygenation [19,20] may mitigate underlying cellular responses [21] (see Additional Reading).

NEUROPLASTICITY: REPAIR AND REGENERATION

Plasticity (the ability to produce and maintain change) is key to repair and regeneration.

- Taking advantage of the limited window of opportunity (up to several months in duration) requires neuroprotection and upregulation of repair molecules, to working with the endogenous repair capacity of the brain and the inhibitory environment.
- Agents to promote endogenous regeneration include trophic factors [22] and signaling targets such as MAPK and Rho-family GTPases [23].

THE FUTURE: SYSTEMIC STABILIZATION, NEUROPROTECTION, NEURORESTORATION/REPAIR

- *Stabilization* is the focus of clinical management and is critical to success of subsequent therapy and outcome.
- *Underlying biochemical and molecular events* should be considered in treatment of an otherwise physiologically stabilized patient. New diagnosis and monitoring tools (e.g., diffusion tensor imaging, biomarkers) may assist in assessing secondary injury.
- *Protection (acute and subacute phase) versus regeneration (chronic phase)*: Current efforts focus on neuroprotection (e.g., progesterone,

antioxidants) [24,25]; regeneration and other pharmacological interventions may hold promise for the future [26].

ADDITIONAL READING

Electronic Reference

Review of TBI pathophysiology: http://faculty.neuroscience.ucla.edu/institution/publication-download?publication_id=144613

Textbook/Chapter

Neurotrauma: New Insights into Pathology and Treatment Edited by: John T. Weber and Andrew I.R. Maas (2007) Progress in Brain Research, Vol. 161 Elsevier B.V ISBN: 9780444530172. Proceedings from the 2006 International & National (US) Societies of Neurotrauma, Roderdam, The Netherlands.

Journal Articles

Beauchamp K, Mutlak H, Smith WR, Shohami E, Stahel PF. Pharmacology of traumatic brain injury: where is the "golden bullet"? *Mol Med.* 2008;14:731–740.

Park E, Bell JD, Baker AJ. Traumatic brain injury: can the consequences be stopped? *CMAJ.* 2008;178:1163–1170.

Veenith T, Goon S, Burnstein RM. Molecular mechanisms of traumatic brain injury: the missing link in management. *World J Emerg Surg.* 2009;4:7.

Yakovlev AG, Faden AI. Mechanisms of neural cell death: implications for development of neuroprotective treatment strategies. *NeuroRx.* 2004;1:5–16.

REFERENCES

1. LaPlaca MC, Simon CM, Prado GR, Cullen DK. CNS injury biomechanics and experimental models. *Prog Brain Res.* 2007;161:13–26.
2. Sun DA, Deshpande LS, Sombati S, et al. Traumatic brain injury causes a long-lasting calcium (Ca^{2+})-plateau of elevated intracellular Ca levels and altered Ca^{2+} homeostatic mechanisms in hippocampal neurons surviving brain injury. *Eur J Neurosci.* 2008;27(7):1659–1672.
3. Lau A, Tymianski M. Glutamate receptors, neurotoxicity and neurodegeneration. *Pflugers Arch.* 2010;460(2):525–542.
4. Cohen AS, Pfister BJ, Schwarzbach E, Grady MS, Goforth PB, Satin LS. Injury-induced alterations in CNS electrophysiology. *Prog Brain Res.* 2007;161:143–169.
5. Foley N, Marshall S, Pikul J, Salter K, Teasell R. Hypermetabolism following moderate to severe traumatic acute brain injury: a systematic review. *J Neurotrauma.* 2008;25(12):1415–1431.
6. Goodman JC, Van M, Gopinath SP, Robertson CS. Pro-inflammatory and pro-apoptotic elements of the neuroinflammatory response are activated in traumatic brain injury. *Acta Neurochir Suppl.* 2008;102:437–439.
7. Hall ED, Vaishnav RA, Mustafa AG. Antioxidant therapies for traumatic brain injury. *Neurotherapeutics.* 2010;7(1):51–61.
8. Chico LK, Van Eldik LJ, Watterson DM. Targeting protein kinases in central nervous system disorders. *Nat Rev Drug Discov.* 2009;8(11):892–909.

9. Serbest G, Burkhardt MF, Siman R, Raghupathi R, Saatman KE. Temporal profiles of cytoskeletal protein loss following traumatic axonal injury in mice. *Neurochem Res.* 2007;32(12):2006–2014.

10. Hovda DA, Becker DP, Katayama Y. Secondary injury and acidosis. *J Neurotrauma.* 1992;9(suppl 1):S47–S60.

11. Kontos HA, Wei EP, Povlishock JT. Pathophysiology of vascular consequences of experimental concussive brain injury. *Trans Am Clin Climatol Assoc.* 1981;92:111–121.

12. Whalen MJ, Carlos TM, Kochanek PM, Heineman S. Blood-brain barrier permeability, neutrophil accumulation and vascular adhesion molecule expression after controlled cortical impact in rats: a preliminary study. *Acta Neurochir Suppl.* 1998;71:212–214.

13. Saatman KE, Creed J, Raghupathi R. Calpain as a therapeutic target in traumatic brain injury. *Neurotherapeutics.* 2010;7(1):31–42.

14. Büki A, Povlishock JT. All roads lead to disconnection?–Traumatic axonal injury revisited. *Acta Neurochir (Wien).* 2006;148(2):181–93; discussion 193.

15. Adibhatla RM, Hatcher JF, Dempsey RJ. Lipids and lipidomics in brain injury and diseases. *AAPS J.* 2006;8(2):E314–E321.

16. Raghupathi R. Cell death mechanisms following traumatic brain injury. *Brain Pathol.* 2004;14(2):215–222.

17. Stoica BA, Faden AI. Cell death mechanisms and modulation in traumatic brain injury. *Neurotherapeutics.* 2010;7(1):3–12.

18. Jaeger PA, Wyss-Coray T. All-you-can-eat: autophagy in neurodegeneration and neuroprotection. *Mol Neurodegener.* 2009;4:16.

19. Minardi J, Crocco TJ. Management of traumatic brain injury: first link in chain of survival. *Mt Sinai J Med.* 2009;76(2):138–144.

20. Rangel-Castilla L, Rangel-Castillo L, Gopinath S, Robertson CS. Management of intracranial hypertension. *Neurol Clin.* 2008;26(2):521–41, x.

21. Park E, Bell JD, Baker AJ. Traumatic brain injury: can the consequences be stopped? *CMAJ.* 2008;178(9):1163–1170.

22. Sun D, Bullock MR, McGinn MJ, et al. Basic fibroblast growth factor-enhanced neurogenesis contributes to cognitive recovery in rats following traumatic brain injury. *Exp Neurol.* 2009;216(1):56–65.

23. Tang BL. Inhibitors of neuronal regeneration: mediators and signaling mechanisms. *Neurochem Int.* 2003;42(3):189–203.

24. Wright DW, Kellermann AL, Hertzberg VS, et al. ProTECT: a randomized clinical trial of progesterone for acute traumatic brain injury. *Ann Emerg Med.* 2007;49(4):391–402, 402.e1.

25. Marklund N, Bakshi A, Castelbuono DJ, Conte V, McIntosh TK. Evaluation of pharmacological treatment strategies in traumatic brain injury. *Curr Pharm Des.* 2006;12(13):1645–1680.

26. Schouten JW, Fulp CT, Royo NC, et al. A review and rationale for the use of cellular transplantation as a therapeutic strategy for traumatic brain injury. *J Neurotrauma.* 2004;21(11):1501–1538.

3

Characterization of Traumatic Brain Injury Severity

Lisa A. Lombard

ISSUES IN CHARACTERIZATION OF TBI

- No universally accepted classification system for all stages of traumatic brain injury (TBI)
- Heterogeneity of characterization scales results in difficulty in interpretation and comparison of research studies and in prognostication for individual patients
- Challenges to the creation of a scale includes difficulty in capturing the wide range of severity of persons with TBI (from concussion to comatose), confounding factors on admission (intoxication, shock, etc.), other physical injuries that may limit function, and potential language deficits that may give inaccurate representation of orientation and command following

CHARACTERIZATION OF INJURY

Glasgow Coma Scale (See Table 1.1)

- Introduced by Teasdale and Jennett [1]; the most commonly used assessment for acute TBI
- Assessment of three domains of eye opening, motor response, and verbal response
- Glasgow Coma Scale (GCS) 3 to 8 is defined to be severe TBI, 9–12 moderate, and 13 to 15 mild
- Limitations:
  - Unable to assess when administered after neuromuscular blockade, and verbal score cannot be obtained when the patient is intubated and is thus recorded as a 1T; this has led to outcome data where those with GCS 4 have a better outcome than with a GCS 3 [2]. These factors may lead to overestimation of brain injury severity and inability to acknowledge worsening neurologic deficit.

- Many different providers may record the GCS in a trauma patient; studies cite inaccuracies in inter-rater reliability more than one-thirds of the time [3].
- As a single factor alone, the GCS has been shown to be only a modest predictor of rehabilitation outcome [4].

Rancho Los Amigos Levels of Cognitive Functioning (Table 3.1)

- Also known as the Levels of Cognitive Functioning Scale (LCFS), it was first outlined in 1972; it describes cognitive functioning after TBI based on interaction with the environment [5].
- Commonly used as a descriptive tool between professionals or for family education, or as a tracking tool for recovery.

Table 3.1 Rancho Los Amigos Cognitive Scale

I. No Response: unresponsive to any stimulus
II. Generalized Response: limited, inconsistent, and nonpurposeful responses—often to pain only
III. Localized Response: purposeful responses; may follow simple commands; may focus on presented object
IV. Confused, Agitated: heightened state of activity; confusion, disorientation; aggressive behavior; unable to perform self-care; unaware of present events; agitation appears related to internal confusion
V. Confused, Inappropriate: nonagitated; appears alert; responds to commands; distractible; does not concentrate on task; agitated responses to external stimuli; verbally inappropriate; does not learn new information
VI. Confused, Appropriate: good directed behavior, needs cuing; can relearn old skills as activities of daily living; serious memory problems, some awareness of self and others
VII. Automatic, Appropriate: appears generally oriented; frequently robot-like in daily routine; minimal or absent confusion; shallow recall; increased awareness of self and interaction in environment; lacks insight into condition; decreased judgment and problem solving; lacks realistic planning for the future
VIII. Purposeful, Appropriate: oriented and responds to the environment but abstract reasoning abilities are decreased relative to premorbid levels

ASSESSMENT OF OUTCOME: THE GLASGOW OUTCOME SCALE (TABLE 3.2)

- One of the earliest scales used to record outcomes from moderate or severe TBI
- Five categories, ranging from dead to good recovery. Some have concerns that the Glasgow Outcome Scale (GOS) oversimplifies patterns of recovery from TBI.
- The GOS-E (extended) increases the categories to eight, splitting each of the categories of severe disability, moderate disability, and good recovery into two each (upper and lower)

Table 3.2 Glasgow Outcome Scale

1: Dead
2: Vegetative state—unable to interact with environment; unresponsive
3: Severe disability—able to follow commands; unable to live independently
4: Moderate disability—able to live independently; unable to return to work or school
5: Good recovery—able to return to work or school

ASSESSMENT OF FUNCTIONAL STATUS

Disability Rating Scale (Table 3.3)

Designed to track changes through the spectrum of severe TBI, from coma to community re-entry [6]

- First three areas are directly from the GCS: eye opening, verbal response, and motor response
- Second section reflects cognitive ability for feeding, grooming, and toileting
- Third section is related to need for assistance and employability
- Scores range from 0 (no disability) to 29 (deep coma)
- Has been validated for self or caregiver reporting and for telephone interviews
- Has been shown to be more sensitive than GOS in measurement of improvement during in-patient rehabilitation as well as 1 year post injury [7]

Functional Independence Measure and the Functional Assessment Measure

- Functional Independence Measure (FIM) [8] is one of the most commonly used measurements of independence in in-patient rehabilitation, and is a frequently used tool in outcomes research.

Table 3.3 Disability Rating Scale

Eye opening
  (0): Spontaneous
  (1): To speech
  (2): To pain
  (3): None
Communication ability
  (0): Orientated
  (1): Confused
  (2): Inappropriate
  (3): Incomprehensible
  (4): None
Motor response
  (0): Obeying
  (1): Withdrawing
  (2): Flexing
  (3): Extending
  (4): None
Feeding (cognitive ability only)
  (0): Complete
  (1): Partial
  (2): Minimal
  (3): None
Toileting (cognitive ability only)
  (0): Complete
  (1): Partial
  (2): Minimal
  (3): None
Grooming (cognitive ability only)
  (0): Complete
  (1): Partial
  (2): Minimal
  (3): None
Level of functioning
  (0): Completely independent
  (1): Independent in a special environment
  (2): Mildly dependent
  (3): Moderately dependent
  (4): Markedly dependent
  (5): Totally dependent
Employability
  (0): Not restricted
  (1): Selected jobs, competitive
  (2): Sheltered workshop, noncompetitive
  (3): Not employable

- Has 18 domains (13 motor/ADL and 5 cognitive/communication), all individually scored from 1 (total dependence) to 7 (complete independence)
- Intended for all types of disabilities that lead to some complaints of it being more weighted toward motor impairments, and thus less sensitive in assessing cognitive issues in persons with TBI
- The Functional Assessment Measure (FAM) adds 12 items to assess more cognitive and psychosocial domains
- Both the FIM and the FAM were found to have good sensitivity to change after TBI, especially in the early stages of recovery [9]
- Both the FIM and FIM+FAM require training to properly score

ASSESSMENT OF POSTTRAUMATIC AMNESIA

- Serves as a measure of TBI severity; objective measurement of orientation can be correlated with outcome in rehabilitation [10] and long-term outcome [11]

Galveston Orientation and Amnesia Test

Ten questions with error points subtracted from 100. Initially designed for mild TBI, critics claim that some of the questions are of little personal significance to severely injured patients, such as mode of transport to the hospital. In addition, there are various point values assigned to questions with no justification for the relative weighting of questions.

Orientation Log (O-Log)

Ten questions focusing on domains of time, place, and condition. Scores on each question range from 0 to 3. It can be used in nonverbal patients, and allows the examiner to use logical cuing to prompt the patient for the correct answer.

ASSESSMENT OF DISORDERS OF CONSCIOUSNESS

- Assessing the patient with a disorder of consciousness (DOC) can be difficult, but the ability to objectively distinguish between minimally conscious state and vegetative state may have significant importance for tracking recovery and establishing appropriate plans of care.

Coma/Near Coma Scale

It was first described in 1982 and uses eight parameters and 11 different stimuli [12]. Scores for responses to individual stimuli range from 0 (normal) to 4 (no response); the composite score is divided by number of items tested to create an average score of 0 to 4. Requires equipment of a bell, a light, noxious olfactory stimulus, and a nasal swab.

JFK Coma Recovery Scale

It was published in 1991 and later revised in 2004 [13]. It is composed of 23 items and six subscales, with each subscale in order of brainstem, subcortical and cortical functions. In a study comparing the diagnostic strengths of this scale with the Disability Rating Scale (DRS) in 80 patients with a severe DOC, the Coma Recovery Scale (CRS) was able to diagnose 10 additional patients who were in a minimally conscious state, who were determined to be in a vegetative state by the DRS [14].

Disorder of Consciousness Scale

It requires a baseline assessment followed by scoring of set stimuli responses in eight subscales. Patients are scored a 0 (no response), 1 (general response), or 2 (localized response) to stimuli. Testing requires a variety of different stimuli, including spoons, pictures, juice, and a television. Some authors cite that the scoring of the DOCS allows for a better assessment of responses in comparison with the CRS, which records presence or absence of responses [15].

ADDITIONAL READING

Electronic Reference
Center for Outcome Measurement in Brain Injury. Retrieved from http://www.tbims.org/combi

Textbooks/Chapters
Arlinghaus KA, Shoaib AM, Price TRP. Neuropsychiatric assessment. In: Sliver JM, McAllister TW, Yudofsky SC, eds. *Textbook of Traumatic Brain Injury.* 1st ed. Arlington, VA: American Psychiatric Publishing; 2005.

Posner JB, Saper CB, Shiff ND, Plum F. *Diagnosis of Stupor and Coma.* 4th ed. New York, NY: Oxford University Press; 2007.

Journal Articles
Hall KM, Hamilton BB, Gordon WA, Zasler ND. Characteristics and comparisons of functional assessment indices: Disability Rating Scale, Functional Independence Measure, and Functional Assessment Measure. *J Head Trauma Rehabilitation.* 1993;8(2):60–74.

REFERENCES

1. Teasdale G, Jennett B. Assessment of coma and impaired consciousness. A practical scale. *Lancet.* 1974;2(7872):81–84.

2. Moskopp D, Stähle C, Wassmann H. Problems of the Glasgow Coma Scale with early intubated patients. *Neurosurg Rev.* 1995;18(4):253–257.

3. Zuercher M, Ummenhofer W, Baltussen A, Walder B. The use of Glasgow Coma Scale in injury assessment: a critical review. *Brain Inj.* 2009;23(5):371–384.

4. Zafonte RD, Hammond FM, Mann NR, Wood DL, Black KL, Millis SR. Relationship between Glasgow coma scale and functional outcome. *Am J Phys Med Rehabil.* 1996;75(5):364–369.

5. Hagen C, Malkmus D, Durham P. *Rancho Los Amigos Levels of Cognitive Functioning Scale.* Downey, CA: Rancho Los Amigos Hospital; 1972.

6. Rappaport M, Hall KM, Hopkins K, Belleza T, Cope DN. Disability rating scale for severe head trauma: coma to community. *Arch Phys Med Rehabil.* 1982;63(3):118–123.

7. Hall K. Overview of functional assessment scales in brain injury rehabilitation. *NeuroRehabilitation.* 1992;2:98.

8. Granger CV, Hamilton BB, Keith RA, Zielezny M, Sherwin FS. Advances in functional assessment for medical rehabilitation. *Top Geriatr Rehabil.* 1986;1(3):59–74.

9. van Baalen B, Odding E, van Woensel MP, Roebroeck ME. Reliability and sensitivity to change of measurement instruments used in a traumatic brain injury population. *Clin Rehabil.* 2006;20(8):686–700.

10. Zafonte RD, Mann NR, Millis SR, Black KL, Wood DL, Hammond F. Posttraumatic amnesia: its relation to functional outcome. *Arch Phys Med Rehabil.* 1997;78(10):1103–1106.

11. Dowler RN, Bush BA, Novack TA, Jackson WT. Cognitive orientation in rehabilitation and neuropsychological outcome after traumatic brain injury. *Brain Inj.* 2000;14(2):117–123.

12. Rappaport M, Dougherty AM, Kelting DL. Evaluation of coma and vegetative states. *Arch Phys Med Rehabil.* 1992;73(7):628–634.

13. Kalmar K, Giacino JT. The JFK Coma Recovery Scale–Revised. *Neuropsychol Rehabil.* 2005;15(3–4):454–460.

14. Giacino JT, Kalmar K, Whyte J. The JFK Coma Recovery Scale-Revised: measurement characteristics and diagnostic utility. *Arch Phys Med Rehabil.* 2004;85(12):2020–2029.

15. Pape TL, Heinemann AW, Kelly JP, Hurder AG, Lundgren S. A measure of neurobehavioral functioning after coma. Part I: Theory, reliability, and validity of Disorders of Consciousness Scale. *J Rehabil Res Dev.* 2005;42(1):1–17.

PART 2

Epidemiology and Primary Prevention

4

Epidemiology of Traumatic Brain Injury

Marie Crandall

DEFINITION

Traumatic brain injury (TBI) occurs when there is a blow or jolt to the head due to rapid acceleration or deceleration or a direct impact. It can also be caused by direct penetrating injury of the brain. Brain function is temporarily or permanently impaired and structural damage may or may not be detectable [1]. Not all blows, bumps, or injuries cause TBI, and the severity of the injury may vary widely.

INCIDENCE AND PREVALENCE

Mortality

Injury is the leading cause of death for all individuals aged 1 to 45, accounting for more than 150,000 deaths every year in the United States, and more than 5 million deaths worldwide [2–4]. Head injury is responsible for the largest proportion of these deaths, contributing to one-third of all injury-related deaths [1,5]. The Center for Disease Control estimates that more than 50,000 people die from TBI every year in the United States [6].

Many patients with TBI will die shortly after their trauma, but mortality depends on a number of factors including age, severity and mechanism of brain injury, and presence of other injuries. The overall mortality of moderate to severe TBI is 21% at 30 days [7], and increases to 50% for severe TBI [8].

Disability

Overview
The overall incidence of TBI is difficult to calculate because of differences in outcome measures, definitions, and reporting [9]. Estimates may include only TBI patients admitted to the hospital and may exclude patients presenting to nontrauma or non–emergency department (ED) practioners, ED

visits that do not lead to admission, and typically do not include individuals who suffer an injury but do not seek medical attention. However, the most recent data from the CDC suggest that 1.7 million people annually suffer a TBI. This can be thought of as a pyramid, with the 52,000 deaths at the top, then the 275,000 hospital admissions, and 1.4 million ED visits. An additional 300,000 people are presumed to suffer injuries that are never reported, although the true incidence of this is unknown [5].

Mild TBI

The presentation and outcomes of TBI vary widely, from a brief loss of consciousness to permanent disability and death. Most TBIs are mild and do not cause permanent or long-term disability; however, all sever-ity levels of TBI have the potential to cause significant, long-lasting dis-ability [10]. The risk of permanent disability is low with mild TBI, with most patients having complete resolution of posttraumatic symptoms by 3 months postinjury. However, up to 10% of patients, typically with a more severely impaired presentation and often with obvious intrac-ranial pathology on imaging, may be more likely to suffer persistent or permanent symptoms [11]. By contrast, permanent disability may be experienced by up to 65% of individuals with moderate TBI, and nearly 100% with severe TBI [12]. Approximately 75% of all brain injuries are concussions or mild TBI [13]. Patients with mild TBI may still suffer symptoms after the incident, including headaches, dizziness, inability to concentrate, and nausea. Up to 30% of patients will report posttrau-matic symptoms, and some patients will have persistent complaints [14], although most of those with persistent symptoms do report improvement by 1 year postinjury [15].

Moderate to Severe TBI

Individuals with moderate to severe TBI may have significant impair-ments, and prognosis depends on the severity of injury [16]. However, up to 90% of patients with moderate TBI will be able to live indepen-dently, although many require assistance with finances, transportation, and more complex tasks [17]. Approximately 30% to 40% of people who have suffered severe TBI will make a good recovery, similar to that of moderate TBI [18]. The remaining patients may have profound and pro-longed disability, existing in a permanent vegetative state or minimally conscious state, or have significant impairments, such as posttraumatic epilepsy. There is also a significant mortality risk, up to 10% at 6 months, mostly because of infectious complications. Prediction of outcomes early after injury is based on logistic regression models including things like age, socioeconomic status, injury severity, biologic markers, and comor-bidities, but these predictors are imperfect. Typically, younger patients, those with insurance, Caucasians, and those with less severe TBI and fewer concomitant injuries will have better outcomes [10,19].

Costs

From a financial perspective, the costs of TBI are prohibitive. In 2000, annual TBI-related costs for acute and chronic care of patients were estimated at $60 billion [20].

DEMOGRAPHICS

Causes

Falls are the leading cause of TBI among all age groups (35.2%), followed by motor vehicle collisions or traffic accidents (17.3%), being struck by/against an object (16.5%), and assaults (10%) [6]. However, causes of TBI fatalities are slightly different. Among all causes of injury, road traffic accidents lead to the most TBI fatalities (31.6%). As another example, the lethality of gunshot wounds to the head is approximately 90%. Because of this, gunshot wounds are a much higher percentage of TBI fatalities than the overall incidence would suggest [13].

Risk Factors

Infants and toddlers up to 4 years of age, older adolescents aged 15 to 19, and adults older than 65 years of age are the highest risk age groups for TBI [12]. This trimodal distribution has been demonstrated for most ethnic and racial groups studied, as well as in global studies of TBI [21–23]. Most studies have found that the highest age-specific incidence is in the young adult years. Injury and debility in this age group also carries significant morbidity, with many more years of potential life lost (YPLL) and lost productivity for injuries incurred in young people. For every age group studied, males are more likely to suffer TBI than females. Among young people, males are up to seven times more likely to suffer a TBI [24]. People of color and those of lower socioeconomic strata also suffer rates of TBI 30% to 50% higher than majority individuals [24,25]. Alcohol is involved in 50% of cases of TBI, either because of intoxicated drivers or pedestrians, increased risk of falls, suicide attempts, or interpersonal violence [26–28].

SUMMARY

TBI is the leading cause of death among the injured, killing more than 50,000 people per year in the United States. Outcomes vary widely depending on mechanism of injury, age, and concomitant injuries or morbidities. Young males, people of color, and the socioeconomically disadvantaged are particularly at risk.

ADDITIONAL READING

Electronic Reference

Traumatic Brain Injury. Center for Disease Control, Atlanta, GA. http://www.cdc.gov/ncipc/factsheets/tbi.htm.

Textbook/Chapter

Silver JM, McAllister TW, Yudofsky SC. *Textbook of Traumatic Brain Injury.* Washington, DC: American Psychiatric Publishing; 2005.

Journal Articles

Bruns J, Hauser WA. The epidemiology of traumatic brain injury: a review. *Epilepsia.* 2003;44(s10):2–10.

Greenwald BD, Burnett DM, Miller MA. Brain injury: epidemiology and pathophysiology. *Arch of Phys Med Rehab.* 2003;84(3 suppl 1):S3–S7.

REFERENCES

1. Parikh S, Koch M, Narayan RK. Traumatic brain injury. *Int Anesthesiol Clin.* 2007;45(3):119–135.
2. World Health Organization. Injury. 2010. http://www.who.int/topics/injuries/en/. Accessed March 18, 2010.
3. Center for Disease Control. Traumatic Brain Injury. 2010. http://www.cdc.gov/traumaticbraininjury/. Accessed March 18, 2010.
4. Center for Disease Control Injury Factbook 2006. http://www.cdc.gov/Injury/publications/FactBook/Introduction-2006-a.pdf. Accessed March 18, 2010
5. Sosin DM, Sacks JJ, Smith SM. Head injury-associated deaths in the United States from 1979 to 1986. *JAMA.* 1989;262(16):2251–2255.
6. Faul M, Xu L, Wald MM, Coronado VG. *Traumatic Brain Injury in the United States: Emergency Department Visits, Hospitalizations, and Deaths.* Atlanta, GA: Centers for Disease Control and Prevention, National Center for Injury Prevention and Control; 2010.
7. Greenwald BD, Burnett DM, Miller MA. Brain injury: epidemiology and pathophysiology. *Arch of Phys Med Rehab.* 2003;84(3 suppl 1):S3–S7.
8. Park E, Bell JD, Baker AJ. Traumatic brain injury: can the consequences be stopped? *CMAJ.* 2008;178(9):1163–1170.
9. Bruns J Jr, Hauser WA. The epidemiology of traumatic brain injury: a review. *Epilepsia.* 2003;44(suppl 10):2–10.
10. Brown AW, Elovic EP, Kothari S, Flanagan SR, Kwasnica C. Congenital and acquired brain injury. 1. Epidemiology, pathophysiology, prognostication, innovative treatments, and prevention. *Arch Phys Med Rehabil.* 2008;89(3 suppl 1):S3–S8.
11. Binder LM, Rohling ML, Larrabee GJ. A review of mild head trauma. Part I: Meta-analytic review of neuropsychological studies. *J Clin Exp Neuropsychol.* 1997;19(3):421–431.
12. Frey LC. Epidemiology of posttraumatic epilepsy: a critical review. *Epilepsia.* 2003;44(suppl 10):11–17.
13. Centers for Disease Control and Prevention. National Center for Injury Prevention and Control. *Report to Congress on Mild Traumatic Brain Injury*

in the United States: Steps to Prevent a Serious Public Health Problem. Atlanta, GA: Centers for Disease Control and Prevention; 2003.

14. De Kruijk JR, Leffers P, Menheere PP, Meerhoff S, Rutten J, Twijnstra A. Prediction of post-traumatic complaints after mild traumatic brain injury: early symptoms and biochemical markers. *J Neurol Neurosurg Psychiatr.* 2002;73(6):727–732.

15. Stålnacke BM, Björnstig U, Karlsson K, Sojka P. One-year follow-up of mild traumatic brain injury: post-concussion symptoms, disabilities and life satisfaction in relation to serum levels of S-100B and neurone-specific enolase in acute phase. *J Rehabil Med.* 2005;37(5):300–305.

16. Rao V, Lyketsos C. Neuropsychiatric sequelae of traumatic brain injury. *Psychosomatics.* 2000;41(2):95–103.

17. Crooks CY, Zumsteg JM, Bell KR. Traumatic brain injury: a review of practice management and recent advances. *Phys Med Rehabil Clin N Am.* 2007;18(4):681–710, vi.

18. Utomo WK, Gabbe BJ, Simpson PM, Cameron PA. Predictors of in-hospital mortality and 6-month functional outcomes in older adults after moderate to severe traumatic brain injury. *Injury.* 2009;40(9):973–977.

19. Shafi S, Marquez de la Plata C, Diaz-Arrastia R, et al. Racial disparities in long-term functional outcome after traumatic brain injury. *J Trauma.* 2007;63(6):1263–8; discussion 1268.

20. Finkelstein E, Corso P, Miller T, et al. *The Incidence and Economic Burden of Injuries in the United States.* New York: Oxford University Press; 2006.

21. Wang CC, Schoenberg BS, Li SC, Yang YC, Cheng XM, Bolis CL. Brain injury due to head trauma. Epidemiology in urban areas of the People's Republic of China. *Arch Neurol.* 1986;43(6):570–572.

22. Tate RL, McDonald S, Lulham JM. Incidence of hospital-treated traumatic brain injury in an Australian community. *Aust N Z J Public Health.* 1998;22(4):419–423.

23. Nell V, Brown DS. Epidemiology of traumatic brain injury in Johannesburg–II. Morbidity, mortality and etiology. *Soc Sci Med.* 1991;33(3):289–296.

24. Jager TE, Weiss HB, Coben JH, Pepe PE. Traumatic brain injuries evaluated in U.S. emergency departments, 1992–1994. *Acad Emerg Med.* 2000;7(2):134–140.

25. Cooper KD, Tabaddor K, Hauser WA, et al. The epidemiology of head injury in the Bronx. *Neuroepidemiology.* 1983;2:70–88.

26. Plurad D, Demetriades D, Gruzinski G, et al. Pedestrian injuries: the association of alcohol consumption with the type and severity of injuries and outcomes. *J Am Coll Surg.* 2006;202(6):919–927.

27. Keenan HT, Runyan DK, Marshall SW, Nocera MA, Merten DF, Sinal SH. A population-based study of inflicted traumatic brain injury in young children. *JAMA.* 2003;290(5):621–626.

28. Bastos ML, Galante L. Toxicological findings in victims of traumatic deaths. *J Forensic Sci.* 1976;21(1):176–186.

5

Prevention of Sports-Related Concussion and Brain Injury

Mayur Jayarao, Lawrence S. Chin, and Robert C. Cantu

GENERAL PREVENTION RECOMMENDATIONS

Sport-specific recommendations exist, but, in general, the following are recommended by the third International Symposia on Concussion in Sport [1] and the National Center for Catastrophic Injury Research (NCCSI) [2,3]:

- All athletes should be required to undergo a preparticipation physical examination.
- All teams should have a qualified trainer; accessible, written emergency procedures; and safe facilities and equipment.
- It is important, whenever possible, for a physician to be on the field of play during game and practice. When this is not possible, arrangements must be made in advance to obtain a physician's immediate services when emergencies arise. Each institution should have a team trainer who is a regular member of the institution's staff and who is qualified in the emergency care of both treating and preventing injuries.
- Coaches should be well trained in physical conditioning, the skills of their sport, and the risks of injury. Coaches should also be able to teach these effectively to athletes.
- Game officials must enforce rules strictly, and coaches should support officials' efforts to conduct safe competitions.
- Fair play and respect should be supported as key elements of sport, with violence and aggression being discouraged.

In addition, if any athlete exhibits any of the features of a concussion, they should be immediately removed from play, evaluated using standard emergency care principles, and monitored for deterioration. A formal assessment of the concussive injury should be made using the Sport Concussion Assessment Tool 2 (SCAT2) [1] or other similar tool.

- Serial monitoring for deterioration is essential over the initial few hours following injury. The appearance of symptoms might be delayed several hours following a concussive episode.
- An athlete diagnosed with a concussion should not be allowed to return-to-play (RTP) on the day of injury nor should they be allowed to operate a vehicle.
- Brief neuropsychological tests such as the Standardized Assessment of Concussion (SAC) [4,5] have been demonstrated to be effective. Standard orientation questions (e.g., time, place, and person) have not been demonstrated as being effective.

There is no clinically significant data available to suggest that protective equipment will prevent concussion, although mouth guards can prevent dental and orofacial injury. Biomechanical studies have demonstrated a reduction in impact forces to the brain with the use of head gear and helmets, but these findings have not been translated to show a reduction in concussion incidence, as yet.

- The use of helmets is, nevertheless, recommended universally, when possible.

Consideration of rule changes may also be indicated, such as those recently suggested for soccer, where studies demonstrated that limb-to-head contact during *heading* challenges accounted for approximately 50% of concussions [6]. Rule changes may also be required in some sports to allow for effective medical assessment to occur without compromising either the athlete or game. In this regard, sport officials can play a critical role.

A more recent concern is that of risk compensation [7], where the use of protective equipment results in dangerous play that can result in a paradoxical increase in injury rates. This is of particular importance in nonadult athletes, in whom injury rates can be higher than that of adults [8].

SPORT-SPECIFIC PREVENTION RECOMMENDATIONS

Football

- Prohibit butt blocking and face tackling, and other techniques in which the helmet and facemask purposely receive the brunt of the initial impact. Keep the head and face out of blocking and tackling. Shoulder block and tackle with the head up.
- Discourage the players from using their heads as battering rams when blocking, tackling, and ball carrying. The rules prohibiting spearing should be enforced in practice and games. Ball carriers should also be taught not to lower their heads when making contact with the tackler.

- All coaches, physicians, and trainers should take special care to see that the players' equipment, particularly the helmet, is properly fitted [9].

Soccer

- Safety measures include anchoring the goals, warning players to avoid climbing on them, and using proper moving, maintenance, and storage techniques.
- Helmets specifically designed for use in soccer are currently a contentious issue. At this time, it is an option.

Ice Hockey

- Current recommendations include the use of a helmet and mouth guard along with strict enforcement of the current rules. In addition, new rules may be required against pushing or checking from behind.

Baseball and Softball (Fast-Pitch)

- Most concussions occur during a head-first slide or when a player is struck with a thrown or batted ball. If the head-first slide is to be allowed, coaches must teach players the safest ways to execute this maneuver.
- Proper protection for batting practice should be provided for the batting practice pitcher and he or she should always wear a helmet.

Lacrosse

- The use of helmets with face shields is required. In addition, the use of mouth guards is also strongly recommended.
- Current rules make it illegal to use the head in contact, as well as striking the opponent on the top of the helmet.

Cheerleading

- Cheerleaders should be trained by a qualified coach with training in gymnastics and partner stunting. This person should also be trained in the proper methods for spotting and other safety factors.
- A qualification system demonstrating mastery of stunts is recommended.
- Coaches should supervise all practice sessions in a safe facility.
- Mini-trampolines and flips or falls off of pyramids and shoulders should be prohibited.

- Pyramids over two high should not be performed. Two high pyramids should not be performed without mats and other safety precautions.
- Cheerleading coaches should have some type of safety certification. The American Association of Cheerleading Coaches and Advisors offers this certification.

Skiing and Snowboarding

- Research suggests that helmets provide protection against head and facial injury and, hence, should be recommended for all participants in these sports [10].

Track and Field

- Track and field concussions are usually limited to athletes who participate in the pole vault, shot put, discus or hammer throw, and javelin throw events.
- For the pole vault event, regulations now require the landing pits to be covered over all sections. Helmets for these athletes are a contentious issue and therefore largely considered optional.
- The risk in the discus or hammer throw, and javelin throw events is usually taken by spectators and other competing athletes who find themselves in the path. Safety regulations require the adjacent areas as well as the back and sides of the circle to be fenced off in order to help eliminate this type of accident.

Other Sports

- In sports such as cycling, ice skating, motor, and equestrian sports, protective helmets may prevent head injury related to falling on hard surfaces.

ADDITIONAL READING

Electronic References
www.sportslegacy.org
www.cdc.gov

Textbook/Chapter
Hoshizake TB. Engineering head protection. In: Cantu RC ed. *Neurologic Athletic Head and Spine Injuries*. Philadelphia, PA: WB Saunders Company; 2000.

Journal Articles

Cantu RC, Mueller FO. The prevention of catastrophic head and spine injuries in high school and college sports. *Br J Sports Med.* 2009;43(13):981–986.

McCrory P, Meeuwisse W, Johnston K, et al. Consensus Statement on Concussion in Sport: the 3rd International Conference on Concussion in Sport held in Zurich, November 2008. *Br J Sports Med.* 2009;43(suppl 1):i76–90.

REFERENCES

1. McCrory P, Meeuwisse W, Johnston K, et al. Consensus Statement on Concussion in Sport: the 3rd International Conference on Concussion in Sport held in Zurich, November 2008. *Br J Sports Med.* 2009;43(suppl 1):i76–i90.

2. Cantu RC, Mueller FO. The prevention of catastrophic head and spine injuries in high school and college sports. *Br J Sports Med.* 2009;43(13):981–986.

3. Cantu RC, Mueller FO. Fatalities and catastrophic injuries in high school and college sports, 1982–1997 lessons for improving safety. *Phys Sportsmed.* 1999;27(8):35–48.

4. McCrea M, Kelly JP, Randolph C, et al. Standardized assessment of concussion (SAC): on-site mental status evaluation of the athlete. *J Head Trauma Rehabil.* 1998;13(2):27–35.

5. McCrea M. Standardized mental status assessment of sports concussion. *Clin J Sport Med.* 2001;11(3):176–181.

6. Andersen TE, Arnason A, Engebretsen L, Bahr R. Mechanisms of head injuries in elite football. *Br J Sports Med.* 2004;38(6):690–696.

7. Hagel B, Meeuwisse W. Risk compensation: a "side effect" of sport injury prevention? *Clin J Sport Med.* 2004;14(4):193–196.

8. Finch CF, McIntosh AS, McCrory P, Zazryn T. A pilot study of the attitudes of Australian Rules footballers towards protective headgear. *J Sci Med Sport.* 2003;6(4):505–511.

9. Cantu RC, Mueller FO. Catastrophic football injuries: 1977–1998. *Neurosurgery.* 2000;47(3):673–675; discussion 675–677.

10. Hagel BE, Pless IB, Goulet C, Platt RW, Robitaille Y. Effectiveness of helmets in skiers and snowboarders: case-control and case crossover study. *BMJ.* 2005;330(7486):281.

6

Prevention of Traumatic Brain Injury Secondary to Modes of Transportation, Falls, and Assaults

Jeffrey Radecki

BACKGROUND

According to the World Health Organization (WHO), traumatic brain injury (TBI) will be the major cause of death and disability by 2020. Worldwide, there are an estimated 57 million individuals living with TBI-related disability [1].

Impact

TBI can result in lifelong consequences affecting physical, emotional, cognitive, and behavioral well-being [2]. More than 5 million Americans live with long-term disability related to TBI [3]. Lifetime costs associated with TBI in the United States total an estimated $60 billion annually, including medical costs and lost productivity [4].

Prevention Strategies

- *Primary prevention*—designed to prevent the injury from occurring. Examples of primary prevention include public awareness of drinking and driving laws, fall-proofing strategies in older persons' homes, and recommendations for gun locks to prevent accidents
- *Secondary prevention*—designed to lessen the damage related to the onset of the injury. Examples include seat belts and air bags in automobiles and helmet use for cyclists
- *Tertiary prevention*—designed to lessen sequelae following the injury. Examples include improved access to trauma centers, educating emergency practitioners in identifying TBI, and availability of comprehensive brain injury rehabilitation facilities

TBI DUE TO FORMS OF TRANSPORTATION
Automobiles

The most common cause of TBI-related fatalities in the United States is motor vehicle accidents (MVAs) [5]. However, at the end of 2009, the number of overall traffic-related fatalities were at the lowest level since 1954. The National Highway Traffic and Safety Administration partially credits the decrease to campaigns supporting seat belt use and preventing drunk driving [6].

Younger Drivers
Although younger drivers aged 15 to 20 make up just 6% of licensed drivers, they account for just below 20% of all US motor vehicle fatalities [7].

A recent decrease in fatalities has been linked to increased seat belt use, alcohol and speeding prevention programs, and probably most notably, provisional license phases for teen drivers, which include several driving restrictions including nighttime driving curfews and passenger restriction, especially riding with other teens. Various younger driver laws are currently in place for 48 states and the District of Columbia [8].

Seatbelts and Airbags
In 2007, seat belts saved an estimated 15,147 lives, with another potential 5000 lives saved if all unrestrained motor vehicle occupants wore seatbelts. The use of a lap-shoulder belt system in conjunction with airbags allows for protection of the head. The important distinction between the seatbelt and airbag system is that seatbelt use is an active function, whereas airbags are passive restraint devices [9]. Side-impact air bags (SABs) are designed specifically to prevent head or head-chest combination injuries in MVAs. If SAB technology were standard equipment in all vehicles, nearly 1000 lives would be saved and another 900 serious injuries could be prevented yearly [10].

Motorcyclists and Helmet Use

Motorcycle helmet use is 37% effective in preventing death and 65% effective in preventing brain injury in crashes. Since a 1995 congressional repeal on federal sanctions against states without helmet laws, there have been numerous states that have chosen to repeal or weaken their helmet laws. By repealing mandatory helmet laws, a dramatic drop in helmet use has been observed [11]. Currently, mandatory helmet laws for all motorcyclists exist in only 20 states and the District of Columbia.

In 2008, 1829 lives were saved by motorcycle helmets. An additional 800 lives could have been saved if all motorcyclists had been helmeted [12].

Bicycling

In the United States in 2003, an estimated 10,700 children were hospitalized for bicycle-related injuries, with TBI occurring in 34% of cases. Of these bicycle-related injuries, MVAs were involved in 84% of cases [13]. Bicycle helmet use is the single most effective strategy in preventing TBI in bicycle accidents. Wearing a bicycle helmet reduces the risk of head injury by up to 88% [14]. However, helmets worn inappropriately or with improper fit are associated with an almost twice greater risk of brain injury [15]. An investigational study found 96% of children and adolescents wore helmets that were either not in good condition or not fitted properly [16]. Teaching programs regarding appropriate helmet wear are key in addressing this issue [17].

FALLS

Falls in Children

Childhood falls have been linked to increased risk of TBI due to larger head to body size ratio, decreased cranial bony protection, vulnerable under-myelinated neural tissue and thus, greater risk of diffuse axonal injury and edema compared to adults [18].

In addition to the bicycle-related prevention measures discussed earlier, playground activities are an important focus of TBI prevention in children. The Consumer Product Safety Commission (CPSC) has developed guidelines intended to reduce the occurrence of playground injuries including TBI [19].

Falls in Older Adults

In adults above 65 years of age, falls are the leading cause of injury-related deaths and emergency department visits [20]. It is estimated that one-third of all adults above the age of 65 fall each year [21]. The older adult population has the highest rate of TBI deaths and hospitalizations among any group [22].

The CDC has developed three resources to help prevent falls and TBI among older adults. The fall prevention strategies focus on encouraging exercise, medication review, vision correction, and safeguarding the home environment against falls. They are as follows:

- *Help seniors live better, longer: Prevent brain injury* [23]

■ *Preventing falls: What works. A compendium of effective community-based interventions from around the world* [24]
■ *Preventing falls: How to develop community-based fall prevention programs for older adults* [24]

Guidelines to improve home safety include improved lighting, removing loose carpets and items that may cause tripping, installing grab bars and nonslip surfaces in bathrooms, and having accessible ways to call for help [25].

VIOLENCE AND ASSAULT

Violence and assaults are a major cause of morbidity and mortality in the United States. A significant number of TBIs are because of handgun use. Targeted prevention programs including community-based education on the proper storage and safeguarding of firearms have met with some success. [26]

ADDITIONAL READING

Electronic References
Center for Disease Control: http://www.cdc.gov/TraumaticBrainInjury/index.html
National Highway Traffic Safety Administration: http://www.nhtsa.dot.gov/

Textbook/Chapter
Zasler ND, Katz DI, Zafonte RD. *Brain Injury Medicine: Principles and Practice.* New York: Demos; 2006.

Journal Articles
Brown AW, Elovic EP, Kothari S, et al. Congenital and acquired brain injury. 1. Epidemiology, pathophysiology, prognostication, innovative treatments, and prevention. *Arch Phys Med Rehabil.* 2008;89(3 suppl 1):S3–S8.
McClure RJ, Turner C, Peel N, Spinks A, Eakin E, Hughes K. Population-based interventions for the prevention of fall-related injuries in older people. *Cochrane Database Syst Rev.* 2005, Issue 1. Art. No.: CD004441.
Rutland-Brown W, Langlois JA, Thomas KE, Xi YL. Incidence of traumatic brain injury in the United States, 2003. *J Head Trauma Rehabil.* 2006;21:544–548.

REFERENCES

1. Murray CJ, Lopez AD. *Global Health Statistics.* Geneva: World Health Organization; 1996.
2. US Department of Health and Human Services. National Institutes of Health. Office of the Director. *Rehabilitation of Persons with Traumatic Brain Injury: NIH Consensus Statement.* October 26–28, 1998;16(1):1–41.

3. Thurman DJ, Alverson C, Dunn KA, Guerrero J, Sniezek JE. Traumatic brain injury in the United States: A public health perspective. *J Head Trauma Rehabil.* 1999;14(6):602–615.

4. Finkelstein E, Corso P, Miller T. *The Incidence and Economic Burden of Injuries in the United States.* New York: Oxford University Press; 2006.

5. Heron, M, Hoyert DL, Murphy SL, et al. *Deaths: Final Data for 2006.* US Department of Health and Human Services, Centers for Disease Control and Prevention, National Center for Health Statistics National Vital Statistics System; 2009;Vol 57, Number 14; http://www.cdc.gov/nchs/data/nvsr/nvsr57/nvsr57_14.pdf

6. NHTSA. *Early Estimate of Motor Vehicle Traffic Fatalities in 2009.* March 2010; DOT HS 811 291 http://www-nrd.nhtsa.dot.gov/Pubs/811291.PDF

7. NHTSA. *Teen Driver Crashes: A Report to Congress.* July 2008. DOT HS 811 005. http://www-nrd.nhtsa.dot.gov/Pubs/811218.PDF

8. Insurance Institute for Highway Safety. (July 2009). *U.S. Licensing Systems for Young Drivers.* www.iihs.org.

9. NHTSA. *Lives Saved in 2007 by Restraint Use and Minimum Drinking Age Laws*; November 2008. DOT HS 811 049. http://www.nhtsa.gov/staticfiles/DOT/NHTSA/NCSA/Content/RNotes/2008/811049r.pdf

10. NHTSA. *Vehicle Shoppers, Air Bags.* www.safercar.gov/Vehicle+Shoppers/Air+Bags/Side-Impact+Air+Bags

11. Mayrose J. The effects of a mandatory motorcycle helmet law on helmet use and injury patterns among motorcyclist fatalities. *J Safety Res.* 2008;39(4):429–432.

12. Traffic Safety Facts: 2008 Data, NHTSA, DOT HS 811159.

13. Shah S, Sinclair SA, Smith GA, Xiang H. Pediatric hospitalizations for bicycle-related injuries. *Inj Prev.* 2007;13(5):316–321.

14. Thompson DC, Rivara FP, Thompson R. Helmets for preventing head and facial injuries in bicyclists. *Cochrane Database Syst Rev.* 1999;Issue 4. Art. No:CD001855.

15. Rivara FP, Astley SJ, Clarren SK, Thompson DC, Thompson RS. Fit of bicycle safety helmets and risk of head injuries in children. *Inj Prev.* 1999;5(3):194–197.

16. Parkinson GW, Hike KE. Bicycle helmet assessment during well visits reveals severe shortcomings in condition and fit. *Pediatrics.* 2003;112(2):320–323.

17. Blake G, Velikonja D, Pepper V, Jilderda I, Georgiou G. Evaluating an in-school injury prevention programme's effect on children's helmet wearing habits. *Brain Inj.* 2008;22(6):501–507.

18. Sookplung P, Vavilala MS. What is new in pediatric traumatic brain injury? *Curr Opin Anaesthesiol.* 2009;22(5):572–578.

19. U.S. Consumer Product Safety Commission. *Public Playground Safety Handbook.* Publication #325, April 2008. Retrieved from http://www.cpsc.gov/cpscpub/pubs/325.pdf

20. Centers for Disease Control and Prevention [CDC]. (). *Web-based injury statistics query and reporting system (WISQARS).* Atlanta, GA: National Center for Injury Prevention and Control, Centers for Disease Control and Prevention; 2005. Available at http://www.cdc.gov/ncipc/wisqars

21. Hausdorff JM, Rios DA, Edelberg HK. Gait variability and fall risk in community-living older adults: a 1-year prospective study. *Arch Phys Med Rehabil.* 2001;82(8):1050–1056.

22. Rutland-Brown W, Langlois JA, Thomas KE, Xi YL. Incidence of traumatic brain injury in the United States, 2003. *J Head Trauma Rehabil.* 2006;21(6):544–548.
23. Center for Disease Control Web site. Accessed 25 August 2010. www.cdc.gov/BrainInjuryinSeniors
24. Center for Disease Control Web site. Accessed 25 August 2010. http://www.cdc.gov/traumaticbraininjury/pdf/blue_book.pdf
25. Center for Disease Control Web site. Accessed 25 August 2010. http://www.cpsc.gov/cpscpub/pubs/705.pdf
26. Coyne-Beasley T, Schoenbach VJ, Johnson RM. "Love our kids, lock your guns": a community-based firearm safety counseling and gun lock distribution program. *Arch Pediatr Adolesc Med.* 2001;155(6):659–664.

PART 3

Mild Traumatic Brain Injury

7

Concussion Versus Mild Traumatic Brain Injury
Is There a Difference?

Grant L. Iverson and Rael T. Lange

INTRODUCTION

A concussion, by definition, is a mild traumatic brain injury (MTBI). Although seemingly a scientific truism, there is not universal agreement in the medical community regarding that statement. In fact, surprisingly, there is ongoing and diverse misunderstanding about the terminology and definitions relating to concussion and MTBI. A list of misunderstandings relating to this terminology is provided in Table 7.1.

DIAGNOSTIC CRITERIA

- There is no universally agreed-upon definition of MTBI. There are three commonly cited definitions developed by (1) the Mild Traumatic Brain Injury Committee of the Head Injury Interdisciplinary Special Interest Group of the American Congress of Rehabilitation Medicine (ACRM MTBI Committee), (2) Center for Disease Control (CDC) working group, and (3) World Health Organization (WHO) Collaborating Centre Task Force on Mild Traumatic Brain Injury. Definitions for sport-related concussion are discussed in a different chapter in this book. The ACRM definition is provided in Table 7.2 [1] (the CDC definition is very similar).
- Obviously, the ACRM definition includes an extraordinarily broad spectrum of injury severity. This definition includes injuries characterized by seconds of confusion to injuries involving up to minutes of traumatic coma, several hours of posttraumatic amnesia (PTA), and a focal contusion visible on day-of-injury computed tomography (CT). Similarly, the WHO definition, reprinted in the following section, includes a broad spectrum of injury.

  MTBI is an acute brain injury resulting from mechanical energy to the head from external physical forces. Operational criteria

TABLE 7.1 Misconceptions in the Medical Community Relating to Concussions and Mild TBIs

Concussions refer only to sport-related injuries

If a person recovers relatively quickly, concussion should be used. If not, then the person has sustained a mild TBI

Concussion, because it is synonymous with brain injury, can be used to describe mild, moderate, and severe traumatic brain injuries

Mild TBI should only be used if there is imaging evidence of brain injury

Mild TBI requires a loss of consciousness

TABLE 7.2 ACRM Definition of Mild Traumatic Brain Injury

A traumatically induced physiological disruption of brain function, as manifested by *at least* one of the following:

1. Any loss of consciousness;
2. Any loss of memory for events immediately before or after the accident;
3. Any alteration in mental state at the time of the accident (e.g., feeling dazed, disoriented, or confused); and
4. Focal neurological deficit(s) that may or may not be transient; but where the severity of the injury does not exceed the following:
   - Loss of consciousness of approximately 30 minutes or less;
   - After 30 minutes, an initial Glasgow Coma Scale (GCS) of 13–15; and
   - Posttraumatic amnesia (PTA) not more than 24 hours

Note: A better conjunction after point 3 should have been "or" as opposed to "and."

From Ref. [1].

for clinical identification include: (i) 1 or more of the following: confusion or disorientation, loss of consciousness for 30 minutes or less, post-traumatic amnesia for less than 24 hours, and/or other transient neurological abnormalities such as focal signs, seizure, and intracranial lesion not requiring surgery; (ii) Glasgow Coma Scale score of 13–15 after 30 minutes post-injury or later upon presentation for healthcare. These manifestations of MTBI must not be due to drugs, alcohol, medications, caused by other injuries or treatment for other injuries (e.g., systemic injuries, facial injuries or intubation), caused by other problems (e.g., psychological trauma, language barrier or coexisting medical conditions) or caused by penetrating craniocerebral injury (p. 115; [2]).

COMPLICATED VERSUS UNCOMPLICATED MTBI

- An important subtype within the MTBI spectrum is an injury characterized by macroscopic damage on day-of-injury CT scan. A *complicated* MTBI is diagnosed if the person has a GCS score of 13 to 15 but shows some trauma-related abnormality (e.g., subarachnoid hemorrhage, intraparenchymal hemorrhage, subdural hematoma, epidural hematoma, and contusion) on a CT or magnetic resonance imaging (MRI) scan. In the original definition, depressed skull fractures (not linear fractures) were also considered characteristic of complicated injuries [3]. Individuals with GCS scores of 13 or 14 are at considerable increased risk for day-of-injury CT abnormalities [4–6]. Moreover, MRI can detect abnormalities missed by CT [7–10].

- Williams and colleagues noted that patients with complicated MTBIs were more likely to have worse cognitive functioning acutely compared with uncomplicated MTBI, and their 6-month functional recovery pattern was more similar to persons with moderate brain injuries. Worse outcome associated with complicated MTBIs has been reported by some [3,11–14], but not all [15–17], researchers.

CLINICAL DIAGNOSIS

- The diagnosis of MTBI is based on injury characteristics, such as LOC, confusion and disorientation, PTA, and neurological signs. Neuroimaging is adjunctive.

- Neuropsychological testing can be used to examine the consequences of a MTBI, but cannot be used as the basis for the initial diagnosis. Neuropsychological test results can be influenced by numerous demographic, situational, preexisting, co-occurring, and injury-related factors.

- The diagnosis of a MTBI is based on a clinical interview, collateral interviews, and review of records. Records from the day of injury (e.g., ambulance crew report and emergency department) and the first few medical contacts can be very helpful for an accurate diagnosis. Clinicians should be careful not to misinterpret PTA for LOC (e.g., a patient who is experiencing PTA and who was walking and talking following injury often incorrectly states that "I woke up in the emergency room").

- A careful and deliberate approach that assesses the presence of loss or altered consciousness, gaps in memory or amnesia (retrograde and posttraumatic), and focal neurological signs should be used [18]. One cannot assume that a very careful and thorough approach was taken by health care providers at the scene or in the emergency department. It can be helpful to use a structured form, such as the one provided in Appendix A, to document injury characteristics.

THEORETICAL CELLULAR NEUROBIOLOGY

The cellular neurobiology of injuries on the milder end of the MTBI severity spectrum has been inferred mostly from the animal literature [19–22]. Giza and Hovda [19,20] described the complex interwoven cellular and vascular changes that occur following concussion as a multilayered neurometabolic cascade. The primary mechanisms include ionic shifts, abnormal energy metabolism, diminished cerebral blood flow, and impaired neurotransmission.

TERMINOLOGY FOR CLINICAL PRACTICE

- In general, concussion is the preferred term in sports, both in clinical practice and in research. The term concussion is frequently used in clinical practice in civilian and military trauma cases, especially for injuries on the milder end of the mild spectrum of injury. As such, many people use the term concussion for most uncomplicated MTBIs.
- In general, we believe that concussion is the preferred term because it is more readily understood by most patients, it is easier to communicate the favorable prognosis associated with this injury, and, hopefully, it is less likely that the patient will have an adverse psychological reaction to learning about his or her injury. However, iatrogenic psychological reactions can arise from the person becoming somatically and psychologically preoccupied with having a MTBI/concussion, regardless of terminology.

ADDITIONAL READING

Electronic References

The Management of Concussion/mTBI Working Group. (2009). *VA/DoD clinical practice guideline for management of concussion/mild traumatic brain injury (mTBI)*: http://www.healthquality.va.gov/mtbi/concussion_mtbi_full_1_0.pdf

Textbooks/Chapters

Iverson GL, Lange RT, Gaetz M, Zasler ND. Mild TBI. In: Zasler ND, Katz HT, Zafonte RD, eds. *Brain injury medicine: Principles and practice.* pp. 333–371. New York: Demos Medical Publishing; 2007.

Iverson GL, Zasler ND, Lange RT. Post-concussive disorder. In: Zasler ND, Katz HT, Zafonte RD, eds. *Brain Injury Medicine: Principles and Practice.* New York, NY: Demos Medical Publishing; 2007:373–405.

McCrea M. *Mild Traumatic Brain Injury and Postconcussion Syndrome: The New Evidence Base for Diagnosis and Treatment.* New York, NY: Oxford University Press; 2007.

Journal Articles

Giza CC, Hovda DA. The neurometabolic cascade of concussion. *J Athl Train.* 2001;36(3):228–235.

Ruff RM, Iverson GL, Barth JT, Bush SS, Broshek DK. Recommendations for diagnosing a mild traumatic brain injury: a National Academy of Neuropsychology education paper. *Arch Clin Neuropsychol.* 2009;24(1):3–10.

REFERENCES

1. Mild Traumatic Brain Injury Committee ACoRM, Head Injury Interdisciplinary Special Interest Group. Definition of mild traumatic brain injury. *J Head Trauma Rehabil.* 1993;8(3):86–87.
2. Carroll LJ, Cassidy JD, Holm L, Kraus J, Coronado VG. Methodological issues and research recommendations for mild traumatic brain injury: the WHO Collaborating Centre Task Force on Mild Traumatic Brain Injury. *J Rehabil Med.* 2004;(43 suppl):113–125.
3. Williams DH, Levin HS, Eisenberg HM. Mild head injury classification. *Neurosurgery.* 1990;27(3):422–428.
4. Gómez PA, Lobato RD, Ortega JM, De La Cruz J. Mild head injury: differences in prognosis among patients with a Glasgow Coma Scale score of 13 to 15 and analysis of factors associated with abnormal CT findings. *Br J Neurosurg.* 1996;10(5):453–460.
5. Borczuk P. Predictors of intracranial injury in patients with mild head trauma. *Ann Emerg Med.* 1995;25(6):731–736.
6. Thiruppathy SP, Muthukumar N. Mild head injury: revisited. *Acta Neurochir (Wien).* 2004;146(10):1075–82; discussion 1082.
7. Uchino Y, Okimura Y, Tanaka M, Saeki N, Yamaura A. Computed tomography and magnetic resonance imaging of mild head injury–is it appropriate to classify patients with Glasgow Coma Scale score of 13 to 15 as "mild injury"? *Acta Neurochir (Wien).* 2001;143(10):1031–1037.
8. Lee H, Wintermark M, Gean AD, Ghajar J, Manley GT, Mukherjee P. Focal lesions in acute mild traumatic brain injury and neurocognitive outcome: CT versus 3T MRI. *J Neurotrauma.* 2008;25(9):1049–1056.
9. Mittl RL, Grossman RI, Hiehle JF, et al. Prevalence of MR evidence of diffuse axonal injury in patients with mild head injury and normal head CT findings. *AJNR Am J Neuroradiol.* 1994;15(8):1583–1589.
10. Topal NB, Hakyemez B, Erdogan C, et al. MR imaging in the detection of diffuse axonal injury with mild traumatic brain injury. *Neurol Res.* 2008;30(9):974–978.
11. van der Naalt J, Hew JM, van Zomeren AH, Sluiter WJ, Minderhoud JM. Computed tomography and magnetic resonance imaging in mild to moderate head injury: early and late imaging related to outcome. *Ann Neurol.* 1999;46(1):70–78.
12. Wilson JTL, Hadley DM, Scott LC, Harper A. Neuropsychological significance of contusional lesions identified by MRI. In: Uzzell BP, Stonnington HH, eds. *Recovery after Traumatic Brain Injury.* Mahway, NJ: Lawrence Erlbaum Associates; 1996:29–50.

13. Temkin NR, Machamer JE, Dikmen SS. Correlates of functional status 3–5 years after traumatic brain injury with CT abnormalities. *J Neurotrauma.* 2003;20(3):229–241.

14. Iverson GL. Complicated vs uncomplicated mild traumatic brain injury: acute neuropsychological outcome. *Brain Inj.* 2006;20(13–14):1335–1344.

15. Hofman PA, Stapert SZ, van Kroonenburgh MJ, Jolles J, de Kruijk J, Wilmink JT. MR imaging, single-photon emission CT, and neurocognitive performance after mild traumatic brain injury. *AJNR Am J Neuroradiol.* 2001;22(3):441–449.

16. Hughes DG, Jackson A, Mason DL, Berry E, Hollis S, Yates DW. Abnormalities on magnetic resonance imaging seen acutely following mild traumatic brain injury: correlation with neuropsychological tests and delayed recovery. *Neuroradiology.* 2004;46(7):550–558.

17. McCauley SR, Boake C, Levin HS, Contant CF, Song JX. Postconcussional disorder following mild to moderate traumatic brain injury: anxiety, depression, and social support as risk factors and comorbidities. *J Clin Exp Neuropsychol.* 2001;23(6):792–808.

18. Ruff RM, Iverson GL, Barth JT, Bush SS, Broshek DK. Recommendations for diagnosing a mild traumatic brain injury: a National Academy of Neuropsychology education paper. *Arch Clin Neuropsychol.* 2009;24(1):3–10.

19. Giza CC, Hovda DA. The pathophysiology of traumatic brain injury. In: Lovell MR, Echemendia RJ, Barth JT, Collins MW, eds. *Traumatic Brain Injury in Sports.* Lisse, The Netherlands: Swets & Zeitlinger; 2004:45–70.

20. Giza CC, Hovda DA. The Neurometabolic Cascade of Concussion. *J Athl Train.* 2001;36(3):228–235.

21. Iverson GL. Outcome from mild traumatic brain injury. *Curr Opin Psychiatry.* 2005;18(3):301–317.

22. Iverson GL, Lange RT, Gaetz M, Zasler ND. Mild TBI. In: Zasler ND, Katz HT, Zafonte RD, eds. *Brain Injury Medicine: Principles and Practice.* New York, NY: Demos Medical Publishing; 2007:333–371.

Appendix A Structured Interview Form for Collecting Head Trauma Event Characteristics

Head Trauma Event Characteristics

Name: _____

Date/Time of injury: _____

Reporter: _____ Patient _____ Parent _____ Spouse _____ Other

1 Injury description

a. Is there evidence of a forcible blow to the head (direct or indirect)?

_____ Yes _____ No _____ Unknown

b. Is there evidence of intracranial injury or skull fracture?

_____ Yes _____ No _____ Unknown

c. Location of impact:

_____ Frontal   _____ Left temporal
_____ Left parietal   _____ Right temporal
_____ Right parietal   _____ Occipital
_____ Neck   _____ Indirect force

2 Cause: _____ MVC   _____ Pedestrian—MVC
_____ Fall   _____ Assault
_____ Sports   _____ Blast
_____ Other (specify) _____

3 Amnesia before (Retrograde)

Are there any events just *before* the injury that you/person has no (even brief) memory of?

_____ Yes   _____ No   _____ Duration _____

4 Amnesia after (Anterograde)

Are there any events just *after* the injury that you/person has no (even brief) memory of?

_____ Yes   _____ No   _____ Duration _____

Appendix A Structured Interview Form for Collecting Head Trauma Event Characteristics

Head Trauma Event Characteristics

5. Loss of consciousness
   Did you/person lose consciousness? _____ Yes _____ No   Duration _____

6. Early signs
   _____ Appears dazed or stunned   _____ Is confused about events
   _____ Answers questions slowly   _____ Repeats questions
   _____ Forgetful (recent info)

7. Were seizures observed?   _____ No   _____ Yes   Detail _____

8. Any deaths/injuries to others that occurred as a result of this event?
   _____ No   _____ Yes

Instructions for collecting injury characteristics information:

Q1   Obtain description of the injury: how injury occurred, type of force, location on the head or body (if force transmitted to head). Different biomechanics of injury result in differential symptom patterns (e.g., occipital blow may result in visual changes, balance difficulties).

Q2   Indicate the cause of injury. Greater forces associated with the trauma are likely to result in more severe presentation of symptoms.

Q3 & 4   Amnesia: Amnesia is defined as the failure to form new memories. Determine whether amnesia has occurred and attempt to determine length of time of memory dysfunction—before (retrograde) and after (anterograde) injury.

Q5   Loss of consciousness (LOC): If occurs, determine length of LOC.

Q6   Early signs: If present, ask the individuals who know the patient (parent, spouse, friend, etc.) about specific signs of the concussion that may have been observed. These signs are typically observed early after the injury.

Q7   Inquire whether seizures were observed or not.

Q8   Deaths or injuries that occur during an event can contribute to the development of mental health symptoms.

Source: Appendix B. The Management of Concussion/mTBI Working Group. (2009). *VA/DoD clinical practice guideline for management of concussion/mild traumatic brain injury (mTBI).* Retrieved April 18, 2010, from http://www.healthquality.va.gov/mtbi/concussion_mtbi_full_1_0.pdf

8

Mild Traumatic Brain Injury
Initial Medical Evaluation and Management

John J. Bruns

The primary objective in the initial evaluation of mild TBI (MTBI) is to determine which patients:

- Have an acute traumatic intracranial, spinal, or other injury
- Have an antecedent medical event or worrisome history
- Can be safely discharged from the acute care setting
- Require referral at acute care discharge

DIAGNOSIS

MTBI may not be apparent during an initial medical and neurological evaluation, because:

- Unconsciousness lasts only briefly or cannot be recognized/verified
- Neurological and/or neuropsychiatric deficits may not be discovered by routine clinical examination [1]
- Symptoms resolve rapidly

Symptoms are often mild and only a minority have any significant sequelae.

RISK FACTORS

Important historical aspects of the injury include:

- Mechanism of injury
- Duration of loss of consciousness (LOC)
- Posttraumatic amnesia
- Other injuries

One potential pitfall in the management of the patient with TBI is to assume that TBI is entirely responsible for the overall clinical picture.

Consideration of an antecedent event such as syncope, transient ischemic attack, orthostasis, or dysrrhythmia leading to TBI is prudent, particularly if the patient is elderly or has multiple comorbidities.

A comprehensive approach in both the emergency department and office setting requires initial consideration of the reversible causes of altered mental status, including, for example, hypoperfusion, hypotension, hypoxemia or hypoglycemia, drug toxicity, polypharmacy, or adverse medication event.

LABORATORY STUDIES

The utility of brain-specific biomarkers in determining the need for neuroimaging and duration of postconcussive symptoms is emerging.

■ There are no laboratory clinical assays helpful in the diagnosis of TBI as of 2011
■ The proteins and molecules released after a brain injury diffuse into the cerebrospinal fluid, cross the blood-brain barrier, and can be measured in the serum. S100B is a serum assay that has the most potential

  • S100B rises and falls within hours after MTBI, making early measurement critical
  • At a cutoff of 0.1 μg/L, the sensitivity is 90% to 100%, but specificity is low at 4% to 65%
  • The 2008 CDC/ACEP MTBI guideline recommends, in MTBI patients without significant extracranial injuries and with a serum S100B level less than 0.1 μg/L measured *within 4 hours of injury,* consideration can be given to not performing a computed tomography (CT)

RADIOGRAPHIC ASSESSMENT

Cervical Spine Evaluation

Acute TBI patients should be considered to have an associated spinal injury until evaluated and excluded.

■ The American Association of Neurological Surgeons guidelines [2] state that radiographic assessment of a cervical spine injury is not required in TBI patients who are awake, alert, not intoxicated, have no neck pain or tenderness, and do not have associated significant distracting injuries (i.e., an injury likely to distract the patient from awareness of neck pain)
■ If these criteria are not met, the patient should have a cervical collar placed immediately
■ Obtain three-view x-rays (anteroposterior, lateral, and odontoid) of the cervical spine
■ Or obtain cervical spine CT (preferable if degenerative joint disease [DJD], elderly, or prior C-spine pathology exists)

Skull Radiography

- Has no role in the evaluation of an adult MTBI patient
- Is neither sensitive nor specific for MTBI

Cerebral Neuroimaging

Head trauma evaluated in the emergency department with a presenting Glasgow Coma Scale (GCS) score of 13 to 15 [3]:

- Up to 15% will have an acute lesion on cranial CT (CCT)
- Less than 1% will require neurosurgical intervention
- Clinical predictors for identifying patients with an abnormal CT have been established (See Journal Articles)
- Patients with a negative CCT are at almost no risk of neurological deterioration

HIGH RISK MILD HEAD INJURY

If *any* of the following are present, cranial CT is indicated [4].

- Persistent GCS < 15 at 2 hours post injury
- Deterioration of GCS during surveillance period
- Focal neurological deficit
- Clinical suspicion of skull fracture
- Prolonged LOC (>5 minutes)
- Prolonged anterograde/retrograde amnesia (>30 minutes)
- Posttraumatic seizure
- Persistent abnormal alertness/behavior/cognition
- Persistent abnormal Abbreviated Westmead Post-Traumatic Amnesia Scale (A-WPTAS) score (<18/18)
- Persistent vomiting (two or more occasions)
- Persistent severe headache
- Known coagulopathy (e.g., warfarin, alcoholic, bleeding diathesis)
- Age > 65 years
- Multisystem trauma
- Dangerous mechanism of injury (e.g., motor vehicle vs. pedestrian)
- Clinically obvious drug or alcohol intoxication
- Neurological impairment
- Delayed presentation or re-presentation

TREATMENT

Guiding Principles

- Obtain a chief complaint-driven methodical history and physical prior to clinical interventions

- Be aware that the condition of patients with TBI may deteriorate rapidly after an apparently innocuous presentation

Primary Survey

The initial evaluation includes an immediate and methodical assessment in accordance with Advanced Trauma Life Support protocols [5].

- Airway (A)
- Respiratory/Breathing (B)
  - Endotrachial intubation may be indicated to ensure adequate:
  - Oxygenation (O_2 Sat > 95%)
  - Ventilation (airway unsecured or hypercarbia)
  - Safely perform cranial or other CT scan
- Circulatory (C): avoid hypotension
- Neurological Deficit (D)

Assessing status while protecting (immobilizing) and evaluating the cervical spine is critical.

If there is an identified abnormality in ABCD or cervical spine:

- EMS system should be activated if unable to provide definitive care. Destination should be:
  - Emergency department or
  - Trauma center if severe TBI is present (GCS < 9)

Secondary Survey

- Following the initial evaluation, a more detailed assessment may ensue
- Try to secure information or corroboration from witnesses or family members
- Patients warranting particular attention include those with intoxication, bleeding diathesis, the elderly, and those with an abnormal neurological baseline

The clinician providing the initial evaluation must decide if further evaluation, neuroimaging, or prolonged observation is indicated.

DISPOSITION AND FOLLOW-UP

Patients with low-risk mild head injury can be discharged home if at 4 hours post injury:

- GCS score 15/15
- A-WPTAS score 18/18
- Normal alertness/behavior/cognition
- Clinically improving after observation

- No "high risk" indication for CT scan
- Responsible adult available to take home and observe

The patient should be discharged with written instructions provided to a responsible adult who will be able to check the patient during the subsequent 24 hours.

- Encourage patients to avoid alcohol and strenuous activities for the next several days.
- Advise patients with MTBI that symptoms may develop and last days to weeks after injury. Provide reassurance that these symptoms are typically transient in nature. Provide guidelines regarding which symptoms merit further medical evaluation (see following section).

Discharge Medications

- Avoid narcotics, sedatives (can cause sedation, interfering with assessment of neurological status), and nonsteroidal anti-inflammatory drugs (NSAIDs)/aspirin (could potentially exacerbate a bleed).
- Muscle relaxants have no role.
- Acetaminophen is preferred for headache.
- Consider antiemetics for nausea.

Discharge Instructions

Go to the nearest hospital or call an ambulance (911) for *any* of the following:

- Fainting or drowsiness—or you cannot wake up
- Acting strange, saying things that do not make sense (change in behavior)
- A constant severe headache or a headache that gets worse
- Vomiting or throwing up more than twice
- Cannot remember new events, recognize people or places (increased confusion)
- Pass out or have a blackout or a seizure (any jerking of the body or limbs)
- Cannot move parts of your body, or clumsiness
- Blurred vision or slurred speech
- Continual fluid or bleeding from the ear or nose

The First 24 to 48 Hours After Injury

- Rest and avoid strenuous activity for at least 24 hours
- You should be checked every 4 hours by someone to make sure that you are alright

- Do not drive for at least 24 hours
- You should not drive until you feel better and can concentrate properly
- Do not drink alcohol, or take sleeping pills or recreational drugs in the next 48 hours
- Do not play sports for at least 24 hours
- Use acetaminophen for pain; *avoid* narcotics and NSAIDs/aspirin
- After 48 hours, gradual resumption of usual activities (work, study, driving)

Follow-Up

- If not feeling back to normal within 2 to 3 days, patients should be evaluated by their primary physician
- Patient with an abnormal A-WPTAS score or significant clinical symptoms, such as headache, nausea, or dizziness, should be routinely medically reviewed within 2 to 3 days
- If necessary, arrange for follow-up with a neurologist or rehabilitation specialist

ADDITIONAL READING

Electronic References

http://www.guideline.gov/content.aspx?id=13116#Section420 (guidelines for neuroimaging in MTBI)

http://www.maa.nsw.gov.au/default.aspx?MenuID=148 (MTBI management guidelines)

Textbook/Chapter

Ma OJ, Cline DM. Head injury. In: *Emergency Medicine Manual*. New York, NY: McGraw-Hill Medical Pub Division; 2003:774–780.

Journal Article

Smits M, Dippel D, de Haan G, et al. External validation of the Canadian CT head rule and the New Orleans criteria for CT scanning in patients with minor head injury. *JAMA*. 2005;294:1519–1525

REFERENCES

1. Gerstenbrandy F, Stepan CH. Mild traumatic brain injury. *Brain Injury*. 2001;15(2):95–97.
2. American Association of Neurological Surgeons/Congress of Neurological Surgeons, Joint Section on Disorders of the Spine and Peripheral Nerves. Radiographic assessment of the cervical spine in asymptomatic trauma patients. *Neurosurgery Volume*. 2002;50(3 suppl):S30–S35.

3. Smits M, Dippel D, de Haan G, et al. External validation of the Canadian CT head rule and the New Orleans criteria for CT scanning in patients with minor head injury. *JAMA*. 2005;294:1519–1525.

4. Motor Accidents Authority NSW. *Guidelines for mild traumatic brain injury following closed head injury*, MAA, Editor. 2008, Sydney. ISBN: 978–1–921422–08–9.

5. American College of Surgeons. *Advanced Trauma Life Support (ATLS) Instructor Manual*. 7th ed. Chicago: American College of Surgeons; 2004.

9

Sports-Related Concussion
Identification and Return-to-Play Decision-Making

Nathan E. Kegel and Mark R. Lovell

BACKGROUND

The American Academy of Neurology (AAN) defines concussion, or mild traumatic brain injury, as "a trauma-induced alteration in mental status that may or may not be accompanied by a loss of consciousness" [1]. The Centers for Disease Control and Prevention estimates an incidence rate of 1.8 to 3.6 million sports and recreational concussions per year [2]. This chapter will discuss current guidelines for identification and management of concussion in sports, with an emphasis on criteria and factors to consider when returning an athlete to the playing field.

Initial Sideline Identification of Signs and Symptoms

The first priority is evaluating an athlete's airway, breathing, and circulation. Once more severe injuries are ruled out (e.g., traumatic neck injury or acute neurosurgical emergency); the evaluation should focus on assessment of mental status. Loss of consciousness (LOC) is rather uncommon in concussion, occurring in less than 10% of injuries [3]. Prolonged LOC (>1–2 minutes) is even less frequent; athletes with LOC are typically unresponsive for only a few seconds [4]. Any athlete demonstrating LOC should be managed conservatively and same day return-to-play is contraindicated.

Confusion and Amnesia

Confusion and amnesia are far more common than LOC. Confusion (i.e., disorientation) represents impaired awareness of and orientation to one's surroundings, and often manifests in athletes as appearing stunned, dazed, or glassy-eyed on the sideline. Confusion often becomes apparent to team-mates before medical staff are notified.

Posttraumatic amnesia (PTA) is characterized by loss of memory for the length of time between the trauma and the point at which the athlete regains normal continuous memory functioning. On-field assessment of PTA can be accomplished via asking the athlete to recall specific events that occurred immediately following the trauma. The presence of PTA is highly predictive of postinjury neurocognitive deficits [4]. Any indication of amnesia should be taken seriously and the athlete should be removed from play.

Headache

Headache occurs in 70% of athletes who sustain a concussion [5]. Most frequently these headaches are described as a sensation of pressure that may be localized to one region of the head or may be generalized in nature. In some athletes, the headache may take the form of a vascular/ migraine headache.

Other Signs and Symptoms

These include blurred vision, changes in peripheral vision, photosensitivity, and difficulty maintaining balance. Athletes may also report increased fatigue, "feeling a step slow," or feeling sluggish. Fatigue is especially common in concussed athletes in the days immediately following the injury. In addition, lingering cognitive symptoms, such as difficulties with attention and concentration, often become apparent in the weeks following the concussion, particularly when the athlete returns to academic or vocational activities. Frequent vomiting or declining mental status following a concussion may indicate a life-threatening situation, necessitating transport to a hospital emergency department and imaging of the brain.

MANAGEMENT OF CONCUSSION

Return-to-Play Guidelines

The concussed athlete should be prohibited from returning to the game during which the concussion took place. The athlete must progress through a graduated return-to-play protocol, beginning with demonstration of an asymptomatic presentation while at rest, and followed by stepwise physical exertion [6]. Each step should, in most circumstances, be separated by 24 hours. Any recurrence of concussive symptoms at a particular level of exertion should result in the athlete dropping back to the previous level. For example, if an athlete is asymptomatic at rest but develops a headache with light exertion, then the athlete should return to complete rest. For an athlete to meet international criteria for return-to-play, he or she must be asymptomatic at full physical exertion and demonstrate baseline neuropsychological test performance, when such data is available [6] (See Table 9.1).

Table 9.1 Return-to-Play Protocol

Initial management following injury

When a player shows any symptoms or signs of a concussion, the following should be applied:

The player should not be allowed to return to play in the current game or practice

The player should not be left alone, and regular monitoring for deterioration is essential over the initial few hours after injury

The player should be medically evaluated after the injury

Return to play must follow a medically supervised stepwise process

A player should never return to play while symptomatic

Return-to-play protocol

It is important to emphasize to the athlete that physical and cognitive rest is required.

The return to play after a concussion follows a stepwise process:

No activity, complete rest. Once asymptomatic, proceed to level 2

Light aerobic exercise such as walking or stationary cycling, no resistance training

Sport specific exercise—for example, skating in hockey, running in soccer; progressive addition of resistance training at steps 3 or 4

Noncontact training drills

Full contact training after medical clearance

Game play

With this stepwise progression, the athlete should continue to proceed to the next level if asymptomatic at the current level. If any postconcussion symptoms occur, the patient should drop back to the previous asymptomatic level and try to progress again after 24 hours. Any medications started for treatment of symptoms directly linked to concussion should be stopped and patient should be asymptomatic following its removal.

Return to Normal Activity Following Concussion

Return to the classroom is a major concern for school-age athletes. Normal school activities such as studying, sitting in class, or eating lunch in a cafeteria can be very difficult following a concussion; these activities may even exacerbate postconcussive symptoms. Teachers, parents, and other adults may not be sensitive to the discomfort of the child and may misattribute declining school performance to laziness or to other factors. Therefore, it is important that specific instructions are provided to the school. It is suggested that health care professionals who regularly evaluate school-age concussed patients use an accommodation form such as the one presented in Table 9.2.

Table 9.2 Return to School Accommodations Form

Student _____ Grade ____ School _____

This student has had a concussion and is likely to experience symptoms such as impaired concentration and memory, headache, light and noise sensitivity, dizziness, and balance problems. These symptoms should improve with rest. Please allow for the following accommodations:

___ Extra time (Child may need additional time to complete assignments)

___ Please allow student to turn in assignments late

___ Please allow student extra time to complete quizzes and tests

___ Please allow student to take breaks if symptoms become worse

___ Please allow student to wear sun glasses while at school

___ Please allow student to wear ear plugs while at school

___ Student should not be required to complete standardized testing until _____

___ This student should not be attending gym or should not be allowed to participate in physical activities during recess.

___ This student can not participate in group sports activities during gym

___ This student can tolerate low level physical activities such as walking

___ This student can participate in physical exertion but not in group activities

___ This student can participate fully in gym

Individual Factors Influencing Return-to-Play Decision-Making

Return-to-play decisions after a concussion are influenced by several factors, including but not limited to an athlete's age, gender, history of prior injury, and particular sport. A brief review of factors that may affect recovery from concussion follows.

Age

Recent research has produced several theories to explain observed age-related differences in recovery from concussion, that is, high school athletes' recovery time may be longer than that of college or professional athletes [7,8].

- Children may experience more prolonged cerebral swelling after traumatic brain injury [9]
- An immature brain may be more sensitive to glutamate [10]

- These factors could lead to a longer recovery period and could increase the likelihood of permanent or severe neurologic deficit should reinjury occur during the recovery period. Furthermore, this provides evidence explaining the occurrence of second impact syndrome exclusively in child and adolescent athletes [11].

Gender

Large-scale epidemiological studies have reported that females have a higher rate of concussion in sports when compared to their male counterparts [12]. The potential reasons for these differences is unclear. Difference in neck strength between males and females is one hypothesis that has been suggested [13]. There may also be gender-specific differences in brain physiology that may contribute to these findings. Further research is needed to better understand the factors involved in these apparent gender differences.

Prior Concussion History

There is a growing body of evidence suggesting detrimental physical and cognitive effects of multiple concussions. A recent retrospective study surveyed a sample of retired National Football League (NFL) athletes and found that those who had experienced three or more concussions were more likely to report persistent symptoms of cognitive impairment and depression [14]. A study examining multiple concussions in college football players [15] found long-term mild deficits in executive functioning and speed of information processing in athletes who sustained two or more concussions. These findings have led to the generally accepted practice of recommending discontinuation of the offending sport/activity if a young athlete demonstrates a lower threshold for injury (e.g., he or she displays concussive symptoms with less provocation), or the athlete demonstrates persistent neurocognitive sequelae or symptoms (e.g., lasting longer than a month). Although some researchers have suggested that three or more concussions should warrant discontinuation from sport, there is still considerable debate regarding this issue.

Time Between Injuries

Although there is currently no formal research examining this factor, most concussion management guidelines contain a provision for restriction of play after multiple concussions within a given season [1,16].

Additional Factors

- The role of genetic factors is postulated to play a role in recovery from injury, largely because of preliminary research in boxers and linkage to the ApoE-4 allele, a marker associated with expression of Alzheimer's disease [17].

■ The role of headache history appears to be a contributory factor in recovery from concussion. Suffering a blow to the head is a well-known trigger for headaches, and a prior history of migraine and other headaches may play a role in protracted recovery from concussion [18,19].

CONCLUSIONS

The management of sports-related concussion begins on the field, rink, or court with the proper identification of the injury, and progresses through the implementation of a systematic return-to-play protocol and return to usual life activities such as school. Proper identification and management of concussion will maximize healthy return-to-play and life activities.

ADDITIONAL READING

Electronic Reference

CDC's Head's Up on Brain Injury: Concussion in Sports. http://www.cdc.gov/concussion/sports/index.html

Textbook/Chapter

Echemendia RJ, ed. *Sports Neuropsychology: Assessment and Management of Traumatic Brain Injury.* New York, NY: Guilford Press; 2006.

Journal Articles

Moser RS, Iverson GL, Echemendia RJ, et al. Neuropsychological evaluation in the diagnosis and management of sports-related concussion. *Arch Clin Neuropsychol.* 2007;8:909–916.

Reddy CC, Collins MW. Sports concussion: management and predictors of outcome. *Curr Sports Med Rep.* 2009;8:10–15.

Van Kampen DA, Lovell MR, Pardini JE, Collins MW, Fu FH. The "value added" of neurocognitive testing after sports-related concussion. *Am J Sports Med.* 2006;34(10):1630–1635.

REFERENCES

1. Quality Standards Subcommittee, American Academy of Neurology. Practice Parameter: the management of concussion in sports. *Neurology.* 1997;48:581–585.
2. Langlois JA, Rutland-Brown W, Wald MM. The epidemiology and impact of traumatic brain injury: a brief overview. *J Head Trauma Rehabil.* 2006;21(5):375–378.
3. Lovell MR, Iverson GL, Collins MW, et al. Measurement of symptoms following sports-related concussion: reliability and normative data for the post-concussion scale. *Appl Neuropsychol.* 2006;13(3):166–174.

4. Collins MW, Iverson GL, Lovell MR, McKeag DB, Norwig J, Maroon J. On-field predictors of neuropsychological and symptom deficit following sports-related concussion. *Clin J Sport Med.* 2003;13(4):222–229.

5. Collins MW, Field M, Lovell MR, et al. Relationship between postconcussion headache and neuropsychological test performance in high school athletes. *Am J Sports Med.* 2003;31(2):168–173.

6. McCrory P, Meeuwisse W, Johnston K, et al. Consensus Statement on Concussion in Sport: the 3rd International Conference on Concussion in Sport held in Zurich, November 2008. *Br J Sports Med.* 2009;43 (suppl 1):i76–i90.

7. Field M, Collins MW, Lovell MR, Maroon J. Does age play a role in recovery from sports-related concussion? A comparison of high school and collegiate athletes. *J Pediatr.* 2003;142(5):546–553.

8. Pellman EJ, Lovell MR, Viano DC, Casson IR. Concussion in professional football: recovery of NFL and high school athletes assessed by computerized neuropsychological testing–Part 12. *Neurosurgery.* 2006;58(2):263–74; discussion 263.

9. Pickels W. Acute general edema of the brain in children with head injuries. *N Engl J Med.* 1950;242:607–611.

10. McDonald JW, Johnston MV. Physiological and pathophysiological roles of excitatory amino acids during central nervous system development. *Brain Res Brain Res Rev.* 1990;15(1):41–70.

11. Cantu R, Voy R. Second impact syndrome: a risk in any sport. *Clin J Sport Med.* 1998;17:37–44.

12. Gessel LM, Fields SK, Collins CL, Dick RW, Comstock RD. Concussions among United States high school and collegiate athletes. *J Athl Train.* 2007;42(4):495–503.

13. Tierney RT, Sitler MR, Swanik CB, Swanik KA, Higgins M, Torg J. Gender differences in head-neck segment dynamic stabilization during head acceleration. *Med Sci Sports Exerc.* 2005;37(2):272–279.

14. Guskiewicz KM, Marshall SW, Bailes J, et al. Recurrent concussion and risk of depression in retired professional football players. *Med Sci Sports Exerc.* 2007;39(6):903–909.

15. Collins MW, Lovell MR, Mckeag DB. Current issues in managing sports-related concussion. *JAMA.* 1999;282(24):2283–2285.

16. Cantu RC. Cerebral concussion in sport. Management and prevention. *Sports Med.* 1992;14(1):64–74.

17. Jordan BD, Relkin NR, Ravdin LD, Jacobs AR, Bennett A, Gandy S. Apolipoprotein E epsilon4 associated with chronic traumatic brain injury in boxing. *JAMA.* 1997;278(2):136–140.

18. Gordon KE, Dooley JM, Wood EP. Is migraine a risk factor for the development of concussion? *Br J Sports Med.* 2006;40(2):184–185.

19. Lau B, Lovell MR, Collins MW, Pardini J. Neurocognitive and symptom predictors of recovery in high school athletes. *Clin J Sport Med.* 2009;19(3):216–221.

The Natural History of Mild Traumatic Brain Injury

Grant L. Iverson and Rael T. Lange

INTRODUCTION

The natural history of mild traumatic brain injury (MTBI) is reasonably well understood. There is a substantial body of evidence suggesting that the symptoms and problems associated with this injury are time-limited and follow a predictable course for most people. The majority of people do not require specific medical treatment. They do, however, benefit from (1) education and reassurance and (2) advice regarding a gradual resumption of activities. A summary of the natural history of MTBI, from a clinical practice guideline prepared by a working group from the US Department of Veterans Affairs and the US Department of Defense, is provided in Table 10.1 [1].

CLINICAL PRESENTATION: SYMPTOMS OF MTBI

- Athletes and trauma patients report diverse physical, cognitive, and emotional symptoms in the initial days and weeks postinjury. In concussed athletes, the most frequently endorsed symptoms in the initial days postinjury are: headaches, fatigue, feeling slowed down, drowsiness, difficulty concentrating, feeling mentally foggy, and dizziness [2].
- Time course for recovery: In very mild injuries, symptomatic recovery typically occurs within 2 weeks. This is illustrated in Figure 10.1 [3]. In a sample of 635 concussed high school and college athletes, 85% recovered symptomatically within the first week postinjury.
- Symptom persistence: It is difficult to predict who will continue to report symptoms several months postinjury. For example, in a well-controlled prospective study of trauma patients, McCauley and colleagues reported that day-of-injury CT abnormalities were not associated with increased risk for the postconcussion syndrome at 3 months postinjury [4].

Table 10.1 Summary of the Natural History, Early Intervention, and Return to Work Following MTBI from the US VA and DoD

Natural history

The vast majority of patients who have sustained an MTBI improve with no lasting clinical sequelae.

Patients should be reassured and encouraged that the condition is transient and full recovery is expected. The term "brain damage" should be avoided. A risk communication approach should be applied[a].

The vast majority of patients recover within hours to days[b], with a small proportion taking longer. In an even smaller minority, symptoms may persist beyond 6 months to a year.

The symptoms associated with postconcussion syndrome are not unique to MTBI. The symptoms occur frequently in day-to-day life among healthy individuals and are also found often in persons with other conditions such as chronic pain or depression.

Early intervention

Early education of patients and their families is the best available treatment for MTBI and for preventing/reducing the development of persistent symptoms.

A primary care model can be appropriate for the management of MTBI when implemented by an interdisciplinary team with special expertise.

Return to work/duty activity

Patients sustaining an MTBI should return to normal (work/duty/school/leisure) activity as soon as possible.

A gradual resumption of activity is recommended.

If physical, cognitive, or behavioral complaints/symptoms re-emerge after returning to previous normal activity levels, a monitored progressive return to normal activity as tolerated should be recommended.

[a] Risk communication involves the exchange of information during patient visits relating to diagnoses, medications, and treatments. A patient-centered approach, based on effective communication, is preferred given the biopsychosocial complexity involved in cases of poor outcome from MTBI. Researchers have reported that the quality of clinician-patient communications can significantly influence the quality of life for patients and improve patient health outcomes.

[b] Author comment: We believe there is a body of evidence to support the statement that the vast majority of concussed athletes recover within the first month and civilian trauma patients recover within the first 6 months.

Source: From Ref. 1. Pages 7–8. This clinical practice guideline was compiled after a comprehensive review of the civilian and military MTBI literature.

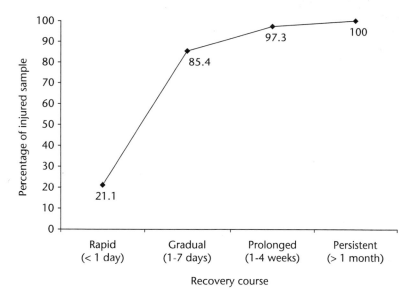

Figure 10.1 Symptom recovery course in 635 concussed high school and college athletes.

Note: The percentage of the injured sample recovered at each interval is based on clinical documentation from physicians and certified athletic trainers on duration of symptoms. Adapted from Ref. [3].

- Evolution into Postconcussion Syndrome: Despite decades of research, the persistent postconcussion syndrome remains controversial. The syndrome is a nonspecific cluster of symptoms that can be mimicked by a number of preexisting or comorbid conditions. Therefore, it is imperative for clinicians to systematically evaluate the possible contribution of many differential diagnoses, comorbidities, and social-psychological factors that may cause or maintain self-reported symptoms long after an MTBI.

COGNITIVE IMPAIRMENT AND RECOVERY

- Initial postinjury presentation: Injured athletes and trauma patients perform more poorly on neuropsychological tests in the initial days postinjury. Injured trauma patients, as a group, perform more poorly on cognitive testing up to the first month following the injury. Neuropsychological deficits typically are not seen in athletes after 1 to 3 weeks and in trauma patients after 1 to 3 months in prospective group studies (see [5] for a review).

- Effect of loss of consciousness: Researchers studying trauma patients have reported that there is no clear association between brief loss of consciousness and short-term neuropsychological outcome (see [3] for a review) or vocational outcome.

- Effect of Posttraumatic Amnesia (PTA): The presence and duration of posttraumatic confusion or amnesia (PTA) has been associated with worse immediate outcome and slower recovery in athletes. PTA in trauma patients also appears to be related to short-term neuropsychological outcome (see 3 for a review). In MTBI, however, the relation between PTA and outcome weakens when outcome is assessed several months postinjury.

- Complicated versus Uncomplicated MTBI [6,7]: Patients with complicated MTBI (i.e., MTBI with abnormalities noted on initial brain imaging) tend to perform more poorly on neuropsychological tests than patients with uncomplicated MTBI in the first 2 months following injury, but only on a small number of tests rather than having globally depressed scores. When differences occur between these two groups, the effect sizes of these differences tend to be medium. At 6 months postinjury, some researchers have not reported differences in neuropsychological test performance between complicated and uncomplicated MTBI patients.

- Meta-Analytic Studies:

  - There are several published meta-analyses [8–11] and reviews [12–14] of the literature relating to cognitive functioning following MTBI which can help put neuropsychological consequences of this injury into context (see Figure 10.2) [15].

  - Meta-analyses can also be used to examine moderator variables. For example, time is a critical moderator variable with MTBI. The effect of sport-related concussion is dramatic in the first 24 hours but small after 7 days have passed. Moreover, the effects of MTBI on cognitive functioning after 1 to 3 months are negligible (comparable to the effects of cannabis). However, when examining patients involved in litigation, the overall effect on cognition is comparable to the effects of moderate-to-severe TBIs (Figure 10.2).

EARLY INTERVENTION

Clinicians should try to prevent poor outcome in people who have suffered an MTBI. Early intervention, as simple as education and reassurance of a likely good outcome, can reduce the number and severity of postconcussion symptoms and increase return to work rates.

In most studies, patients participating in early intervention programs consisting of educational materials plus various additional treatments and/or assessments (e.g., neuropsychological testing, meeting with a therapist, reassurance, access to a multidisciplinary team) report fewer

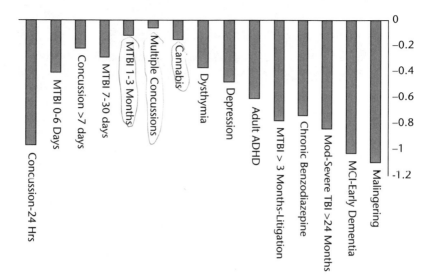

Figure 10.2 Meta-analytic effect sizes: neuropsychological functioning.

Figure reprinted from: Ref. 15. Effect sizes typically are expressed in pooled, weighted standard deviation units. However, across studies, there are some minor variations in the methods of calculation. By convention, effect sizes of 0.2 are considered small, 0.5 medium, and 0.8 large. This is from a statistical, not necessarily clinical, perspective. For this figure, the overall effect on cognitive or neuropsychological functioning is reported. Effect sizes less than 0.3 should be considered very small and difficult to detect in individual patients because the patient and control groups largely overlap.

postconcussion symptoms at 3 months postinjury [16] and at 6 months postinjury [17,18] compared to patients who received standard hospital treatment (see 3 for a review). Educational brochures or sessions typically provide information regarding common symptoms, likely time course of recovery, reassurance of recovery, and suggested coping strategies following MTBI.

ADDITIONAL READING

Electronic Reference
http://www.dvbic.org/images/pdfs/Providers/VADoD-CPG---Concussion-mTBI.aspx

Textbooks/Chapters
McCrea M. *Mild Traumatic Brain Injury and Postconcussion Syndrome: The New Evidence Base for Diagnosis and Treatment*. New York, NY: Oxford University Press; 2007.

Iverson GL, Lange RT, Gaetz M, Zasler ND. Mild TBI. In: Zasler ND, Katz HT, Zafonte RD, editors. *Brain Injury Medicine: Principles and Practice.* New York: Demos Medical Publishing; 2007:333–371.

Iverson GL, Zasler ND, Lange RT. Postconcussive disorder. In: Zasler ND, Katz HT, Zafonte RD, eds. *Brain Injury Medicine: Principles and Practice.* New York: Demos Medical Publishing; 2007:373–405.

Journal Articles

Bigler ED. Neuropsychology and clinical neuroscience of persistent post-concussive syndrome. *Journal of the International Neuropsychological Society.* 2008;14(1):1–22.

Dikmen SS, Corrigan JD, Levin HS, Machamer J, Stiers W, Weisskopf MG. Cognitive outcome following traumatic brain injury. *Journal of Head Trauma Rehabilitation.* 2009;24(6):430–438.

Dikmen S, Machamer J, Fann JR, Temkin NR. Rates of symptom reporting following traumatic brain injury. *Journal of the International Neuropsychological Society.* 2010;16(3):401–411.

REFERENCES

1. The Management of Concussion/mTBI Working Group. VA/DoD clinical practice guideline for management of concussion/mild traumatic brain injury (mTBI). April 18, 2009. http://www.healthquality.va.gov/mtbi/concussion_mtbi_full_1_0.pdf. Accessed April 18, 2010.

2. Lovell MR, Iverson GL, Collins MW, et al. Measurement of symptoms following sports-related concussion: reliability and normative data for the post-concussion scale. *Appl Neuropsychol.* 2006;13(3):166–174.

3. McCrea M, Iverson GL, McAllister TW, et al. An integrated review of recovery after mild traumatic brain injury (MTBI): implications for clinical management. *Clin Neuropsychol.* 2009;23(8):1368–1390.

4. McCauley SR, Boake C, Levin HS, Contant CF, Song JX. Postconcussional disorder following mild to moderate traumatic brain injury: anxiety, depression, and social support as risk factors and comorbidities. *J Clin Exp Neuropsychol.* 2001;23(6):792–808.

5. Iverson GL, Lange RT, Gaetz M, Zasler ND. Mild TBI. In: Zasler ND, Katz HT, Zafonte RD, eds. *Brain Injury Medicine: Principles and Practice.* New York: Demos Medical Publishing; 2007:333–371.

6. Iverson GL. Complicated vs uncomplicated mild traumatic brain injury: acute neuropsychological outcome. *Brain Inj.* 2006;20(13–14):1335–1344.

7. Williams DH, Levin HS, Eisenberg HM. Mild head injury classification. *Neurosurgery.* 1990;27(3):422–428.

8. Belanger HG, Curtiss G, Demery JA, Lebowitz BK, Vanderploeg RD. Factors moderating neuropsychological outcomes following mild traumatic brain injury: a meta-analysis. *J Int Neuropsychol Soc.* 2005;11(3):215–227.

9. Belanger HG, Vanderploeg RD. The neuropsychological impact of sports-related concussion: a meta-analysis. *J Int Neuropsychol Soc.* 2005;11(4):345–357.

10. Binder LM. A review of mild head trauma. Part II: Clinical implications. *J Clin Exp Neuropsychol.* 1997;19(3):432–457.

11. Schretlen DJ, Shapiro AM. A quantitative review of the effects of traumatic brain injury on cognitive functioning. *Int Rev Psychiatry.* 2003;15(4):341–349.

12. Ruff R. Two decades of advances in understanding of mild traumatic brain injury. *J Head Trauma Rehabil.* 2005;20(1):5–18.

13. Carroll LJ, Cassidy JD, Peloso PM, et al.; WHO Collaborating Centre Task Force on Mild Traumatic Brain Injury. Prognosis for mild traumatic brain injury: results of the WHO Collaborating Centre Task Force on Mild Traumatic Brain Injury. *J Rehabil Med.* 2004;(43 suppl):84–105.

14. Iverson GL. Outcome from mild traumatic brain injury. *Curr Opin Psychiatry.* 2005;18(3):301–317.

15. Iverson GL. Mild traumatic brain injury meta-analyses can obscure individual differences. *Brain Inj.* 2010;24(10):1246–1255.

16. Ponsford J, Willmott C, Rothwell A, et al. Impact of early intervention on outcome following mild head injury in adults. *J Neurol Neurosurg Psychiatr.* 2002;73(3):330–332.

17. Mittenberg W, Tremont G, Zielinski RE, Fichera S, Rayls KR. Cognitive-behavioral prevention of postconcussion syndrome. *Arch Clin Neuropsychol.* 1996;11(2):139–145.

18. Wade DT, King NS, Wenden FJ, Crawford S, Caldwell FE. Routine follow up after head injury: a second randomised controlled trial. *J Neurol Neurosurg Psychiatr.* 1998;65(2):177–183.

11

Cumulative Effects of Repeated Mild Traumatic Brain Injury

Gentian Toshkezi, Lawrence S. Chin, and Robert C. Cantu

INTRODUCTION

Repeated mild traumatic brain injuries (MTBIs) may occur in a variety of contexts, most commonly in athletics, and can have significant long-term neurologic impact. This chapter will specifically focus on the cumulative effects of MTBI in sports, but the same concepts are applicable regardless of the mechanism of injury.

In some sports such as boxing, where the goal is to cause repeated blows to the head, or football, where frequent head contact is inevitable, the study of this disease is of prime importance. Furthermore, there is often a culture of toughness that predisposes participants to continue playing through minor head injuries, putting the athlete at risk for repeated trauma. Repeated injuries may also be seen in other sports such as soccer, ice hockey, lacrosse, rugby, equestrian events, and skiing because of the high incidence of collisions, falls, or striking the ball [1,2]. Repetitive MTBI can cause long-lasting neurologic symptoms. It is reported that 17% of cases develop a condition called chronic traumatic encephalopathy, previously known as dementia pugilistica (see following section) [1].

EPIDEMIOLOGY

In a prospective cohort study done on 2905 US collegiate football players from 1999 to 2001, 6.5% of the players had more than one MTBI within the same season, and 1.6% presented with three or more concussions within the same season [3]. In another study, certified athletic trainers who worked with high school and collegiate football players were surveyed; of 17,549 players, 5.1% presented with at least one concussion per year, and of these concussed players, 14.7% had more than one concussion in the same season [4]. Players with a history of more than three concussions were in turn three times more likely to have a repeat concussion than players with no history of brain trauma.

Although the cumulative effect of two concussions results in little or no difference in symptoms compared to suffering a single concussion, patients with multiple concussions often experience a longer recovery period [5]. Both the increased risk for future injury and slower recovery are signs of potential increased neuronal vulnerability following recurrent concussive brain injuries.

PHYSIOPATHOLOGY

Studies of the cortical silent period (CSP), defined as the time between stimulation of the cortex and resulting muscle activity on electromyography (EMG), show that there is an altered CSP even in asymptomatic athletes who score normally on neuropsychologic tests following a concussion [6]. Furthermore, athletes with multiple concussions tend to report more severe symptoms, and abnormalities of cortical functioning, based on duration of the CSP, persist far beyond the acute phase of the injury. It is hypothesized that the neurophysiologic substrate of the CSP is related to altered GABA-B receptor sensitivity, which renders the brain more vulnerable to subsequent traumatic events [6]. Animal studies show a disrupted neuronal metabolic cascade resulting in accelerated glycolysis and increased lactate levels following concussion. Downstream effects include an increase in intracellular calcium, mitochondrial dysfunction, impaired oxidative metabolism, axonal disconnection, impaired neurotransmission, and delayed cell death. These metabolic changes following concussions make neurons more vulnerable to secondary ischemic injury and perhaps repeat injury [3].

These pathologic mechanisms may be similar to those that cause brain degeneration in Alzheimer's disease (AD) [7]. Boxers with dementia pugilistica show β-amyloid protein–containing diffuse plaques and neurofibrillary tangles that are similar to findings seen in AD. Unlike AD, however, the neurofibrillary tangles of dementia pugilistica are located in superficial rather than deep layers of the neocortex and occur without neuritic plaques [1,8].

CLINICAL MANIFESTATIONS

The severity of concussion-related symptoms may worsen with successive injuries even when a time lag exists between injuries [4]. The cumulative effect of MBTI most dramatically affects cognitive function, particularly planning and memory. Athletes with three or more concussions also appear to have more significant loss of consciousness, anterograde amnesia, and confusion [2,9–12].

DIAGNOSIS

A detailed history and physical is critical for the evaluation of a patient presenting with cumulative effects of MTBI. The standard diagnostic tool is neuropsychological testing. Brain computed tomography (CT) and magnetic resonance imaging (MRI) are less helpful in the diagnosis of cumulative effects of MTBI. Functional MRI of the brain may detect frontal lobe hyperperfusion seen in repeated concussions, but at this stage is still investigational [13]. Testing for the CSP via transcranial magnetic stimulation may one day prove to be a valuable sensitive diagnostic exam, capable of detecting brain abnormalities in repeated concussion even in asymptomatic athletes or when neuropsychologic tests are negative [6]; at present, it is still solely an experimental modality, however.

CHRONIC TRAUMATIC ENCEPHALOPATHY

Background

In 1928, Martland introduced the term punch-drunk to describe neurologic symptoms related to repeated blows to the head; this later came to be known as dementia pugilistica because it was found often in boxers [1,9].

Pathophysiology

The currently favored term, chronic traumatic encephalopathy (CTE), is associated with atrophy of cerebral hemispheres, mesial temporal lobes, thalamus, mammillary bodies and brainstem, as well as dilatation of the ventricular system and cavum septum pellucidum, and scarring and neuronal loss of cerebellar tonsils [1,4,14,15]. Pathognomonic neuropathologic signs include preferential involvement of superficial cortical layers; irregular and patchy distribution in the frontal and temporal cortex; a propensity for sulcal depths, perivascular, periventricular, and subpial distribution; and accumulation of tau-immunoreactive astrocytes. Tau deposition in CTE is seen preferentially in layer II and upper third of layer III in the neocortex, and is more dense than that seen in AD. Also unlike AD, the deposition of β-amyloid in plaques is not consistently present. These key neuropathologic findings distinguish CTE from other tauopathies [1].

Clinical Manifestations and Diagnosis

Patients with CTE present with headaches, dizziness, unsteady gait, fatigue, and dysarthria, as well as psychosocial and neurocognitive symptoms such as memory loss, attention deficit, difficulty in concentration, slow information processing, confusion, loss of judgment, irritability, emotional distress, and inability to keep employment. In severe cases, there is a progressive slowing of movement, a propulsive gait, tremor, masked facies, deafness, dysarthria, dysphagia, ptosis, and other ocular abnormalities [1].

Clinical deterioration in CTE occurs in three stages [1,16]:

Stage 1—affective disturbances and psychotic symptoms
Stage 2—social instability, erratic behavior, memory loss, and initial symptoms and signs of Parkinsonism
Stage 3—general cognitive dysfunction, progression of dementia, speech and gait abnormalities, or full blown Parkinsonism

Presently, there are no biomarkers for the diagnosis of CTE.

RECOMMENDATIONS AND CONCLUSIONS

The obvious solution to preventing cumulative effects of MTBI is to avoid injury in the first place. Limiting the risk of brain injury with effective headgear is mandatory, and further research to improve helmet design should be supported. Adherence to strict "return-to-play" guidelines should be adopted. Physicians, nurses, trainers, coaches, and athletes should be better educated about TBI and its consequences. Finally, a cultural change must occur that puts the health of the athlete ahead of all other factors in decisions regarding participation. Only then will the safeguards and guidelines being established for prevention of brain injury be fully realized.

ADDITIONAL READING

Electronic Reference
www.sportslegacy.org

Textbook/Chapter
Cantu RC, Cantu RV. Head injuries. In: Delee JC, Drez D, Miller MD, eds. *Orthopaedic Sports Medicine Principles and Practice*. 3rd ed. Philadelphia, PA: Saunders Elsevier; 2009:657–663.

Journal Article
Cantu RC, Gean AD. Second-impact syndrome and a small subdural hematoma: an uncommon catastrophic result of repetitive head injury with a characteristic imaging appearance. *J Neurotrauma*. 2010;27:1557–1564.

REFERENCES

1. McKee AC, Cantu RC, Nowinski CJ, et al. Chronic traumatic encephalopathy in athletes: progressive tauopathy after repetitive head injury. *J Neuropathol Exp Neurol*. 2009;68(7):709–735.
2. Slemmer JE, Matser EJ, De Zeeuw CI, Weber JT. Repeated mild injury causes cumulative damage to hippocampal cells. *Brain*. 2002;125(Pt 12):2699–2709.

3. Guskiewicz KM, McCrea M, Marshall SW, et al. Cumulative effects associated with recurrent concussion in collegiate football players: the NCAA Concussion Study. *JAMA*. 2003;290(19):2549–2555.

4. Echemendia JR, Julian JL. Mild traumatic brain injury in sports: neuropsychology's contribution to a developing field. *Neuropsychol Rev*. 2001;11(2):69–88.

5. Iverson GL, Brooks BL, Lovell MR, Collins MW. No cumulative effects for one or two previous concussions. *Br J Sports Med*. 2006;40(1):72–75.

6. De Beaumont L, Lassonde M, Leclerc S, Théoret H. Long-term and cumulative effects of sports concussion on motor cortex inhibition. *Neurosurgery*. 2007;61(2):329–36; discussion 336.

7. Kutner KC, Erlanger DM, Tsai J, Jordan B, Relkin NR. Lower cognitive performance of older football players possessing apolipoprotein E epsilon4. *Neurosurgery*. 2000;47(3):651–7; discussion 657.

8. Ardila A, Mendez MF. Dementia pugilistica. In: Gilman S, ed. *MedLink Neurology*. San Diego, CA: MedLink Corporation; 2005.

9. Cantu RC. Chronic traumatic encephalopathy in the National Football League. *Neurosurgery*. 2007;61(2):223–225.

10. Gronwall D, Wrightson P. Cumulative effect of concussion. *Lancet*. 1975;2(7943):995–997.

11. Matser JT, Kessels AG, Lezak MD, Troost J. A dose-response relation of headers and concussions with cognitive impairment in professional soccer players. *J Clin Exp Neuropsychol*. 2001;23(6):770–774.

12. Moser RS, Schatz P, Jordan BD. Prolonged effects of concussion in high school athletes. *Neurosurgery*. 2005;57(2):300–6; discussion 300.

13. Lovell MR, Pardini JE, Welling J, et al. Functional brain abnormalities are related to clinical recovery and time to return-to-play in athletes. *Neurosurgery*. 2007;61(2):352–9; discussion 359.

14. Jordan BD. Neurologic aspects of boxing. *Arch Neurol*. 1987;44(4):453–459.

15. Stiller J, Weinberger DR. Boxing and chronic brain damage. *Psychiatric Clinics of North America*. 1985;2:87–89.

16. Corsellis JA, Bruton CJ, Freeman-Browne D. The aftermath of boxing. *Psychol Med*. 1973;3(3):270–303.

12

Second Impact Syndrome

Gary Goldberg and Brian Steinmetz

GENERAL PRINCIPLES

Definition

Second impact syndrome (SIS) is a rare condition in which the brain swells rapidly when a person suffers a second mild traumatic brain injury (MTBI) before an earlier MTBI has completely resolved [1]. The second injury is generally not severe, with the consequent brain effect being well out of proportion to the apparent head trauma.

Epidemiology

Exact incidence is unknown—SIS appears to be a relatively rare occurrence. Much of the work on SIS has been done in sport-related head injuries. From 1980 to 1993 the National Center for Catastrophic Sports Injury Research in Chapel Hill, NC, identified 35 probable cases among American football players [2]. A more recent study of American high school and college football players demonstrated 94 catastrophic head injuries (with significant intracranial bleeding or edema) over a 13-year period [3]. Seventy-one percent of high school players suffering such injuries had a previous concussion in the same season, with 39% known to have been playing with some residual postconcussion symptoms.

True SIS is rare; 17 cases have been fully published and, according to one literature review, only five reflected a probable case of SIS [4]. SIS has been described most often in young males engaged in contact sports such as boxing, football, and ice hockey.

Although the number of published cases of confirmed SIS is quite small [4,5], and one might view this as somewhat encouraging, the scenario in which a young, previously healthy individual succumbs suddenly and dramatically to this condition indicates that SIS must still be taken as a very serious potentially avoidable consequence of head trauma. The outcome from this condition is often death or severe disability.

Pathophysiology

SIS is thought to be due to sensitization of the brain to the effects of subsequent trauma as a result of an initial head injury. Initial response to a significant concussion can involve transient development of cerebral edema, which is constrained by activation of autoregulatory mechanisms that respond to the induced physiologic stress of the trauma. This initial acute response to the trauma involves vasoconstriction and a reduction in cerebral blood flow, which can contribute to ischemia.

A subacute phase then involves a state of altered cerebral metabolism that may last for several days, involving decreased protein synthesis and reduced oxidative capacity [6]. This alteration in brain metabolism makes the brain more vulnerable to the pathologic effects of a second insult. Fischer and Vaca [7] have thus proposed that when the patient sustains a "second impact" to the head while in this vulnerable subacute state, the brain loses its ability to autoregulate cerebral perfusion pressures and blood flow. This can then lead to rapid-onset massive cerebral edema precipitating transtentorial brain herniation. Death has been reported to occur in a matter of 2 to 5 minutes in true SIS, usually without time to stabilize or transport an athlete from the playing field to the emergency department.

Experiments in concussed rats demonstrated significantly prolonged abnormalities in brain metabolism and behavior when a second impact to the animal's head was administered at 3 days after an initial impact. Such abnormalities were not seen with impacts delivered 2 days before and after day 3 [8,9], implying that there may be a metabolic window of susceptibility to a second impact during the recovery from an initial head injury. A second impact occurring within this window could lead to more dramatic and prolonged symptoms.

DIAGNOSIS

History

- SIS is definitively established through documentation of two separate sequential head injury events with unresolved symptoms of the first head injury persisting through to the second head injury. Most stringent diagnostic criteria for SIS require that the initial head injury be witnessed and medically assessed with confirmed symptomatology persisting through to the second witnessed impact
- History of rapid neurologic deterioration following a witnessed second head injury
- SIS is distinguished from repetitive head injury syndrome (RHIS), or chronic traumatic encephalopathy (CTE), in which a person sustains several repeated minor head injuries spread out over time and, as a result, experiences a gradual decline in cognitive, affective, and behavioral function (see Chapter 13)

- SIS is generally seen in individuals under the age of 18, whereas RHIS/CTE is typically seen in adults [10,11,12].

Physical Examination

- In the unconscious athlete, prompt assessment and stabilization of airway, breathing, and circulation, placement of a cervical collar and spine precautions is essential.
- Careful neurologic examination is done including assessment of brainstem function and Glasgow Coma Scale score.
- Examine for evidence of elevated intracranial pressure (pupillary response, papilledema, obtundation, etc.).

Radiographic Assessment

- Computed tomography (CT) scan: rule out structural damage such as intracranial hemorrhage [13].
- Vascular studies (CT perfusion or CT angiography): can detect vascular pathology and evidence of abnormal cerebral blood flow patterns including vascular congestion.
- Magnetic resonance imaging: offers more structural detail to aid in detecting subtle structural changes.

Autopsy Findings

- Diagnosis is definitively made at autopsy: the brain shows diffuse and extensive cerebral edema, often with evidence of transtentorial herniation.

TREATMENT

- Treatment must be intensive and cannot be delayed.
- Patient should be immediately stabilized with special emphasis on airway management, and neurosurgery consulted.
- Rapidly intubate and institute measures to reduce elevated intracranial pressure.
- Treatment of impaired autoregulation of cerebral vasculature in true SIS may be difficult or impossible. Surgery is generally not effective.
- Prognosis is generally poor. Mortality rate approaches 50%, with remaining survivors uniformly left with significant residual neurologic disability.

PREVENTION OF SECOND IMPACT SYNDROME IN SPORTS

- The best way to prevent SIS is to reduce the overall incidence of concussion in contact sports through protective headgear, education, and enforcement of rules designed to reduce the likelihood of producing a significant injury (see Chapter 5).

■ Any athlete who remains symptomatic following a concussion should not be allowed to return to play. If unsure about status of symptom resolution remember: "When in doubt, sit them out."

■ Multiple clinical guidelines have been published advising on the timing of return to play and level of participation following a first concussion. Such guidelines exist, at least in part, to prevent SIS [14,15,16,17].

■ Physicians with experience in concussion recognition and management should be consulted to evaluate athletes before return to play is authorized.

■ There is a tendency for athletes to minimize and under-report persisting postconcussion symptoms, particularly under circumstances where there are significant competitive stakes involved. Preseason education for the athlete and family members is essential. Education for officials and coaching staff is also very important.

ADDITIONAL READING

Electronic References
http://en.wikipedia.org/wiki/Second-impact_syndrome
http://espn.go.com/video/clip?id=3651929&categoryid=null
http://www.thinkfirst.ca/index.aspx

Textbook/Chapter
Collins MW, Pardini JE. Concussion. In: McMahon PJ, ed. *Current Diagnosis and Treatment in Sports Medicine*. New York, NY: McGraw-Hill Professional; 2007:180–193.

Journal Articles
McCrory P. Does second impact syndrome exist? *Clin J Sport Med.* 2001;11:144–149.

Bey T, Ostick B. Second impact syndrome. *Western J Emerg Med.* 2009;10:6–10.

REFERENCES

1. Saunders RL, Harbaugh RE. The second impact in catastrophic contact-sports head trauma. *JAMA*. 1984;252(4):538–539.
2. Cantu RC. Second-impact syndrome. *Clin Sports Med*. 1998;17(1):37–44.
3. Boden BP, Tacchetti RL, Cantu RC, Knowles SB, Mueller FO. Catastrophic head injuries in high school and college football players. *Am J Sports Med*. 2007;35(7):1075–1081.
4. McCrory PR, Berkovic SF. Second impact syndrome. *Neurology*. 1998;50(3):677–683.

5. Poirier MP. Concussions: assessment, management and recommendations for return to activity. *Clin Ped Emergency Med.* 2003;4:179–185.

6. Hovda DA, Yoshino A, Kawamata T, Katayama Y, Becker DP. Diffuse prolonged depression of cerebral oxidative metabolism following concussive brain injury in the rat: a cytochrome oxidase histochemistry study. *Brain Res.* 1991;567(1):1–10.

7. Fischer J, Vaca F. Sport-related concussions in the emergency department. *Top Emerg Med.* 2004;26:260–266.

8. Vagnozzi R, Tavazzi B, Signoretti S, et al. Temporal window of metabolic brain vulnerability to concussions: mitochondrial-related impairment—part I. *Neurosurgery.* 2007;61:379–388; discussion 388–389.

9. Tavazzi B, Vagnozzi R, Signoretti S, et al. Temporal window of metabolic brain vulnerability to concussions: oxidative and nitrosative stresses—part II. *Neurosurgery.* 2007;61:390–395; discussion 395–396.

10. Lovell MR, Fazio V. Concussion management in the child and adolescent athlete. *Curr Sports Med Rep.* 2008;7(1):12–15.

11. McKee AC, Cantu RC, Nowinski CJ, et al. Chronic traumatic encephalopathy in athletes: progressive tauopathy after repetitive head injury. *J Neuropathol Exp Neurol.* 2009;68(7):709–735.

12. Omalu BI, DeKosky ST, Minster RL, Kamboh MI, Hamilton RL, Wecht CH. Chronic traumatic encephalopathy in a National Football League player. *Neurosurgery.* 2005;57(1):128–34; discussion 128.

13. McCrory P, Berkovic S, Cordner S. Deaths due to brain injury among footballers in Victoria, from 1968 to 1998. *Med J Aust.* 2000;172:217–220.

14. Cantu RC. Guidelines for return to contact sports after a cerebral concussion. *Phys Sportsmed.* 1986;14:75–83.

15. Colorado Medical Society School and Sports Medicine Committee. Guidelines for the management of concussion in sports. *Colorado Med.* 1990;87:4.

16. Practice parameter: the management of concussion in sports (summary statement). Report of the Quality Standards Subcommittee. *Neurology.* 1997;48:581–585.

17. McCrory P, Meeuwisse W, Johnston K, et al. Consensus statement on concussion in sport—The 3rd international conference on concussion in sport held in Zurich, November 2008. *PM & R.* 2009;1(5):406–420.

13

Brain Imaging in Mild Traumatic Brain Injury

Jeffrey David Lewine

BACKGROUND

- Almost 85% of brain injuries are classified as mild in nature. Anatomic evidence of injury is generally lacking in these cases because traditional neuroimaging examinations are usually negative, even in the setting of persistent symptoms.
- When computed tomography (CT) or magnetic resonance imaging (MRI) are positive for acute trauma-related structural pathology in the setting of mild traumatic brain injury (MTBI), the injury is classified as a *complicated* MTBI.
- Advanced structural and functional brain imaging methods can sometimes provide objective evidence of MTBI in the absence of findings on conventional imaging.

IMAGING ASSESSMENTS

Types of Imaging

There are two main categories of imaging—those that look explicitly at brain structure, and those that look at various aspects of brain function.

Brain Structure

In the acute care setting, structural imaging is warranted whenever there has been a trauma-related alteration in consciousness or a change in neurological status. Such imaging is needed to rule out potentially life-threatening problems [1,2].

- *CT*—uses x-rays to make tomographic images of the body. CT is generally the first brain imaging method to be employed in the emergency medical management of patients with head trauma, because it provides rapid identification of critical pathology including skull fractures and intracranial bleeds [2] (see Chapter 10 for further discussion of this topic.)

- *MRI*—By examining how magnetic field gradients and systematically applied radiofrequency pulses alter the behavior of the hydrogen protons of water molecules, MRI provides detailed information on the soft tissues of the body. In general, MRI is inferior to CT for identification of skull fractures, but it is superior to CT for the identification of intra-parenchymal abnormalities. T1, T2-FLAIR and T2-weighted gradient echo sequences are especially useful in the clinical evaluation of TBI [2]. Diffusion tensor imaging (DTI) and associated fiber-tractography may be additionally useful for identification of trauma-induced abnormalities in white matter pathways [3] (see Figure 13.1). MRI is warranted if subjective complaints persist beyond the acute injury phase, or if there is any deterioration in clinical status [1,2].

Brain Function

Functional imaging methods generally are not indicated for the identification of acute life-threatening lesions associated with trauma. Rather, functional methods become useful when looking for evidence of brain

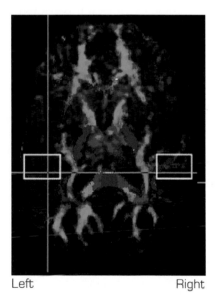

Left   Right

FIGURE 13.1 Diffusion tensor imaging and fiber tractography in mild head trauma. Data are from A 17-year-old male with a history of multiple sports-related concussions. Imaging shows a reduction in the density and number of fibers in the left superior temporal region compared to the right (note image is left-on-left). *Source*: From Ref. [15].

injury in cases where structural imaging is negative. Evidence of a functional disruption of the brain can be valuable in guiding medical management during subacute and chronic phases of injury.

There are two general classes of functional imaging methods—those that examine biochemical, metabolic, and hemodynamic functions, and those that directly assess brain electrophysiology. The main biochemical/metabolic/hemodynamic methods are: positron emission tomography (PET), single photon emission computed tomography (SPECT), functional MRI (fMRI), and magnetic resonance spectroscopy (MRS). The main electrophysiological methods are electroencephalography (EEG) and magnetoencephalography (MEG) [4].

- *PET*—uses compounds labeled with positron-emitting radionucleotides to assess brain biochemistry and metabolism. Brain injury evaluations usually use fluorodeoxyglucose (FDG), and thereby measure regional metabolism, an indirect measure of neuronal activity. Studies may collect data while the brain is "at rest" or during the performance of working memory or attention tasks [5].

  - *Findings in MTBI*: Even in cases without gross structural damage, PET images are usually reported to be abnormal, based on visual inspection of data. However, both hypo- and hypermetabolic regions have been reported, with a general lack of correlation between specific PET findings and neuropsychological profile [5].

- *SPECT*—similar to PET except that relevant radionucleotides emit single photons (γ rays) rather than positrons. As such, the spatial resolution of SPECT is slightly poorer than that of PET. On the other hand, the dose of radioactivity is lower for SPECT, so it is possible to perform resting and activation studies on successive days. Most trauma studies use technitium-labeled hexamethylpropyleneamine oxime (Tc-HMPAO), with images providing information on regional bloodflow, an indirect measure of regional metabolism.

  - *Findings in MTBI*: Even in cases without gross structural damage, visual inspection of SPECT data identifies abnormalities in the majority of cases, especially during activation procedures. Frontal and temporal hypoperfusion along with basal ganglia hypoperfusion are most commonly reported, with conflicting reports on the consistency of relationships between the location of SPECT anomalies and specific clinical profiles [5]. As is the case with PET, few studies have examined diagnostic specificity with respect to normal comparison subjects or subjects with nontrauma related cognitive compromise.

- *fMRI*—The magnetic properties of oxygenated and deoxygenated blood are slightly different, so it is possible to use echo-planar, blood oxygen-level dependent (BOLD) MRI to examine regional blood flow. Most fMRI studies are task dependent, that is, activity profiles during a resting state are compared with those during performance of a cognitive task.

- *Findings in MTBI*: Several investigative teams have shown, in group-averaged data, reduced activation during cognitive challenges related to working memory [6] or attention [7]. Diagnostic applicability to individual subjects remains to be determined.

- *MRS*—The local microenvironment influences the resonance frequency of protons, so it is possible to use MR technology to measure regional concentrations of certain metabolites including N-acetylaspartate (NAA, a neuron-specific metabolic marker), creatine (Cr, which is related to energy metabolism), and choline (Cho, a cell membrane marker).

  - *Findings in MTBI*: Some studies have identified altered metabolite concentrations and reduced NAA/Cho and NAA/Cr ratios following mild trauma, suggesting perturbed metabolic activity in the regions measured [8,9]. Clinical applicability is still under investigation.

- *EEG*—uses contact electrodes applied to the scalp to measure electrical potential patterns that are directly caused by changing patterns of current within brain cells. Clinical EEG involves visual inspection of data from 19+ electrodes arrayed about the head. Quantitative EEG (QEEG) evaluation may also be performed. QEEG involves a statistical comparison of the patient's data with data within a normative database.

  - *Findings in MTBI*: Clinical EEG abnormalities are seen in less than 25% of patients with MTBI, and usually consist of nonspecific diffuse slowing. In contrast, QEEG has been reported to have a high sensitivity in the identification of MTBI [10], but the discriminants used in these studies have variable reliability [11] and specificity.

- *MEG*—uses special superconducting sensors to detect the weak neuromagnetic signals generated by the brain's electrical activity [12,13–15]. There are two fundamental differences between EEG and MEG signals. First, the skull acts as an electrical barrier that smears and distorts the electrical signals measured by EEG, but magnetic signals pass through the skull without significant attenuation or distortion. MEG, therefore, provides better spatial resolution of brain activity. Second, whereas EEG is sensitive to both radial and tangential currents (i.e., those flowing perpendicular and parallel to the skull, respectively), MEG is sensitive to only tangential currents. The MEG is essentially a filtered version of EEG. Most MEG laboratories collect simultaneous EEG data to take advantage of the complimentary nature of the methods.

  - *Findings in MTBI:* Focal dipolar slow wave activity can be seen in normal appearing tissue following MTBI, especially if there are persistent cognitive symptoms (see Figures 13.2 and 13.3). The presence of this activity appears to track symptom severity, with the

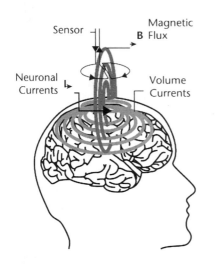
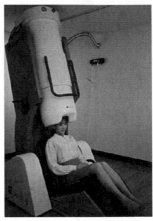

Right Anterior Temporal Sensors—Normal Comparison Subject

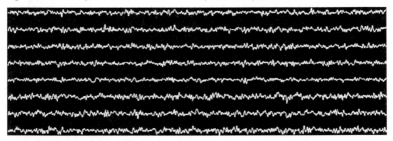

Right Anterior Temporal Sensors—MILD+PCS Patient

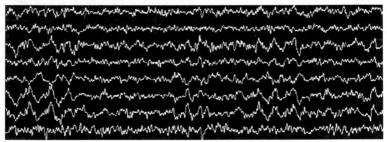

Figure 13.2 MEG involves measurement of the weak magnetic signals generated by neuronal currents. The super-cooled MEG sensors are contained within an insulated dewar with the sensors arrayed about the head. The output of each sensor is a signal showing how the local magnetic flux changes in time. Waveforms show 5 seconds of data. For the patient with a history of mild head trauma and persistent postconcussive symptoms (PCS), large amplitude slow waves are seen. The neuronal generators of the slow wave activity can be localized and plotted on spatially aligned MR images (see Figure 13.3).

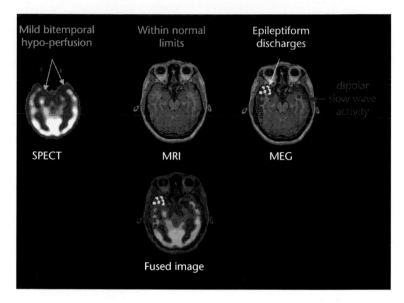

FIGURE 13.3 Data are shown for a 23-year-old female subject who suffered a mild head trauma in a motor vehicle accident. She reported only a brief <1 minute loss of consciousness and her GCS was 15 at the time of hospital admission. MRI performed at the time of admission was interpreted to be within normal limits. Nevertheless, she reported a chronic postconcussive syndrome characterized by documented memory and attention problems and some general cognitive decline. Follow-up MRI, 21 months post trauma, was within normal limits. SPECT revealed mild bitemporal hypoperfusion. MEG revealed right and left temporal focal slow waves and additional left parietal slowing. MEG also showed rare left temporal epileptiform spikes (with source locations indicated by yellow dots) even though the subject had never been reported to show a clinical seizure. Subsequent to these studies, the patient was placed on valproic acid (Depakote). Follow-up neuropsychological testing conducted 6 months after initiation of Depakote revealed a significant improvement in memory function, although attention skills and general processing speed did not improve.

slow waves resolving when symptoms resolve. If cognitive symptoms persist, dipolar slow waves also persist [14]. Available data indicate that focal ischemia and/or damage to underlying white matter pathways is associated with postconcussive dipolar slow wave activity [12,15]. Certain auditory and somatosensory event-related responses in MEG may also be abnormal following MTBI. While MEG is generally viewed an investigational tool in the study of brain injury, select centers with requisite expertise have begun to explore using MEG as a clinical diagnostic tool for TBI as well.

SUMMARY

Structural Imaging

Even mild trauma can lead to life-threatening injury. CT is warranted whenever there is a posttraumatic alteration in consciousness or perturbation of neurological status (see Chapter 10 for a detailed discussion of this topic). MRI can be useful as a compliment to CT, especially if symptoms persist after the immediate acute phase of injury. In some cases, other structural methods, including diffusion tensor analysis, are of value (e.g., in patients with persistent symptoms), as they may offer objective evidence of TBI-related pathology.

Functional Imaging

Functional methods may be of particular value during subacute and chronic phases, when objective evidence of brain dysfunction (in the absence of gross structural lesions) can influence medical management, return-to-work decisions, and medical-legal matters.

Limitations of functional methods include restricted access to relevant equipment and personnel for data processing and interpretation. Other problems with some of the methods include (1) over-reliance on visual inspection and "clinical-expertise," rather than quantitative metrics and (2) results for some imaging modalities that are based mostly on the analysis of group-averaged data, rather than data from individuals. Finally, most functional imaging studies are not routinely used in clinical practice, and their routine application in a clinical setting is not presently recommended.

Additional Considerations

Although functional imaging methods may appear to be very sensitive to detecting lesions even in the setting of mild trauma, there is a general lack of specificity of findings. Just as none of the somatic, psychiatric, or cognitive symptoms that are associated with traumatic injury are specific for

TBI, hypometabolism, hypoperfusion, abnormal metabolic and biochemical markers, and slowing on EEG and MEG can all be seen in a wide range of clinical conditions. As such it is not enough to show that imaging is abnormal relative to normal comparison subjects. To date, studies of the differential diagnostic specificity of most of the imaging modalities are lacking, so the linkage between the objective functional imaging findings of brain dysfunction and a history of trauma must be based on clinical insight, knowledge of premorbid status, and patient history and symptoms.

ADDITIONAL READING

Electronic Reference

Jagoda AS, Bazarian JJ, Bruns JJ Jr, et al. Clinical policy: neuroimaging and decisionmaking in adult mild traumatic brain injury in the acute setting. *Ann Emerg Med.* 2008;52:714–748. www.acep.org/workarea/downloadasset.aspx?id=8814

Textbook/Chapter

Ricker JH, Arenth P. Functional neuroimaging of TBI. In: Zasler ND, Katz DI, Zafonte RD, eds. *Brain Injury Medicine: Principles and Practice.* New York, NY: Demos Medical Publishing; 2006:149–156.

Journal Articles

Belanger HG, Vanderploeg RD, Curtiss G, Warden DJ. Recent neuroimaging techniques in mild traumatic brain injury. *J Neuropsychiat Clin Neurosci.* 2007;19:5–20.

Jagoda AS, Bazarian JJ, Bruns JJ Jr., et al. Clinical policy: neuroimaging and decisionmaking in adult mild traumatic brain injury in the acute setting. 2008;52:714–748.

Lewine JD, Davis JT, Bigler E, et al. Multimodal brain imaging in mild head trauma: integration of MEG, SPECT, and MRI. *J Head Trauma Rehab.* 2007;23:141–155.

REFERENCES

1. Jagoda AS, Bazarian JJ, Bruns JJ Jr., et al. Clinical policy: neuroimaging and decisionmaking in adult mild traumatic brain injury in the acute setting. *Ann Emerg Med.* 2008;52:714–748.
2. Orrison WW, Lewine JD. Neuroimaging in closed head injury. In: Rizzo M, Tranel D, eds. *Head Injury and Post-concussive Syndrome.* New York, NY: Churchill Livingstone; 1995:71–88.
3. Mayer AR, Ling J, Mannell MV, et al. A prospective diffusion tensor imaging study in mild traumatic brain injury. *Neurology.* 2010;74:643–650.
4. Orrison WW Jr., Lewine JD, Sanders JA, Hartshorne MF. *Functional Brain Imaging.* St. Louis, MO: Mosby Year Book; 1995.
5. Belanger HG, Vanderploeg RD, Curtiss G, Warden DJ. Recent neuroimaging techniques in mild traumatic brain injury. *J Neuropsychiat Clin Neurosci.* 2007;19:5–20.

6. McAllister TW, Sparling MB, Flashman LA, Guerin SJ, Mamourian AC, Saykin AJ. Differential working memory load effects after mild traumatic brain injury. *Neuroimage.* 2001;14:1004–1012.

7. Mayer AR, Mannell MV, Ling J, et al. Auditory orienting and inhibition of return in mild traumatic brain injury: a FMRI study. *Hum Brain Map.* 2009;30:4152–4166.

8. Brooks WM, Friedmann SD, Gasparovic C. Magnetic resonance spectroscopy in traumatic brain injury. *J Head Trauma Rehabil.* 2001;16:149–164.

9. Gasparovic C, Yeo R, Mannell G, et al. Neurometabolite concentrations in gray and white matter in mild traumatic brain injury: an H-magnetic resonance spectroscopy study. *J Neurotrauma.* 2009;26:1635–1643.

10. Thatcher RW, Walker RA, Gerson I, Geisler FH. EEG discriminant analyses of mild head trauma. *Electroencephalogr Clin Neurophysiol.* 1998;73:93–106.

11. Nuwer MR, Hovda DA, Schrader LM, Vespa PM. Routine and quantitative EEG in mild traumatic brain injury. *Clin Neurophysiol.* 2005;116:2001–2025.

12. Lewine JD, Davis JT, Bigler E, et al. Multimodal brain imaging in mild head trauma: integration of MEG, SPECT, and MRI. *J Head Trauma Rehab.* 2007;23:141–155.

13. Lewine JD, Orrison WW, Sloan JH, Kodituwakku PW, Davis JT. Neuromagnetic assessment of pathophysiological brain activity induced by minor head trauma. *AJNR Am J Neuroradiol.* 1999;20:857–866.

14. Lewine JD, Sloan JH, Orrison WW, et al. Neuromagnetic evaluation of brain dysfunction in post-concussive syndromes associated with mild head trauma. In: Uzzell B, Stonnington H, Doronzo J, eds. *Recovery After Traumatic Brain Injury.* Mahwah, NJ: Lawrence Erlbaum Associates; 1996:7–28.

15. Huang M, Theilmann RJ, Robb A, et al. Integrated imaging approach with MEG and DTI to detect mild traumatic brain injury in military and civilian patients. *J Neurotrauma.* 2009;26:1213–1226.

Somatic Manifestations of Mild Traumatic Brain Injury

Michael Henrie and Elie P. Elovic

Common somatic manifestations of mild traumatic brain injury (MTBI) include balance deficits, dizziness, fatigue, headache, nausea, visual disturbances, tinnitus, slurred speech, dysesthesias, weakness, and musculoskeletal complaints such as cervical spine injury and whiplash-associated disorders (WADs). In general, the initial symptoms associated with TBI occur as a result of neurometabolic processes [1]. One must also consider that some symptoms may result from the associated cranial injury that often accompanies MTBI. The most important of these manifestations that are not discussed elsewhere in this text are discussed in the following sections.

FATIGUE

Definition

Fatigue is defined as (1) that state following a period of mental or bodily activity, characterized by a lessened capacity for work and reduced efficiency of accomplishment, usually accompanied by a feeling of weariness, sleepiness, or irritability; (2) sensation of boredom and lassitude due to absence of stimulation, monotony, or lack of interest in one's surroundings [2].

Classification

Fatigue can be classified as (1) central fatigue, resulting from supratentorial structures, and (2) peripheral fatigue, which has a physical, metabolic, or muscular origin. It can be further subdivided as either physical or mental/cognitive. There is substantial overlap between central and peripheral processes governing fatigue [3]. In addition, excessive daytime sleepiness is common following TBI [4] and should be viewed as a separate but related construct; it should be differentiated from fatigue, although they often coexist.

Epidemiology

Twenty-one percent of individuals with MTBI complain of fatigue [5]. It is one of the most common postconcussion symptoms, and may remain even after other symptoms have resolved [6].

Pathophysiology

Centrally mediated fatigue results from direct injury to central structures such as the reticular activating system and basal ganglia. A number of other factors that may contribute to fatigue include depression, decreased levels of the amino acids tryptophan and tyrosine, and alterations in cholinergic, serotonergic, and histaminergic pathways [3]. Endocrine disease, including deficiencies in growth hormone, cortisol, testosterone, and thyroid hormones, can also produce fatigue [7]. In addition, there is evidence to suggest that the injured brain is subject to fatigue because it needs to "work harder" in order to compensate for cognitive impairments such as decreased processing speed and attention [8].

Diagnosis

Clinical Presentation
Fatigue can affect an individual's cognitive function, ability to successfully perform activities of daily living, quality of life, and employment. When obtaining a history, the line of questioning should help differentiate between fatigue and sleepiness and should include identification of possible psychologic, neurologic, or endocrine abnormalities.

Examination and Laboratory Assessment
Several subjective scales have been used to measure fatigue in brain-injured patients—Fatigue Severity Scale, Visual Analog Scale for Fatigue, Fatigue Impact Scale, Barrow Neurological Institute (BNI) Fatigue Scale, and Cause of Fatigue (COF) Questionnaire. The BNI and COF Questionnaire were designed specifically for brain-injured patients [3,9]. In their consensus statement on hypopituitarism and TBI, Ghigo et al. recommend systematic screening for endocrine dysfunction in all patients with TBI [7].

Treatment

Nonpharmacologic management of fatigue includes the following: Establish a routine home exercise program with the goal of optimizing cardiovascular health and improving physical well-being. Follow good dietary habits with the goal of weight reduction to improve energy efficiency. Educate patients on appropriate sleep hygiene and address any treatable sleep disorders. Address depression if present. Introduce compensatory activities and activity modification to conserve energy [3]. Pharmacologic management should be initiated if conservative measures fail. Management includes discontinuation or appropriate substitution of any medications with the potential to cause fatigue. One of the most common problems is the inappropriately prolonged use of anticonvulsants. If posttraumatic epilepsy is present, the least sedating medication should be used.

Few well-designed studies have looked at the use of stimulants in the management of Posttraumatic fatigue. However, a number of papers have shown efficacy of stimulants for treatment of decreased cognition (processing speed, alertness, etc.) in TBI [10]. In other populations these agents have demonstrated a positive effect on fatigue. The dopaminergic agents methylphenidate and dextroamphetamine have demonstrated benefit in treating HIV-related fatigue [11]. These agents can be dosed to coincide with periods of important activity during the day. Modafinil, a nondopaminergic agent, thought to work through histaminergic pathways, has been reported to be of benefit in stroke, multiple sclerosis, and depression [12]. *Ginkgo biloba*, an over-the-counter agent also has some evidence for its efficacy in the treatment of chronic fatigue syndrome [13]. Endocrine deficiencies requiring immediate treatment include: diabetes insipidus, adrenal insufficiency, and secondary thyroid insufficiency. Replacement of gonadal and growth hormone deficiencies should be postponed until the need for such therapy is confirmed by appropriate retesting, typically at least 1 year after injury [7].

BALANCE AND DIZZINESS

Definition

The term dizzy is nonspecific and can refer to presyncopal lightheadedness or a sense of an impeding fainting episode, vertigo or the illusion of movement, a sense of imbalance, or multisensory dizziness, which occurs with pathology affecting multiple organ systems [14].

Classification

Dizziness following brain injury can be broadly categorized by etiology as vestibular and nonvestibular.

Epidemiology

Dizziness may affect up to 20% to 50% of individuals with mild to moderate TBI. It is also one of the five most common complaints that distinguish postconcussive patients from healthy controls [15].

Pathophysiology

The balance system is complex and consists of multiple sensory inputs including the visual, somatosensory, and proprioceptive systems in addition to the vestibular end organs. Injury to any of the components can lead to complaints of dizziness and imbalance [16]. In addition, injury to the head, which does not necessarily result in TBI, may account for the symptoms. Vestibular causes are thought to result from ischemia, hemorrhage, or direct trauma to one or more components of the vestibular system. The more common causes are benign positional vertigo that may result from displacement of calcium crystals from the otoliths into the semicircular canal, and labyrinthine concussion caused by violent head movements. Labyrinthine concussion can occur in the absence of a temporal bone fracture and is often used to describe the spectrum of inner ear symptoms that occur following brain injury. Decreased processing speed, migraine headache, and concomitant injuries to the visual system or musculoskeletal system should also be considered as potentially affecting the vestibular system's output [14]. Less common vestibular causes of dizziness and poor balance include perilymphatic fistula and posttraumatic Menier's syndrome. There is little information available in the literature regarding nonvestibular causes of dizziness following TBI. Causes likely include positional orthostasis, cervical spine injury, medications such as antihypertensives and anticonvulsants, hyponatremia, and rarely vestibular epilepsy [14].

Diagnosis

Clinical Presentation
Symptoms are often poorly or vaguely described. Common complaints include lightheadedness, feeling drunk, a spinning or rotating sensation, and balance problems [14]. This condition may contribute to balance difficulty, falls, problems with transfers and ADLs, as well as psychological distress [14]. A detailed neurotologic history is the most important factor in determining treatment course, and therefore must be accurately obtained [16].

Examination
Metrics used to assess physical functioning include both objective and self-reported measures with the *Dynamic Gait Index* and *measures of*

gait velocity being examples of the former; and the *Dizziness Handicap Inventory, Vertigo Handicap Questionnaire, and Vertigo Symptom Scale* being examples of the latter [14]. Balance can also be measured with metrics such as the *Balance Error Scoring System* [17]. If benign positional vertigo is suspected, the Dix-Hallpike test should be performed [16].

Laboratory and Radiologic Assessment
Formal audiometric testing should be obtained, given the anatomic relationship between the peripheral vestibular and auditory systems. Radiographic evaluation and laboratory vestibular/balance testing can confirm a lesion site, but are less likely to drive treatment decisions [16].

Treatment

The most common use of medications is the short-term use of vestibular suppressants. Vestibular suppressants include anticholinergics (scopolamine), antihistamines (meclizine and promethazine), benzodiazapines, and phenothiazine. Vestibular suppressants have an effect that can significantly slow the body's natural compensation process, and can exacerbate cognitive complaints; they should only be used on a short-term "as needed" basis. Chronic medication use has little benefit, unless directed at treatment of secondary causes of dizziness/poor balance such as migraine headaches or psychologic disorders. Surgery is generally reserved for cases involving temporal bone fracture or perilymphatic fistula. Balance rehabilitation therapy (BRT), also known as vestibular rehabilitation, is the most frequently used form of treatment for dizziness and vestibular disorders [14,16]. Vestibular rehabilitation employs balance exercises that enhance central nervous system compensation for vestibular dysfunction. Although a few studies have looked at BRT in TBI, some with encouraging results, it is still unclear if this intervention is effective [14].

WHIPLASH-ASSOCIATED DISORDERS

Definition

The Quebec Task Force on WAD defines whiplash as "...an acceleration-deceleration mechanism of energy transfer to the neck. It may result from rear-end or side-impact motor vehicle collisions, but can also occur during diving or other mishaps. The impact my result in a variety of clinical manifestations" [18].

Classification

The Quebec Task Force developed the following classification taxonomy [19]:

Grade 0	No complaint or physical sign
Grade 1	Neck complaint (pain, stiffness, or tenderness) without physical signs
Grade 2	Neck complaint with musculoskeletal signs (ROM loss or tenderness)
Grade 3	Neck complaint and neurologic signs
Grade 4	Neck complaint and fracture or dislocation

Epidemiology

The literature regarding whiplash disorders associated with MTBI is limited. However, a recent study found all hockey players sustaining concussion complained of symptoms of WAD [20]. The incidence of claims for whiplash in the general population is 1 to 6 per 1000 people per year. Most patients recover quickly with only 15% to 20% of patients remaining symptomatic after 12 months [18].

Pathophysiology

Whiplash is associated with an acceleration-deceleration event. Common associated injuries include articular pillar fracture and subchondral plate fracture, annulus fibrosus tear and endplate avulsion/fracture, hemarthrosis of the facet joint, contusion of the intra-articular meniscus of the facet joint, rupture of the joint capsule, and anterior longitudinal ligament injury [21].

Diagnosis

Clinical Presentation

Head, neck, and upper thoracic pain typically dominate the clinical picture, but patients may also complain of dizziness, tinnitus, and blurred vision. Symptoms are often poorly explained. Initial symptoms are often delayed for several hours after the injury.

Examination

A comprehensive biomechanical and neurological examination should be performed. The area of tissue injury and pain generator should be identified. Look for areas of kinetic chain dysfunction and biomechanical overload and any adaptive mechanisms.

Radiologic Assessment

The American College of Radiology's "Appropriateness Criteria for Imaging and Treatment Decisions" state that in acutely symptomatic patients, with or without neurologic deficit, initial cervical spine imaging is indicated. If there is radiographic evidence of instability or focal neurologic deficits, more advanced imaging should be obtained [22].

Treatment

Acute care consists of reassurance, activity modification, and pain control. Recommendations of the Quebec Task Force include the following:

- No medications for grade I injury and short-term use of nonsteroidal anti-inflammatory drugs (NSAIDs) and non-narcotic analgesics for grades II and III injury.
- Narcotics should not be prescribed for grades I and II, but can be used for a limited time in grade III injury.
- Muscle relaxants should not be used in the acute phase of treatment.

Although the literature regarding medical management of whiplash injury is sparse [23], low back pain treatment has been more extensively studied and may offer additional treatment options. Muscle relaxants have been shown to be effective in treating muscle spasm associated with acute low back pain, but are cognitively sedating. Gabapentin and tricyclic antidepressants have been used effectively to treat radicular pain [23]. Rehabilitation should focus on identifying and correcting biomechanical deficits and adaptive patterns in the kinetic chain [19].

ADDITIONAL READING

Electronic Reference
http://www.cdc.gov/concussion/what_to_do.html

Textbooks/Chapters
Fellus J, Elovic E. Fatigue: assessment and treatment. In: Zasler ND, Katz DI, Zafonte RD, eds. *Brain Injury Medicine: Principles and Practice*. New York, NY: Demos Medical Publishing; 2007:545–556.

Shepard N, Clendaniel RA, Ruckenstein M. Balance and dizziness. In: Zasler ND, Katz DI, Zafonte RD, eds. *Brain Injury Medicine: Principles and Practice*. New York, NY: Demos Medical Publishing; 2007:491–510.

Journal Articles
Chamelian L, Feinstein A. Outcome after mild to moderate traumatic brain injury: the role of dizziness. *Arch Phys Med Rehabil*. 2004;85(10):1662–1666.

Ghigo E, Masel B, Aimaretti G, et al. Consensus guidelines on screening for hypopituitarism following traumatic brain injury. *Brain Inj*. 2005;19(9):711–724.

Maskell F, Chiarelli P, Isles R. Dizziness after traumatic brain injury: overview and measurement in the clinical setting. *Brain Inj.* 2006;20(3):293–305.

Spitzer WO, Skovron M, Salmi L, et al. Scientific monograph of the Quebec Task Force on Whiplash-Associated Disorders: redefining "whiplash" and its management. *Spine.* 1995;20(8 suppl):1S–73S.

Stulemeijer M, van der Werf S, Bleijenberg G, Biert J, Brauer J, Vos PE. Recovery from mild traumatic brain injury: a focus on fatigue. *J Neurol.* 2006;253(8):1041–1047.

REFERENCES

1. Iverson GL, Lange RT, Gaetz M, Zasler ND. Mild TBI. In: Zasler ND, Katz DI, Zafonte RD, eds. *Brain Injury Medicine: Principles and Practice.* New York, NY: Demos Medical Publishing; 2007:333–372.

2. *Stedmans Medical Dictionary.* Baltimore: Lippincott, Williams, and Wilkins; 2006.

3. Fellus JL, Elovic EP. Fatigue: assessment and treatment. In: Zasler ND, Katz DI, Zafonte RD, eds. *Brain Injury Medicine: Principles and Practice.* New York, NY: Demos Medical Publishing; 2007:545–556.

4. Watson NF, Dikmen S, Machamer J, Doherty M, Temkin N. Hypersomnia following traumatic brain injury. *J Clin Sleep Med.* 2007;3(4):363–368.

5. Middleboe T, Andersen HS, Birket-Smith M, Friis ML. Minor head injury: impact on general health after 1 year. A prospective follow-up study. *Acta Neurol Scand.* 1992;85(1):5–9.

6. Stulemeijer M, van der Werf S, Bleijenberg G, Biert J, Brauer J, Vos PE. Recovery from mild traumatic brain injury: a focus on fatigue. *J Neurol.* 2006;253(8):1041–1047.

7. Ghigo E, Masel B, Aimaretti G, et al. Consensus guidelines on screening for hypopituitarism following traumatic brain injury. *Brain Inj.* 2005;19(9):711–724.

8. Cantor JB, Ashman T, Gordon W, et al. Fatigue after traumatic brain injury and its impact on participation and quality of life. *J Head Trauma Rehabil.* 2008;23(1):41–51.

9. Belmont A, Agar N, Hugeron C, Gallais B, Azouvi P. Fatigue and traumatic brain injury. *Ann Readapt Med Phys.* 2006;49(6):370–374.

10. Whyte J, Vaccaro M, Grieb-Neff P, Hart T. Psychostimulant use in the rehabilitation of individuals with traumatic brain injury. *J Head Trauma Rehabil.* 2002;17(4):284–299.

11. Breitbart W, Rosenfeld B, Kaim M, Funesti-Esch J. A randomized, double-blind, placebo-controlled trial of psychostimulants for the treatment of fatigue in ambulatory patients with human immunodeficiency virus disease. *Arch Intern Med.* 2001;161(3):411–420.

12. Rammohan KW, Rosenberg JH, Lynn DJ, Blumenfeld AM, Pollak CP, Nagaraja HN. Efficacy and safety of modafinil (Provigil) for the treatment of fatigue in multiple sclerosis: a two centre phase 2 study. *J Neurol Neurosurg Psychiatr.* 2002;72(2):179–183.

13. Logan AC, Wong C. Chronic fatigue syndrome: oxidative stress and dietary modifications. *Altern Med Rev.* 2001;6(5):450–459.

14. Maskell F, Chiarelli P, Isles R. Dizziness after traumatic brain injury: overview and measurement in the clinical setting. *Brain Inj.* 2006;20(3):293–305.
15. Chamelian L, Feinstein A. Outcome after mild to moderate traumatic brain injury: the role of dizziness. *Arch Phys Med Rehabil.* 2004;85(10):1662–1666.
16. Shepard NT, Clendaniel RA, Ruckenstein M. Balance and dizziness. In: Zasler ND, Katz DI, Zafonte RD, eds. *Brain Injury Medicine: Principles and Practice.* New York, NY: Demos Medical Publishing; 2007:491–510.
17. Iverson GL, Kaarto ML, Koehle MS. Normative data for the balance error scoring system: implications for brain injury evaluations. *Brain Inj.* 2008;22(2):147–152.
18. Teasell R, Shapiro A. The clinical picture of whiplash injuries. In: Malanga GA, Nadler SF, eds. *Whiplash.* Philadelphia: Hanley and Belfus Inc; 2002.
19. Liebenson C, Skaggs C. The role of chiropractic treatment in whiplash injury. In: Malanga GA, Nadler SF, eds. *Whiplash.* Philadelphia: Hanley and Belfus Inc; 2002.
20. Hynes LM, Dickey JP. Is there a relationship between whiplash-associated disorders and concussion in hockey? A preliminary study. *Brain Inj.* 2006;20(2):179–188.
21. Barnsley L, Lord SM, Bogduk N. The pathophysiology of whiplash. In: Malanga GA, Nadler SF, eds. *Whiplash.* Philadelphia: Hanley and Belfus Inc; 2002. 41–77.
22. Fortin J, Weber E. Imaging of whiplash injuries. In: Malanga GA, Nadler SF, eds. *Whiplash.* Philadelphia: Hanley and Belfus Inc; 2002.
23. Nadler S, Malang G. Medications in the treatment of whiplash-associated disorders. In: Malanga GA, Nadler SF, eds. *Whiplash.* Philadelphia: Hanley and Belfus; 2002.

15

Cognition in Mild Traumatic Brain Injury
Neuropsychological Assessment

Theodore Tsaousides, Kristen Dams-O'Connor, and
Wayne A. Gordon

GENERAL PRINCIPLES

Definition

Neuropsychological assessment (NPA) is the quantitative and qualitative evaluation of cognitive, emotional, and behavioral function. Changes after mild traumatic brain injury (MTBI) can be subtle or pronounced, temporary or persistent. NPA is essential for accurate diagnosis and treatment of MTBI [1].

Purpose

The purposes of a NPA following MTBI include:

- Identifying/describing the nature and extent of any cognitive deficits and emotional changes
- Determining the need for treatment and informing the development of an individualized treatment plan to address the cognitive, emotional, and behavioral deficits (e.g., cognitive rehabilitation, psychotherapy, medication)
- Evaluating the effectiveness of interventions in terms of their immediate and long-term impact on proximal (e.g., specific cognitive problems) or distal goals (e.g., return to work, social integration)

COMPREHENSIVE NPA

A comprehensive NPA following MTBI consists of a thorough clinical interview and several hours of testing that may include verbal and nonverbal tests, paper and pencil tests, motor and constructional tasks, and self-report questionnaires. The following are essential components to comprehensive NPA.

Clinical Interview

A thorough clinical history provides context for understanding the neuropsychological test data and the functional impact of injury-related changes on daily living. Important issues to address during a clinical interview following MTBI include:

- Description of the injury—Determine how the injury occurred, duration of any alteration in mental status (i.e., confusion, posttraumatic amnesia), or loss of consciousness. Inquire about symptoms that have begun since the injury occurred [2].
- Comprehensive TBI history—In addition to information about the current injury, it is important to determine if a person has sustained multiple MTBIs, as the effects of these injuries can be additive.
- Review of imaging studies—Inquire about what tests were done in the emergency room and whether the results are available. Studies show that only a small percentage of patients with MTBI show positive findings on CT scans [3].

Neuropsychological Testing

The data gathered in a NPA comes from standardized tests designed to quantify cognitive, emotional, and behavioral functioning.

- Domains—Domains to be assessed following MTBI include attention/concentration, speed of information processing, learning/encoding of new information, motor speed, memory, reading speed and comprehension, verbal fluency and language use, and executive functions (problem-solving, planning, organization, decision-making, prioritizing, etc.). Assessment of dysexecutive behaviors such as impulsivity, apathy, risk-taking, irritability, and daily blunders should also be included.
- Instrument selection—Select tests that are sensitive to the subtle cognitive changes that are characteristic of MTBI. Tests with a low ceiling or intended for use as screening tools (i.e., mini mental status examinations) are not useful in assessing persistent changes related to MTBI, as these gross measures are unlikely to detect the impairments in higher-order cognitive abilities that are characteristic of MTBI.
- Assessment of mood—Emotional distress may exacerbate the person's perceptions of the extent of their cognitive deficits and compound their functional impairments [2]. Individuals with MTBI commonly

experience depression, anxiety, and emotional dysregulation. These changes in mood may be related to the injury event itself, or may be secondary to functional impairments (e.g., absence from work or school), physical injuries, pain, and fatigue. Posttraumatic stress disorder (PTSD) can co-occur with MTBI, particularly when the circumstances leading to the injury were traumatic or combat-related [4].

- Functional relevance—Select tests to evaluate cognitive and behavioral domains that are particularly important for an individual's day-to-day functioning. For example, it may be important to assess reading efficiency in college students, math calculation skills in accountants, sustained attention in truck drivers, and so on.

Interpretation of NPA Data

Comprehensive NPA data should be interpreted in the context of an individual's educational, vocational, and social functioning.

- Quantitative versus qualitative data—Diagnostic and treatment planning decisions following MTBI should rely both on scores obtained from standardized tests, as well as detailed clinical observations. While quantitative test scores allow comparisons of an individual's abilities to normative samples and estimates of preinjury function, qualitative data gained through clinical observation provide rich information that can support the interpretation of objective test scores. For example, an individual's inability to arrive on time for a testing session may provide information that supplements tests of executive functioning [1].

- Relative versus absolute impairments—*Absolute* impairments are indicated by very low test scores. In contrast, *relative* impairments are reductions in functioning relative to the individual's levels of premorbid functioning. Estimates of premorbid function are based on educational and vocational history and on tests designed to assess premorbid cognitive ability (e.g., Wechsler Adult Reading Test, Test of Premorbid Function, and National Adult Reading Test). Relative impairments are not necessarily reflected in objectively low (i.e., below average) test scores. However, both absolute and relative impairments may have significant impact on daily functioning, as well as occupational and social-role performance. Individuals with MTBI may show no absolute impairments, but show relative impairments that considerably affect their ability to function. For example, a person who performs within the "average" range following MTBI may have performed in the "high average" or "superior" range prior to their injury. Thus, this person's current "average" range score does not reveal the extent of his or her current impairments [1].

- Mitigating factors—Performance on NPA following MTBI can be affected by physical, cognitive, and emotional factors. For example, headaches, dizziness, fatigue, visual impairments, and drowsiness due to medication may interfere with test performance. Anxiety, depression, and low motivation may affect test performance negatively. Incentive to manifest disability for secondary gain is an additional mitigating factor that may affect test performance. Effort and malingering tests should be included in NPAs, especially when there is current or future potential for secondary gain [1].

Feedback and Recommendations Following the Assessment

- Feedback—It is appropriate to provide feedback to the client and his or her family about the findings of NPA. Feedback should be provided in language that is understandable to the client/family members. Allow the client and family the opportunity to ask questions.
- Recommendations

    - *Treatment planning*—Use the results of the NPA to identify appropriate interventions, based on the cognitive strengths and weaknesses revealed in the assessment. Cognitive rehabilitation, which provides training and education to maximize cognitive functioning and minimize the functional consequences of neurocognitive impairments, is usually the treatment of choice following MTBI.

    - *Assist with vocational/educational planning*—Use the data to assess an individual's ability to return to their prior occupational or educational pursuits and whether previously identified career goals are attainable in light of the individual's profile of deficits.

    - *Accommodations*—For individuals able to return to work or school, use the data gathered from the NPA to assess the type and degree of accommodations needed in order to optimize success. Examples of accommodations include extended time allowance during exams, frequent rest breaks, or use of a computerized calendar with embedded reminders and cues to improve organization and time management.

- Referrals for further evaluation or diagnostic testing—Determine whether the observed sequelae of MTBI require additional diagnostic evaluations by another specialist and make appropriate referrals.

OTHER TYPES OF ASSESSMENT FOLLOWING MTBI

Brief Cognitive Assessments

Brief cognitive assessments are routinely performed by a variety of health professionals (physicians, nurses, physical therapists, occupational therapists, speech pathologists, etc.) to assess presence of cognitive deficits. Several brief screening instruments exist (e.g., Mini Mental Status Exam, Montreal Cognitive Assessment, Clock Drawing Test). Although these instruments may be useful in detecting gross impairments, they are unlikely to detect the subtle changes in cognitive functioning. Indeed, most individuals with MTBI will perform these assessments without any difficulty despite having demonstrable impairments when given more extensive NPA. Therefore, clinicians should not rely on brief assessments to identify post-MTBI cognitive deficits or changes in cognitive function.

Computerized Assessments

Several computerized cognitive tests (CCTs) have been developed to assess changes in cognition. CCTs are used widely for assessing sports-related injuries. Examples of popular CCTs include the Cambridge Neuropsychological Test Automated Battery (CANTAB), the Automated Neuropsychological Assessment Metrics (ANAM), and the Immediate Postconcussion Assessment and Cognitive Testing (ImPACT).

- Advantages—Availability of alternate forms, good test-retest reliability, minimal practice effects, output that provides performance and variability-in-performance indices, shorter administration time, accessibility, and automation of administration, scoring, and data storage.
- Disadvantages—Little normative data exist for CCTs and the reliability and validity of these assessments has not been adequately demonstrated. Test results still require interpretation by a trained clinician. The relationship between test scores and functional impact is not always evident [5].

ISSUES RELATED TO NPA FOLLOWING MTBI

Timing of NPA

Given the nature of MTBI, a different clinical profile is likely to emerge as a function of the time since injury, as well as the number of injuries.

- Immediate assessment (0 to 3 months post injury)—Acute symptoms are assessed with brief screening tools that can be administered soon after the injury, for example, on the sidelines after sports-related concussion, bedside in an emergency room or physician's office. These brief assessments typically examine orientation, posttraumatic amnesia, reaction time, verbal comprehension, and recall. In addition, the presence of physical symptoms, such as headaches, dizziness, or imbalance should be evaluated [6].

- Assessment more than 3 months post injury—MTBI may result in cognitive and emotional changes that persist for months and even years post injury. Cognitive domains affected may include attention, reaction time, learning and memory, executive dysfunction, and verbal fluency [7–10].

Examiner Qualifications

Formal graduate school training in neuropsychology, clinical and cognitive psychology, and supervised training in NPA is required.

Repeated Testing

Comprehensive NPAs should not be repeated in intervals of less than 12 months, because practice effects secondary to frequent testing with similar measures can threaten the validity of subsequent NPAs. Moreover, physicians and rehabilitation clinicians should avoid using common neuropsychological measures to conduct "check-up" cognitive evaluations during office visits, because this provides another threat to measurement validity in subsequent NPAs.

ADDITIONAL READING

Electronic References

Mount Sinai Brain Injury Research Center. http://www.mssm.edu/research/programs/rehabilitation-research-and-training-in-tbi-intervention/projects-and-grants

http://www.biausa.org/_literature_51031/Family_News_and_Views_Neuropsychological_Assessment

Textbooks/Chapters

Lezak M, Howieson DB, Loring DW. *Neuropsycological Assessment.* New York, NY: Oxford University Press; 2004.

Strauss E, Sherman EMS, Spreen O. *A Compendium of Neuropsychological Tests.* New York, NY: Oxford University Press; 2006.

Tate RL. *A Compendium of Tests, Scales and Questionnaires.* New York, NY: Psychology Press; 2010.

Journal Articles

Guskiewicz KM, Marshall SW, Bailes J, et al. Association between recurrent concussion and late-life cognitive impairment in retired professional football players. *Neurosurgery.* 2005;57(4):719–726.

Tsaousides T, Gordon WA. Cognitive rehabilitation following traumatic brain injury: assessment to treatment. *Mt Sinai J Med.* 2009;76(2):173–181.

Wilson BA, Rous R, Sopena S. The current practice of neuropsychological rehabilitation in the united kingdom. *Appl Neuropsychol.* 2008;15(4):229–240.

REFERENCES

1. Lezak M, Howieson DB, Loring DW. *Neuropsycological Assessment*. New York, NY: Oxford University Press; 2004.
2. Crooks CY, Zumsteg JM, Bell KR. Traumatic brain injury: a review of practice management and recent advances. *Phys Med Rehabil Clin N Am.* 2007;18(4):681–710, vi.
3. Cushman JG, Agarwal N, Fabian TC, et al.; EAST Practice Management Guidelines Work Group. Practice management guidelines for the management of mild traumatic brain injury: the EAST practice management guidelines work group. *J Trauma.* 2001;51(5):1016–1026.
4. Stein MB, McAllister TW. Exploring the convergence of posttraumatic stress disorder and mild traumatic brain injury. *Am J Psychiatry.* 2009;166(7):768–776.
5. Collie A, Darby D, Maruff P. Computerised cognitive assessment of athletes with sports related head injury. *Br J Sports Med.* 2001;35(5):297–302.
6. Sheedy J, Geffen G, Donnelly J, Faux S. Emergency department assessment of mild traumatic brain injury and prediction of post-concussion symptoms at one month post injury. *J Clin Exp Neuropsychol.* 2006;28(5):755–772.
7. Belanger HG, Vanderploeg RD, Curtiss G, Warden DL. Recent neuroimaging techniques in mild traumatic brain injury. *J Neuropsychiatry Clin Neurosci.* 2007;19(1):5–20.
8. Dikmen SS, Corrigan JD, Levin HS, Machamer J, Stiers W, Weisskopf MG. Cognitive outcome following traumatic brain injury. *J Head Trauma Rehabil.* 2009;24(6):430–438.
9. Johansson B, Berglund P, Rönnbäck L. Mental fatigue and impaired information processing after mild and moderate traumatic brain injury. *Brain Inj.* 2009;23(13–14):1027–1040.
10. Vanderploeg RD, Curtiss G, Belanger HG. Long-term neuropsychological outcomes following mild traumatic brain injury. *J Int Neuropsychol Soc.* 2005;11(3):228–236.

16

Cognition in Mild Traumatic Brain Injury
Is There a Risk of Late Development of Dementia?

William B. Barr

GENERAL PRINCIPLES

Mild traumatic brain injury (MTBI) is associated with short-lived altera-tions in attention, processing speed, and memory retrieval. Results of meta-analyses demonstrate that MTBI has little or no effect on cogni-tive functioning beyond the first 3 months following the initial injury [1]. Findings regarding a role for MTBI as a risk factor for dementia are inconclusive, although this remains a topic of heavy debate among health care professionals.

Definitions

Dementia is commonly defined as a neurodegenerative condition charac-terized by decreased intellectual functioning, memory impairment, and decrements in other cognitive domains including language, executive functions, or visual perception.

Classification

Multiple forms of dementia are linked to TBI.

- **Alzheimer's disease (AD)** is a common neurodegenerative disor-der, which accounts for approximately 50% to 60% of all age-related dementia. It afflicts 8% to 10% of the population above the age of 65 and almost 50% above the age of 85 [2]. The relationship between TBI and AD remains inconclusive. Several case control and epidemiologic studies indicate that TBI is a general risk factor for developing AD and report odds ratios ranging from 3.5 to 13.75 [3]. Other studies have, however, failed to replicate these findings.

- **Mild cognitive impairment (MCI)** is a preclinical phase of dementia characterized by memory impairment with a preservation of global cognitive functions and daily living skills. Individuals with this condition progress to an onset of AD at a much higher rate than their peers. Studies of professional athletes have suggested a fivefold increase in the rate of MCI in those with a history of two or more occurrences of MTBI [4]. The link between MCI and MTBI has not been explored adequately in larger scale epidemiologic studies.
- **Chronic traumatic encephalopathy (CTE)** is a long-term consequence of repetitive MTBIs. It has been estimated that CTE develops in 20% of all professional boxers [5]; there have also been a number of reports that it occurs in professional football players [6]. A growing number of investigators believe that this condition may be more prevalent than originally thought.

Etiology

- TBI is thought to provide one of the major environmental factors responsible for the development of AD. Many investigators believe that the majority of cases of MCI are caused by the same factors responsible for AD [2].
- Frequent MTBIs are considered the major etiological factor in CTE. Genetics, including the APOE genotype might also play a role in the development of CTE, particularly in those with years of exposure to TBI [7].

Pathophysiology

- Brain changes in AD are characterized by widespread cell loss, particularly in the hippocampus, entorhinal cortex, and adjacent neocortex. The disease is also characterized by the presence of neuritic plaques and neurofibrillary tangles, which are primarily the result of extracellular deposition of β-amyloid and the intracellular aggregation of tau protein, respectively [8]. The pathological process underlying MCI is thought to resemble an early evolving form of AD.
- There is experimental and postmortem evidence that production and accumulation of β-amyloid occurs within hours of a TBI [9]. Findings suggesting an interaction between head injury and APOE ε4 are consistent with a hypothesis that head injury enhances the production of neuritic plaques by increasing the expression of APOE. Other mechanisms linking TBI to AD include neuronal loss, persistent inflammation, and cytoskeletal pathology.
- The pathological characteristics of CTE include cerebral atrophy, septal and hypothalamic anomalies, cerebellar changes, degeneration of the substantia nigra, and a dense regional occurrence of neurofibrillary tangles. CTE shares many features with AD pathology, with

tau-immunoreactive neurofibrillary tangles seen most prominently. Neuritic plaques are present in less than half of the cases.

DIAGNOSIS

A confirmed diagnosis of AD or CTE can only be made postmortem. Diagnoses provided antemortem are limited to the classification of "probable" forms of dementia based on a combination of history, clinical presentation, and neuroimaging findings.

Risk Factors

- Age is the strongest risk factor for development of AD with the likelihood of developing the condition doubling every 5 years after age 65. By the age of 85, the risk approaches 50%. Risk is increased in patients diagnosed with MCI. Inheritance is another strong risk factor for AD, consistent with the genetic model. First-degree relatives of individuals with late onset AD have a 50% chance of developing the disorder. There is also some evidence that the condition appears more often in males. Individuals who are healthy and mentally active are thought to be less susceptible to developing AD as are those with stronger intellectual functioning and higher levels of educational attainment [10]. Brain injury survivors with lower levels of education are known to develop dementia sooner than age-matched cohorts.
- Age, combined with degree of exposure (i.e., number of MTBIs) appear to be the greatest known risk factors for developing CTE.

Clinical Presentation

- The clinical features of AD typically develop in a slow and insidious manner, although symptoms developing over years might appear to have arisen abruptly in the context of a medical illness or in response to radical environmental changes. Memory impairment (difficulty retaining new information) is the major feature of AD; memory for information from events occurring years ago remains relatively intact. Difficulties with language are also observed, often initially characterized by a tendency to grope for words. Paucity of speech is observed during later stages of the illness. Other cognitive difficulties include problems with executive function and higher-order visual skills. Behavioral and affective features are also prominent. Symptoms of depression are seen in approximately 25% of AD patients [11]. Some may develop agitation and a tendency to wander secondary to confusion. Motor symptoms, such as gait changes, can be seen in latter stages of the illness. There is no known difference in the signs seen in AD patients with versus without a history of TBI [3].

- CTE also begins with subtle cognitive changes in addition to more prominent motor symptoms than AD [5]. Cognitive impairments involve attention, memory, and executive dysfunction. The classical presentation is similar to what has been associated with a "subcortical" form of dementia. Early motor symptoms include balance difficulties, tremor, and dysarthria, followed by ataxia and signs of parkinsonism. Behavioral features include irritability and general disinhibition. Affected individuals may show signs of the disorder during the later stages of their playing careers, with nearly half developing symptoms within 4 years of their retirement.

Physical Examination

- A detailed physical and neurological examination, and routine laboratory testing is recommended in patients with suspected AD or CTE to rule out "reversible" causes of dementia, such as hypothyroidism, vitamin B_{12} deficiency, central nervous system infection, or toxic effects of alcohol or drugs. It is also important to rule out basic disorders of visual acuity or auditory perception that might affect one's ability to encode new information.

Diagnostic Evaluation

- There is no definitive biological marker for AD or CTE. Neuropsychological testing is helpful in documenting impairment in cognitive function at the early stage of all forms of dementia. Standardized neuropsychological methods also provide an objective means of tracking the course of these disorders through serial testing.

Neuroradiographic Assessment

- Structural imaging using computerized tomographic (CT) scan or magnetic resonance imaging (MRI) in patients with suspected AD will commonly demonstrate generalized atrophy. However, these findings are nonspecific to the effects of AD. Studies using functional brain imaging methods such as fluorodeoxyglucose-positron emission tomography (FDG-PET) or single photon emission computed tomography (SPECT) have indicated that decreased metabolism and perfusion of the parietal lobes and medial temporal regions are a sensitive indicator of AD [11]. Imaging findings are not helpful in making the distinction between MCI and AD, and their application remains largely experimental.
- Many of the structural imaging findings demonstrated in AD are also found in CTE. Identification of a *cavum septum pellucidum* is an additional finding from structural imaging that appears to be relatively

specific to CTE [6]. MRI is generally considered more sensitive than CT for detecting cerebral contusions, small subdural hematomas, and white matter abnormalities. Diffusion tensor imaging (DTI) may be used to assess large-scale axonal integrity in CTE. Functional imaging studies have demonstrated more abnormalities in frontal and temporal regions in CTE than is commonly seen in AD [6].

TREATMENT

- The primary pharmacological strategy for treating memory disturbance in AD involves the use of cholinesterase inhibitors such as donepezil, rivastigmine, or galantamine [11]. Studies focusing on treatment of mild-to-moderate forms of AD have shown marginal benefits in cognition and behavior. Side effects include nausea, dizziness, gastrointestinal irritation, and weight loss. Memantine, an N-methyl-D-aspartic acid (NMDA) receptor agonist, has been shown to be effective as an add-on medication in moderate to severe AD. The existence of more severe behavioral issues including aggression and psychotic symptoms might necessitate additional treatment with antipsychotic medications such as olanzapine.
- Empirical evidence for treating CTE is lacking. Strategies for treating the cognitive and behavioral components of CTE generally follow those applied in treatment of AD. The major exception is that a number of individuals with CTE also exhibit signs of parkinsonism, which can be treated with dopamine agonists such as carbidopa/levodopa.

ADDITIONAL READING

Electronic Reference

Boston University Center for the Study of Traumatic Encephalopathy website. http://www.bu.edu/cste/

Textbook/Chapter

Jordan BD. Chronic traumatic brain injury. In Bailes JE, Lovell MR, Maroon JC, eds. *Sports-Related Concussion*. St. Louis, MO: Quality Medical Publishing; 1999:52–64.

Journal Articles

Bazarian JJ, Cernak I, Noble-Haeusslein L, et al. Long-term neurologic outcomes after traumatic brain injury. *J Head Trauma Rehabil*. 2009;24(6):439–451.

Gavett BE, Stern RA, Cantu RC, et al. Mild traumatic brain injury: a risk factor for neurodegeneration. *Alzheimer's Research and Therapy*. 2010;2(18):1–3.

Johnson VE, Stewart W, Smith DH. Traumatic brain injury and amyloid-β pathology: a link to Alzheimer's disease? *Nature Reviews: Neuroscience*. 2010;11:1–10.

Van Den Heuvel C, Thornton E, Vink R. Traumatic brain injury and Alzheimer's disease: a review. *Prog Brain Res*. 2007;161:303–316.

REFERENCES

1. Belanger HG, Curtiss G, Demery JA, Lebowitz BK, Vanderploeg RD. Factors moderating neuropsychological outcomes following mild traumatic brain injury: a meta-analysis. *J Int Neuropsychol Soc.* 2005;11(3):215–227.
2. Cummings JL, Cole G. Alzheimer disease. *JAMA.* 2002;287(18):2335–2338.
3. Lye TC, Shores EA. Traumatic brain injury as a risk factor for Alzheimer's disease: a review. *Neuropsychol Rev.* 2000;10(2):115–129.
4. Guskiewicz KM, Marshall SW, Bailes J, et al. Association between recurrent concussion and late-life cognitive impairment in retired professional football players. *Neurosurgery.* 2005;57(4):719–26; discussion 719.
5. Jordan BD. Chronic traumatic brain injury associated with boxing. *Semin Neurol.* 2000;20(2):179–185.
6. McKee AC, Cantu RC, Nowinski CJ, et al. Chronic traumatic encephalopathy in athletes: progressive tauopathy after repetitive head injury. *J Neuropathol Exp Neurol.* 2009;68:709–735.
7. Kutner KC, Erlanger DM, Tsai J, Jordan B, Relkin NR. Lower cognitive performance of older football players possessing apolipoprotein E epsilon4. *Neurosurgery.* 2000;47(3):651–7; discussion 657.
8. Duyckaerts C, Delatour B, Potier MC. Classification and basic pathology of Alzheimer's disease. *Acta Neuropathologica.* 2009;118:5–36.
9. Magnoni S, Brody DL. New perspectives on amyloid-beta dynamics after acute brain injury: moving between experimental approaches and studies in the human brain. *Arch Neurol.* 2010;67(9):1068–1073.
10. Stern Y. Cognitive reserve. *Neuropsychologia.* 2009;47(10):2015–2028.
11. Mayeux R. Clinical practice. Early Alzheimer's disease. *N Engl J Med.* 2010;362(23):2194–2201.

17

Postconcussion Syndrome
Diagnostic Characteristics and Clinical Manifestations

Erica Wang and Felise S. Zollman

[Note that throughout this text you will see the terms Post Concussion Syndrome (PCS) and Post Concussion Disorder (PCD) used interchangeably. While there is some controversy as to which term is more appropriate, both are presented here based on author preference and the specific context of the information provided.]

GENERAL PRINCIPLES

Definition

Although there is no universally accepted definition of postconcussion syndrome (PCS), the *Diagnostic and Statistical Manual of Mental Disorders*, fourth edition (DSM-IV) [1] and the *International Classification of Diseases*, 10th Revision (ICD-10) [2], each have established criteria for the diagnosis of PCS.

DSM-IV Criteria

- A history of head trauma that causes "significant cerebral concussion"
- Objective evidence (e.g., neuropsychological testing) of deficits in attention or memory
- A minimum of three of the eight following symptoms must be present and persist for *at least 3 months*:
  - Easily fatigued
  - Disordered sleep
  - Headache
  - Vertigo or dizziness
  - Easily provoked irritability or aggression
  - Anxiety, depression, or emotional lability
  - Apathy or lack of spontaneity, motivation, or initiation
  - Personality changes or inappropriate behavior
- Symptoms begin or worsen after brain injury
- Significant decline from previous level of functioning as demonstrated by interference in social, occupational, or academic functioning
- Symptoms do not meet criteria for dementia due to head trauma and are not better accounted for by another disorder

ICD-10 Criteria

- A history of head trauma with loss of consciousness
- At least one symptom from three of the following six groupings:
  - Headache, dizziness, general malaise, excessive fatigue, or noise intolerance
  - Irritability or emotional lability that is easily provoked; may be accompanied by depression and/or anxiety
  - Subjective complaints of difficulty with concentration, memory, or performing mental tasks without clear objective evidence of impairment
  - Insomnia
  - Reduced tolerance of alcohol, stress, or emotional excitement
  - Preoccupation with symptoms, fear of permanent brain damage and/or adoption of sick role

In every circumstance, before diagnosing PCS, one must first ascertain that a precipitating traumatic brain injury (TBI) did in fact occur. This is based on identifying (1) a mechanism of injury likely to have resulted in a TBI, and (2) a temporally associated change in neurologic function or onset/exacerbation of neurologic symptoms. In the absence of this, the occurrence of a TBI cannot be asserted and therefore PCS cannot be diagnosed.

Epidemiology

The literature widely cites estimation that 1 year after injury, approximately 10% to 20% of persons will have persistent symptoms of PCS [3]. However, accurate incidence and prevalence of PCS truly has not been established despite decades of research, largely because of limitations in subject recruitment (i.e., not all persons who suffer a MTBI come to medical attention) [4].

Pathophysiology

The initial symptom constellation reflects the neurometabolic cascade that occurs immediately following a mild traumatic brain injury (MTBI). Symptom persistence, however, is influenced by a variety of factors that ultimately affect how persons perceive their symptoms after MTBI. Such confounding factors include personality traits, affective disorders, chronic pain disorders, medication side effects, diagnosis threat, exaggeration, and malingering, among others [5] (see Figure 17.1).

Selected factors are discussed in more detail in the following:

- Personality
  - Five personality traits are considered vulnerable to poor outcome: the overachieving, the dependent, the insecure, the grandiose, and those with borderline personality characteristics [6].

- Social-psychological
    - Nocebo effect—symptoms are caused by expectation of experiencing certain symptoms and problems after injury
    - Diagnosis threat—adverse effect on task performance by highlighting history of head injury [7].
    - Stereotype threat—negative stereotype associated with having an injury adversely affects task performance
    - Good-old-days bias—overestimation in difference between pre- and postinjury symptoms/functioning [8].
- Symptom exaggeration—amplification of symptom or sign that has true physiological or psychological basis; most commonly seen in cases involving personal injury litigations, Worker's Compensation claims, and disability evaluations [9].
- Malingering—intentional exaggeration of symptoms or feigning symptoms for an external reward; less common than symptom exaggeration

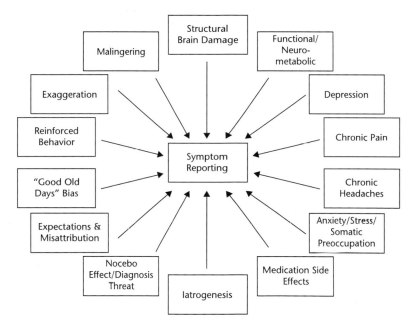

Figure 17.1 Factors which may influence symptom persistence post MTBI.

DIAGNOSIS

Clinical Presentation

- Most common early symptoms include fatigue, headache and dizziness/lightheadedness. Other common symptoms include blurry/

double vision, irritability, poor concentration, impairment in memory and attention, sensitivity to light/noise, and sleep disturbance [10].

- Diagnosis of PCS is based on symptom presentation and is nonspecific. Healthy persons as well as persons with a variety of conditions (e.g., depression, fibromyalgia, chronic pain, posttraumatic stress disorder, orthopedic injuries, whiplash) frequently report symptom constellations that can meet criteria for PCS in the absence of head injury [11] (see Table 17.1).

Table 17.1 Percentages of Subjects Endorsing Symptoms at a Mild or Moderate-Severe Level (British Columbia Post-concussion Symptom Inventory.)

Items	Healthy Community Volunteers		Patients With Depression		Patients With Fibromyalgia	
	Mild	Moderate-Severe	Mild	Moderate-Severe	Mild	Moderate-Severe
Headaches	19.6	3.2	59.4	28.1	72.2	37.0
Dizziness/light-headed	11.4	1.3	31.2	10.9	37.0	7.4
Nausea/ feeling sick	133	0.0	40.6	10.9	35.2	18.5
Fatigue	27.8	5.1	85.6	57.8	96.3	79.6
Extra sensitive to noises	11.4	1.3	50.0	18.8	68.5	44.4
Irri lab It-	21.5	5.1	76.6	35.9	53.7	25.9
Sadness	18.4	1.3	76.6	56.3	55.6	33.3
Nervous or tense	16.5	1.3	65.6	35.9	59.3	33.3
Temper problems	15.8	5.1	37.5	15.6	27.8	7.4
Poor concentration	16.5	3.2	78.1	46.9	75.9	44.4
Memory problems	13.3	3.8	70.3	42.2	74.1	44.4
Difficulty reading	*8.2*	1.9	40.6	23.4	48.1	24.1
Poor sleep	22.8	5.1	78.1	53.1	87.0	59.3

Healthy adults (N = 158), patients with depression (N = 64), and patients with fibromyalgia (N = 54). Patients with depression were diagnosed by their family physician or psychiatrist., and their diagnosis was confirmed using the SC1D-I. Their average age was 41.1 years (SD = 12.5). and their average education was 14.6 years (SD = 3.2). Approximately 71% of the sample was female. The patients with fibromyalgia were mostly women (94%). Their average age was 51.4 years (SD = 12.8, Range = 17–75). Their average education was 13.5 years (SD = 2.4, Range = 7–20)

Evaluation

- Because the clinical presentation of PCS is nonspecific, PCS should be considered a diagnosis of exclusion.
- Obtain a detailed history of the injury, ascertaining that an inciting TBI did in fact occur, and a description of the onset and progression of symptoms.
- Neuropsychological testing may be beneficial in more thoroughly characterizing the nature/extent of cognitive/behavioral/affective deficits, if any, in establishing a baseline, and as an educational tool regarding areas of strength and weakness. Caution must be exercised in interpreting results, however, because many of the aforementioned confounding factors (e.g., mood disorder, medication use, and malingering) can result in significant abnormal test results even in the absence of TBI (see Figure 10.2).
- Differential diagnosis includes, but is not limited to, cervical injuries and whiplash-associated disorders (resulting in headaches), chronic pain syndromes, depression/dysthymia, anxiety disorders, posttraumatic stress disorder, and iatrogenesis/medication side effects. Before concluding that the patient's symptoms are due to PCS, the provider must evaluate and treat confounding problems that may account for the clinical presentation (e.g., pain, insomnia, mood disorder, and medication side effects).

TREATMENT

Management of PCS is discussed in detail in the following chapter. Basic principles include (1) addressing and treating confounding factors, (2) education/reassurance, (3) introduction of behavioral modifications/lifestyle changes if indicated, and (4) judicious, modest use of medication where appropriate.

ADDITIONAL READING

Electronic Reference

http://www.sciencedirect.com/science?_ob=MImg&_imagekey=B6VDJ-4K7WJ56-1-1&_cdi=5984&_user=10&_pii=S0887617706000497&_origin=search&_coverDate=05%2F31%2F2006&_sk=999789995&view=c&wchp=dGLzVtb-zSkWA&md5=2bd9753e2ed7bab5ffdfc05deaac4610&ie=/sdarticle.pdf

Textbook/Chapter

McCrea MA. *Mild Traumatic Brain Injury and Post-Concussive Syndrome: The New Evidence Base for Diagnosis and Treatment.* New York: Oxford University Press; 2008.

Journal Articles

Alexander MP. Mild traumatic brain injury: pathophysiology, natural history, and clinical management. *Neurology.* 1995;45(7):1253–1260.

Mittenburg W, Strauman S. Diagnosis of mild head injury and the post-concussion syndrome. *J Head Trauma Rehabil.* 2000;15(2):783–791.

Ryan LM, Warden DL. Post-concussion syndrome. *Int Rev Psychiatry.* 2003;15:310–316.

REFERENCES

1. American Psychiatric Association. *Diagnostic and Statistical Manual of Mental Disorders, Text Revision (DSM IV-TR).* 4th ed. Washington, DC; 2000: Appendix B:760–764.

2. World Health Organization. *The ICD-10 Classification of Mental and Behavioral Disorders: Clinical Descriptions and Diagnostic Guidelines.* Geneva, Switzerland: version 2007:63–64.

3. Rutherford WH, Merrett JD, McDonald JR. Symptoms at one year following concussion from minor head injuries. *Injury.* 1979;10(3):225–230.

4. McCullagh S, Feinstein A. Outcome after mild traumatic brain injury: an examination of recruitment bias. *J Neurol Neurosurg Psychiatr.* 2003;74(1):39–43.

5. Iverson GI, Zasler ND, Lange RT. Post-concussive disorder. In: Zasler ND, Katz DI, Zafonte RD, eds. *Brain Injury Medicine: Principles and Practice.* New York: Demos Medical Publishing; 2007:393–394.

6. Kay T, Newman B, Cavallo M, Ezrachi O, Resnick M. Toward a neuropsychological model of functional disability after mild traumatic brain injury. *Neuropsychology.* 1992;6(4):371–384.

7. Suhr JA, Gunstad J. Further exploration of the effect of "diagnosis threat" on cognitive performance in individuals with mild head injury. *J Int Neuropsychol Soc.* 2005;11(1):23–29.

8. Gunstad J, Suhr JA. "Expectation as etiology" versus "the good old days": postconcussion syndrome symptom reporting in athletes, headache sufferers, and depressed individuals. *J Int Neuropsychol Soc.* 2001;7(3):323–333.

9. Weissman HN. Distortion and deceptions in self presentation: effects of protracted litigation on personal injury tests. *Behav Sci Law.* 1990;8:67–74.

10. Dischinger PC, Ryb GE, Kufera JA, Auman KM. Early predictors of postconcussive syndrome in a population of trauma patients with mild traumatic brain injury. *J Trauma.* 2009;66(2):289–96; discussion 296.

11. Iverson GI, Zasler ND, Lange RT. Post-concussive disorder. In: Zasler ND, Katz DI, Zafonte RD, eds. *Brain Injury Medicine: Principles and Practice.* New York: Demos Medical Publishing; 2007:377–379.

18

Postconcussion Syndrome
Symptom Management

William C. Walker and Richard D. Kunz

TREATMENT OF POSTCONCUSSION SYNDROME

Introduction

A "miserable minority" of patients who sustain mild traumatic brain injury (MTBI; concussion) have symptoms that persist beyond several months. Such lingering symptoms are termed postconcussion syndrome (PCS), which is further defined in Chapter 19. The focus of this chapter is the treatment of PCS; for the treatment of MTBI refer to Chapter 10. Evidence to guide treatment of PCS in the form of randomized controlled trials is lacking, but review of the literature reveals a relative expert consensus concerning appropriate treatment principles. This chapter will review these principles along with author recommendations on specific interventions.

General Principles of PCS Management

- Management of postconcussion symptoms should focus on promoting recovery and avoiding harm.
- Patients with prolonged symptoms are suffering, distressed, and in need of guidance, education, support, and understanding.
- A patient-centered approach should be used to provide the needed reassurance and motivation.
- Treatment of somatic complaints (e.g., insomnia, dizziness/incoordination, nausea, alterations of smell/taste, appetite problems, vision/hearing changes, numbness, and fatigue) should be based on individual factors and symptom presentation.
- Any medications added for symptom control must be carefully prescribed after consideration of sedating properties or other side effects.
- In patients with persistent postconcussion symptoms (PPCS) that have been refractory to treatment, consideration should be given to

other factors including psychiatric, psychosocial support, and issues of compensation/litigation.

- One effective semiquantitative way to monitor the course of PCS and success of applied treatments is by quantifying the number and intensity of individual symptoms using one of the available standardized inventories such as the Postconcussion Syndrome Checklist [1], Rivermead Post Concussion Symptoms Questionnaire [2], or Concussion Symptom Checklist [3].

Education

Education is the mainstay of PCS treatment. Bell et al., [4] recently reported a randomized controlled trial in which patients with concussion who received telephone counseling, focused on education and symptom management, showed significantly less PCS symptoms at 6 months post injury compared to patients who received standard hospital discharge materials.

- Assure the patient that symptoms are part of the normal recovery process, and not signs of permanent brain dysfunction.
- Noncontact, aerobic, and recreational activities should be encouraged within the limits of the patient's symptoms; increased headache or irritability suggests that this level has been exceeded.
- Encourage resumption of occupational, educational, and social responsibilities in a graded fashion to avoid the perception of stress or fatigue.
- Ascertain current sleep/wake cycle and provide counseling regarding appropriate sleep hygiene (see Table 18.1).
- Provide printed and verbal material.

TABLE 18.1 Education for Sleep Hygiene

Good sleep hygiene:
Avoid going to bed too early in the evening
Avoid stimulants, caffeinated beverages, power drinks, and nicotine during the evening
Avoid stimulating activities before bedtime (e.g., exercise, video games, TV)
Avoid alcohol
Restrict the nighttime sleep period to about 8 hours
Wake up at a regular time in the morning (e.g., 7 AM)
Arise from bed at a regular time in the morning (e.g., by 8 AM)
Reduce (to less than 30 minutes) or abolish daytime naps
Engage in daytime physical and mental activities (within the limits of the individual's functional capacity)

Physical Rehabilitation

- A general exercise program that includes strength training, core stability, aerobic activities, and range of motion is ideal.
- Gradually increase duration and intensity to accommodate the activity intolerance and fatigue that is commonly associated with PCS.
- Targeted vestibular, visual, and proprioceptive therapeutic exercise is recommended for persistent dizziness, disequilibrium, and spatial disorientation impairments based on evidence of efficacy in different populations with vestibular disorders [5–7].
- Patients with vestibular disorders who received customized programs showed greater improvement than those who received generic exercises [6].
- Targeted therapeutic exercise is also recommended for any persisting focal musculoskeletal impairments.
- If a person's normal activity involves significant physical activity, exertional testing (i.e., stressing the body) should be conducted before permitting full resumption.

Psychological Treatment

- Psychological treatment early after sustaining MTBI may protect against developing PCS. Meta-analysis of the literature suggests that patients who receive brief psychological treatment after MTBI have a significantly reduced incidence of persisting PCS compared to patients who receive standard acute care [8].
- Treatment typically includes additional education, reassurance, and cognitive restructuring—the reattribution of symptoms to benign causes.
- Efficacy data is lacking once PCS is established, but physicians often include psychologist referral in their treatment plan [9]. In these authors' opinion, referral to a neuropsychologist or psychologist with expertise in PCS is indicated when there is failure to respond to initial treatments, worsening stress, deterioration in function, or impairment in vocational or social function.

Cognitive Rehabilitation

Patients who have cognitive symptoms that do not resolve or have been refractory to treatment should be considered for referral for neuropsychological assessment. Individuals with memory, attention, and/or executive function deficits that do not respond to initial treatment (e.g., reassurance, management of sleep dysfunction, mood disorders, and somatic complaints) may benefit from cognitive therapy (e.g., speech and language pathology, neuropsychology, or occupational therapy) for compensatory training (e.g., use of external memory aids such as a personal digital assistant [PDA] or pocket notebook).

PHARMACOLOGIC MANAGEMENT OVERVIEW

Postconcussion symptoms are frequently treated with medications despite the paucity of randomized controlled trials. A survey by Evans et al. [8] of treatments prescribed by a representative sample of physicians showed that nonsteroidal anti-inflammatory analgesics were most often recommended. Antidepressant medications were the second most commonly prescribed overall, and the treatment preferred by neurologists. Where evidence-based data exists to direct pharmacotherapeutic decision-making, it will be presented; where such data is not presented, the recommendations made represent the opinions of the author.

Thorough medication reconciliation is crucial. The existing medication list should be reviewed for agents that can cause neurologic abnormalities (centrally acting medications, pain medications, etc.). If a medication with neurologic side effects is identified, consider discontinuing or decreasing dose and re-evaluate after 1 week.

Headache Pharmacologic Management

Headache is the most common PCS symptom. Management should be tailored to the subtype of headache (see Chapter 55 for a detailed discussion of this subject).

Mood Disorders Pharmacologic Management

- Anxiety and depression symptoms can be treated with a variety of medications. The choice is usually dictated by comorbid symptoms and the side effect profile of the various agents.
- In general, selective serotonin reuptake inhibitors (SSRIs; e.g., sertraline, citalopram, fluoxetine, paroxetine) are preferred first line agents because of their relatively benign side effect profiles and lower cost generic availability. Serotonin-norepinephrine reuptake inhibitors (SNRIs; e.g., duloxetine, venlafaxine) and atypicals (e.g., mirtazapine, bupropion) may also be considered.
- In the authors' experience, irritability and anger also often respond to the aforementioned antidepressants. The antiepileptic mood stabilizers (e.g., valproic acid and carbamazepine) may also be acceptable options, especially if neither depression nor anxiety is prominent.

Fatigue Pharmacologic Management

- Fatigue symptoms may be secondary to comorbid conditions. After conditions such as depression, insomnia, and sleep apnea have been ruled out or treated, stimulant medications may be appropriate.

- An activating antidepressant (e.g., flouxetine) is a reasonable agent to try initially. If the patient is already on an antidepressant medication, consider switching to one with a less sedating profile.
- Amphetamine-like stimulants (e.g., methylphenidate and dexedrine) may be beneficial, although careful monitoring is needed given their abuse potential.
- Modafinil, a medication approved by FDA for narcolepsy and shift work sleep syndrome, is a higher cost alternative. However, a study of 53 patients on an average of 6 years after TBI severe enough to require inpatient rehabilitation showed no consistent benefit for fatigue or excessive daytime sleepiness [10].
- Amantadine has mixed evidence of efficacy for fatigue symptoms in multiple sclerosis and is considered by some to be an option for PCS-related fatigue.

Sleep Dysfunction

- Primary sleep disorders should be considered and ruled out with a sleep study as indicated.
- Additional behavioral interventions should be considered and are preferred over pharmacotherapy, including meditation, relaxation training, and white noise devices.
- Benzodiazepines should be avoided.
- Additional management recommendations can be found in Chapter 54.

Dizziness and Disequilibrium

- Medication review and reconciliation is crucial because numerous medications have dizziness as a potential side effect.
- Vestibular suppressants (e.g., meclizine) might be helpful during the acute period of several vestibular disorders but have not been shown to be effective in chronic dizziness after concussion [11].
- The mainstays of treatment for persisting symptoms are the aforementioned vestibular exercises in combination with habituation and coping strategies.
- Specific treatments may be indicated for some subtypes (e.g., Semont and modified Epley maneuvers for benign paroxysmal positional vertigo).

ADDITIONAL READING

Electronic Reference

http://emedicine.medscape.com/article/292326-treatment

Textbook/Chapter

McAllister TW. Mild brain injury and the postconcussion syndrome. In: Silver JM, McAllister TW, Yudofsky SC, eds. *Textbook of Traumatic Brain Injury.* 2nd ed. Washington, DC: American Psychiatric Pub; 2005:279–308.

Journal Articles

De Groot MH, Phillips SJ, Eskes GA. Fatigue associated with stroke and other neurologic conditions: implications for stroke rehabilitation. *Arch Phys Med Rehabil.* 2003;84(11):1714–1720.

Mittenberg W, Canyock EM, Condit D, Patton C. Treatment of post-concussion syndrome following mild head injury. *J Clin Exp Neuropsychol.* 2001;23(6):829–836.

REFERENCES

1. Gouvier WD, Cubic B, Jones G, Brantley P, Cutlip Q. Postconcussion symptoms and daily stress in normal and head-injured college populations. *Arch Clin Neuropsychol.* 1992;7(3):193–211.

2. King NS, Crawford S, Wenden FJ, Moss NE, Wade DT. The Rivermead Post Concussion Symptoms Questionnaire: a measure of symptoms commonly experienced after head injury and its reliability. *J Neurol.* 1995;242(9):587–592.

3. Miller LJ, Mittenberg W. Brief cognitive behavioral interventions in mild traumatic brain injury. *Appl Neuropsychol.* 1998;5(4):172–183.

4. Bell KR, Hoffman JM, Temkin NR, et al. The effect of telephone counselling on reducing post-traumatic symptoms after mild traumatic brain injury: a randomised trial. *J Neurol Neurosurg Psychiatr.* 2008;79(11):1275–1281.

5. Herdman SJ, Clendaniel RA, Mattox DE, Holliday MJ, Niparko JK. Vestibular adaptation exercises and recovery: acute stage after acoustic neuroma resection. *Otolaryngol Head Neck Surg.* 1995;113(1):77–87.

6. Shepard NT, Telian SA. Programmatic vestibular rehabilitation. *Otolaryngol Head Neck Surg.* 1995;112(1):173–182.

7. Yardley L, Burgneay J, Andersson G, Owen N, Nazareth I, Luxon L. Feasibility and effectiveness of providing vestibular rehabilitation for dizzy patients in the community. *Clin Otolaryngol Allied Sci.* 1998;23(5):442–448.

8. Evans RW, Evans RI, Sharp MJ. The physician survey on the post-concussion and whiplash syndromes. *Headache.* 1994;34(5):268–274.

9. Mittenberg W, Canyock EM, Condit D, Patton C. Treatment of post-concussion syndrome following mild head injury. *J Clin Exp Neuropsychol.* 2001;23(6):829–836.

10. Jha A, Weintraub A, Allshouse A, et al. A randomized trial of modafinil for the treatment of fatigue and excessive daytime sleepiness in individuals with chronic traumatic brain injury. *J Head Trauma Rehabil.* 2008;23(1):52–63.

11. Zee DS. Perspectives on the pharmacotherapy of vertigo. *Arch Otolaryngol.* 1985;111(9):609–612.

19

Confounding Factors in Postconcussive Disorders

Nathan D. Zasler

INTRODUCTION

The diagnosis of postconcussive disorders may be complicated by a number of confounding factors. The purpose of this chapter is to identify some of these issues and provide guidelines for addressing them. Even if a concussion (i.e., mild traumatic brain injury [MTBI]) is diagnosed based on neurological criteria at the time of an accident, one cannot necessarily conclude that symptoms ascribed to the event at the time of subsequent examination are in fact causally related, nor for that matter that physical findings are attributable to the claimed concussive injury. The temporal onset of symptoms, as well as their nature, severity, frequency, and response to treatment must be considered in assessing both causality and apportionment in the context of differential diagnosis after claimed MTBI. Clinicians need to consider all potential confounding issues that make assessing and managing this group of patients so challenging [1,2].

NOMENCLATURE

- Cerebral concussion (Latin: *commotion cerebri*) is a phraseology that has been used since the time of Hippocrates, although not always to reference mild forms of brain insult. There remains some confusion and debate as to whether concussion and MTBI are analogous.
- The phrases "brain injury" and "head injury" are often used interchangeably, although these are two distinct terms. The former describes insult/trauma to the cerebrum and the latter connotes traumatic injury to the cranium or its surrounding structures.
- Postconcussion syndrome (PCS)—by common medical parlance, a syndrome is a consistent set of signs and/or symptoms that occur together to define a condition; however, the use of the phrase PCS is really a misnomer because the signs and symptoms that follow concussion are inconsistent across patients.

- Postconcussion disorder (PCD)—this term was introduced in the psychiatric literature in the American Psychiatric Association's *Diagnostic and Statistical Manual of Mental Disorders* (DSM); however, there is no evidence-based literature to support all the criteria endorsed in the definition (see following section) nor any consensus on the use of the definition outside of psychiatry. The terms PCS and PCD are used interchangeably in clinical practice.

DIAGNOSTIC CRITERIA

Although there are no internationally agreed upon diagnostic criteria for concussion, there are a plethora of definitions [1]:

- The World Health Organization's International Statistical Classification of Diseases and Related Health Problems (ICD-10) proposed a set of research based criteria for PCS, which required head trauma and loss of consciousness (LOC) preceding the onset of symptoms by a period of up to 4 weeks, and having symptoms in at least three of six symptom categories. There are a number of problems with this criteria including the assumptions that the six symptom categories actually occur reliably as symptom clusters (as opposed to being empirically grouped), that subjective cognitive complaints have any substantive positive correlation with objectively measured ones, and that the various symptoms included in the six categories are pathognomonic for MTBI.

- The American Congress of Rehabilitation Medicine (ACRM) defined MTBI as 30 minutes or fewer of LOC, 24 hours or fewer of posttraumatic amnesia (PTA), and a Glasgow Coma Scale (GCS) score of 13 or more. The criteria have been criticized for not being more formalized, the inclusion of a broad range of injury severity, and the over-reliance on subjective patient report.

- In 1994, the American Psychiatric Association's DSM defined MTBI using PTA and LOC; however, this definition uses terminology inconsistently (e.g., closed head injury and cerebral concussion) and includes seizures as an injury severity marker, although seizures in MTBI occur at about the same rate as de novo epilepsy in the general population.

- The Centers for Disease Control Working Group developed a conceptual definition for MTBI in 2003 that more thoroughly addressed the nature of the injury, delineated common observed and/or self-reported symptoms but also qualified that the diagnosis could not be made in the absence of alteration in consciousness at the time of the initial injury.

- The most recent attempt at formulating guidelines for assessment and management was in 2008 in Zurich, Switzerland and was organized by the International Olympic Committee Medical Commission and other sports federations [3]. The panel members did not analogize MTBI with concussion but did provide a definition of concussion that is probably the most complete and well thought out of the definitions currently available (see http://www.sportconcussions.com/html/Zurich%20Statement.pdf)

DIFFERENTIAL DIAGNOSTIC ISSUES

The aim of evaluation following a claimed concussion should be to appropriately understand the preinjury, injury, and postinjury history to facilitate accurate diagnosis of concussion and/or PCS. Thorough and appropriate differential diagnosis requires pursuing differential etiologies for the presenting symptoms and/or signs and understanding the myriad "pathologies" that might produce symptoms attributed to concussion but that in fact have noncerebral etiologies [4–6].

History

Obtaining a detailed history about preinjury, injury, and postinjury symptoms and signs can be very helpful in elucidating the true nature of the patient's current complaints and their accurate apportionment [2]. Interviewing other parties who may have knowledge of the patient prior to the injury in question and/or were present at the scene of the accident and after may provide key information relating to the nature and cause of the current clinical presentation.

Physical Examination

Subtle neurological findings may be seen in persons after concussion, including smell or hearing loss, vestibular dysfunction, higher-level balance impairment, kinetic tremor, slowed reaction time, and frontal motor impairments [1].

Diagnostic Assessments

A few of the more commonly used and more sensitive testing approaches include neuroimaging, electrophysiological, neuro-otological, chemosensory, and neuropsychological testing. It is critical for clinicians to also understand the appropriate applications and limitations of such tests, as well as their sensitivity and specificity [2,7–9].

Pathologies That May Produce Signs and Symptoms Parallel to Those of Concussion

Cranial Trauma

Trauma to the cranium can produce an array of symptoms that parallel postconcussive symptoms without having any concurrent brain injury

[1,8]. Some of the problems commonly seen after these types of injuries include headache, tinnitus, hearing loss, hyperacusis, vestibulopathies, olfactory impairments, and visual dysfunction.

Cervical Injuries

Injuries to the neck, such as through acceleration/deceleration or direct trauma, may produce an array of problems that may be mistaken for PCS, including referred cervicogenic headache, tinnitus, cervical vertigo, visual problems, and retro-orbital pain.

Chronic Pain

Posttraumatic pain disorders are an often-overlooked concomitant of cranial and cervical trauma. When pain becomes chronic (i.e., more than 6 months duration), it typically becomes more challenging to separate problems that are due to pain from other posttrauma conditions including PCS. Pain also tends to have adverse consequences on sleep, cognition, and behavior, which further complicate both assessment and treatment [10,11].

Affective Issues

Patients often develop secondary reactive psychological states after trauma. Clinicians working with such patients should be familiar with anxiety spectrum disorders including posttraumatic stress disorder (PTSD), depression, and adjustment disorders. Occasionally, patients may present with affective lability, similar to a pseudobulbar affective disorder with a propensity to become easily tearful [1].

Comorbidities

Patients often have multiple contributors to symptomatology following concussion. One cannot automatically assume that symptoms are attributable to an MTBI/concussion [1,2,8,12].

IATROGENESIS

The phenomenon of iatrogenesis can work in two directions, neither of which, ultimately, is in the best interest of the patient. Doctors who dismiss symptoms that are truly neurological following concussion clearly do the patient a disservice. They further promulgate potential for adverse adaptive responses, including anxiety, depression, insomnia, stress and worsening of pain, as well as protract impairment and any related functional disability by not treating the real problem. On the other hand, clinicians who over-diagnose concussion-related impairments may actually be producing a nocebo effect; that is, they are instilling negative expectancies, which may ultimately manifest into maladaptive behaviors, reinforce disability (which in fact may not be present), and perpetuate inappropriate diagnostic labels, as well as lead to ineffective and clinically unnecessary treatment [13,14]).

OTHER FACTORS TO CONSIDER

Clinicians should be aware of the literature examining the impact of personality, psychosocial factors, stress and litigation on symptom reporting, clinical presentation, prognosis, and treatment response [15,16].

Another important area of clinical assessment is that of response bias testing. In the context of postconcussion assessment, response bias testing allows the practitioner to determine the response style of the patient relative to whether they are providing unbiased responses or coloring them in a particular direction (i.e., symptom minimizing versus symptom magnifying). In this latter context, practitioners need to be aware of how stress, litigation, and psychological factors may affect both response style and effort in order to fully evaluate the validity of interview data and diagnostic testing results [17,18].

CONCLUSIONS

Practitioners must take an array of confounding variables into consideration when assessing and treating persons following concussive brain injuries. Comprehensive assessment of preinjury, injury, and postinjury history, and a well-informed knowledge of concussion guidelines and current MTBI science will result in optimizing diagnostic accuracy and treatment outcomes.

ADDITIONAL READING

Electronic References
http://www.cdc.gov/concussion/index.html
http://www.cdc.gov/ncipc/pub-res/tbi_toolkit/physicians/mtbi/mtbi.pdf

Textbooks/Chapters
Iverson GL, Lange RT, Gaetz M, Zasler N. Mild traumatic brain injury. In: Zasler ND, Katz DI, Zafonte R, eds. *Brain Injury Medicine: Principles and Practice.* New York: Demos; 2007.

Iverson GL, Zasler ND, Lange RT. Post-concussive disorders. In: Zasler ND, Katz DI, Zafonte R, eds. *Brain Injury Medicine: Principles and Practice.* New York: Demos; 2007.

McCrea M. *Mild Traumatic Brain Injury and Post-concussion Syndrome: The New Evidence Base for Diagnosis and Treatment (AACN Workshop Series).* New York: Oxford University Press; 2007.

Journal Articles

Iverson GL. Clinical and methodological challenges with assessing mild traumatic brain injury in the military. *J Head Trauma Rehabil.* 2010;25(5):313–319.

McCrory P, Meeuwisse W, Johnston K, et al. Consensus statement on concussion in sport—the Third International Conference on Concussion in Sport held in Zurich, November 2008. *Phys Sportsmed.* 2009;37(2):141–159.

Ruff RM, Iverson GL, Barth JT, et al. Recommendations for diagnosing a mild traumatic brain injury: a National Academy of Neuropsychology Education Paper. *Arch Clin Neuropsychol.* 2009;24:3–10.

REFERENCES

1. Iverson GL, Zasler ND, Lange RT. Post-concussive disorders. In: Zasler ND, Katz DI, Zafonte R, eds. *Brain Injury Medicine: Principles and Practice.* New York: Demos; 2007.

2. Iverson GL, Lange RT, Gaetz M, Zasler N. Mild traumatic brain injury. In: Zasler ND, Katz DI, Zafonte R, eds. *Brain Injury Medicine: Principles and Practice.* New York: Demos; 2007.

3. McCrory P, Meeuwisse W, Johnston K, et al. Consensus statement on concussion in sport—the Third International Conference on Concussion in Sport held in Zurich. *Phys Sportsmed.* 2008;37(2):141–159.

4. Zasler ND. Neuromedical diagnosis and treatment of post-concussive disorders. In: Horn LJ, Zasler ND, eds. *Rehabilitation of Post-Concussive Disorders.* Philadelphia: Hanley & Belfus; 1992:33–68.

5. Ruff RM, Iverson GL, Barth JT, et al. Recommendations for diagnosing a mild traumatic brain injury: a National Academy of Neuropsychology Education Paper. *Arch Clin Neuropsychol.* 2009;24:3–10.

6. McCrea M, Iverson GL, McAllister TW, et al. An integrated review of recovery after mild traumatic brain injury (MTBI): implications for clinical management. *Clin Neuropsychol.* 2009;23(8):1368–1390.

7. Sbordone RJ. Neuropsychological tests are poor at assessing the frontal lobes, executive functions and neurobehavioral symptoms of traumatically brain injured patients. *Psychol Inj Law.* 2010;3:25–35.

8. Horn LJ, Zasler, ND, eds. *Rehabilitation of Post-Concussive Disorders. State of the Art Reviews in Physical Medicine and Rehabilitation.* Philadelphia: Hanley and Belfus; 1992.

9. Heilbronner RL, Sweet JJ, Morgan JE, et al. American Academy of Clinical Neuropsychology Consensus Conference Statement on the neuropsychological assessment of effort, response bias and malingering. *Clin Neuropsychol.* 2009;23(7):1093–1129.

10. Iverson GL, McCracken LM. 'Postconcussive' symptoms in persons with chronic pain. *Brain Inj.* 1997;11:783–790.

11. Hart RP, Martelli MF, Zasler ND. Chronic pain and neuropsychological functioning. *Neuropsychol Rev.* 2000;10(3):131–149.

12. Satz PS, Alfano MS, Light RF, et al. Persistent post-concussive syndrome: a proposed methodology and literature review to determine the effects, if any, of mild head and other bodily injury. *J Clin Exp Neuropsychol.* 1999;21:620–628.

13. Benson H. The nocebo effect: history and physiology. *Prev Med.* 1997;26:612–615.
14. Mittenberg W, DiGiulio DV, Perrin S, Bass AE. Symptoms following mild head injury: expectation as aetiology. *J Neurol Neurosurg Psychiatry.* 1992;55:200–204.
15. Paniak C, Reynolds S, Toller-Lobe G, Melnyk A, Nagy J, Schmidt D. A longitudinal study of the relationship between financial compensation and symptoms after treated mild traumatic brain injury. *J Clin Exp Neuropsychol.* 2002;24:187–193.
16. Machulda MM, Bergquist TF, Ito V, Chew S. Relationship between stress, coping, and post concussion symptoms in a healthy adult population. *Arch Clin Neuropsychol.* 1998;13:415–424.
17. Carroll LJ, Cassidy JD, Peloso PM, et al. Prognosis for mild traumatic brain injury: results of the WHO collaborating centre task force on mild traumatic brain injury. *J Rehabil Med.* 2004;36:84–105.
18. Martelli MF, Nicholson K, Zasler ND. Assessment of response bias. In: Zasler N, Katz D, Zafonte R, eds. *Brain Injury Medicine: Principles and Practice.* New York: Demos; 2007.

20

Recognizing Manifestations of Posttraumatic Stress Disorder in Patients With Traumatic Brain Injury

Eric B. Larson

BACKGROUND

Definition

Posttraumatic stress disorder (PTSD) is psychiatric syndrome characterized by persistent symptoms of anxiety after exposure to a traumatic
event. In patients with traumatic brain injury (TBI), PTSD is sometimes
confused with postconcussion disorder, adjustment disorder, personality
change due to TBI, and with dementia due to TBI.

Diagnostic Criteria

Problems from each of the following six categories must be observed
[1]: (1) history of exposure to trauma, (2) trauma is persistently
re-experienced, (3) engaging in avoidant behavior or experiencing
numbing of general responsiveness, (4) increased autonomic arousal,
(5) duration of symptoms is more than 1 month, and (6) significant
distress or functional impairment results from these symptoms.

Epidemiology

In the general population, lifetime prevalence of PTSD is 7.8%. In patients
with mild TBI, estimates of prevalence range from 10% to 27%. Prevalence
of PTSD has been shown to be the same among mild TBI patients as it is
among patients with other traumatic injuries [2]. In patients with severe
TBI, the best estimate of prevalence is 3%, although self-report of symptoms is much higher [3].

Etiology

A Behavioral Account

Most forms of anxiety are a result of appraisal of an impending (future) threat. PTSD involves processing a *past* trauma as a current threat, possibly because of activation of implicit memories of the traumatic events. Discrimination between current experience and past implicit memories may be more difficult because the latter are more vaguely defined than are explicit memories [4].

A Neurobiological Account

The implicit learning involved in PTSD may be mediated by neural circuits that are routed through the amygdala. It is proposed this system is distinct from the explicit learning that occurs via the hippocampus [5].

Pathophysiology

Inconsistent evidence of atrophy in the hippocampus and in the anterior cingulate cortex has been reported in PTSD patients. Some have proposed these are stress-induced changes, but twin studies suggest that reduced volume in these structures is a pretrauma vulnerability factor [6].

DIAGNOSIS

Risk Factors

Knowledge of characteristics that leave patients vulnerable to PTSD can help determine if that disorder in present in a TBI survivor with an ambiguous clinical presentation.

- Pretrauma risk factors—Sex and marital status are the strongest demographic predictors of PTSD. Women and previously married (e.g., divorced or widowed) individuals have the highest risk for PTSD [7].
- Trauma-related risk factors—For men, the highest risk for PTSD is for those who have been in combat and for those who have witnessed someone being killed or severely injured. For women, the highest risk is associated with rape or sexual molestation.
- Posttrauma risk factors—A lack of subsequent social support and experience of additional life stressors are both stronger predictors of PTSD than pretrauma risk factors [8].
- Poor cognitive function [9]—A pretrauma cognitive deficit may leave an individual less able to cope with stressors, which may make them more vulnerable to PTSD.
- TBI patients are at increased risk for PTSD at 6 months after injury if they experienced acute stress disorder after their injury, if they

exhibited symptoms of depression and anxiety within 1 week of injury, if they had a previous history of psychiatric disorder, or if they had memory for the traumatic event [10].

Clinical Presentation

In mild TBI, PTSD patients often present symptoms of trauma-related emotional distress along with symptoms of postconcussion disorder. Symptoms observed in both disorders include noise sensitivity, fatigue, anxiety, insomnia, poor concentration, poor memory, and irritability. The presence of these symptoms alone is not diagnostic of either disorder because all have high base rates in the general population as well.

Symptoms

- Recurrent intrusive distressing recollections of the traumatic event. Such memories are sudden, unwanted, and disruptive to one's activities
- Recurrent distressing dreams of the event (nightmares)
- Sudden acting or feeling as if the traumatic event were recurring. This involves perception that the trauma is happening in the present and differs from remembering the traumatic event as a past occurrence. Contact with present reality is greatly diminished. This may involve hallucinations or dissociative experience (i.e., a "flashback")
- Intense psychological distress at exposure to trauma-related cues
- Physiological reactivity on exposure to trauma-related cues
- Efforts to avoid thoughts or feelings associated with the trauma
- Efforts to avoid activities or situations that arouse recollections of trauma (e.g., appointment cancelations, failed appointments, and tardiness to treatment sessions)
- Inability to recall an important aspect of the trauma, only if determined not to be because of posttraumatic amnesia
- Markedly diminished interest in significant activities that are still available despite physical disability
- Feeling of detachment or estrangement from others
- Restricted range of affect
- Sense of foreshortened future
- Difficulty falling or staying asleep
- Irritability or outbursts of anger
- Difficulty concentrating
- Hypervigilance—This does not necessarily exclude situations in which an individual's perception of threat is justified by actual danger in their environment
- Exaggerated startle response

Evaluation

- Symptom checklists—Questionnaires that rely on self-report like the PTSD Checklist [11] require little time to complete (5 minutes or less) and may be used as screening measures but should not be used for diagnosis given their poor specificity. Further, in TBI patients, self-report is notoriously inaccurate.
- Structured interviews—The "gold standard" for PTSD diagnosis, clinician interviews require extended time to complete (30 to 120 minutes). They also require formal training to assure inter-rater reliability. Measures include the Clinician-Administered PTSD Scale for DSM-IV [12] and the Structured Clinical Interview for the DSM-IV Axis I Disorders [13].
- Neuropsychological evaluation—Standardized psychological assessment provides a detailed description of the nature of cognitive impairment and emotional distress. However, in cases where it is unclear whether a patient has sustained a mild TBI, identifying cognitive impairment does not assist with differential diagnosis, because such impairment can be seen in individuals with PTSD alone [14].

Controversies

It has been suggested that TBI does not produce PTSD because the disturbance of consciousness that must occur in the former interferes with formation of memories of trauma, which is presumably the cause of symptoms in the latter [15]. Although some evidence supports this conclusion, other studies show that PTSD exists in individuals who lost consciousness at the time of their injury [10,16]. The formation of implicit memories (that may not require clear consciousness at the time of trauma and that may exist in the absence of explicit recall) has been offered as an explanation for this counterintuitive finding.

TREATMENT

Guiding Principles

Exposure and Avoidance

Treatment that increases exposure to trauma-related stimuli in a supportive, controlled environment is effective at reducing symptoms. Avoidance of stimuli that provoke distress results in increased anxiety when those triggers can no longer be escaped.

Medication and Cognition

Some pharmacological interventions are effective at short-term management of anxiety but can result in iatrogenic cognitive impairment, which makes them bad choices for TBI survivors.

Initial Management

- Reliance on psychopharmacology is necessary primarily in cases where cognitive impairment makes psychotherapy unrealistic.
- Use of medications that affect serotonergic and noradrenergic pathways can be specifically useful in control of hyperarousal.
- Selective serotonin reputake inhibitors (SSRIs) are more effective than older antidepressants for most symptoms of PTSD; trazodone can be helpful in reducing nightmares and daytime anxiety.
- Prazosin, a centrally acting noradrenergic α1 blocker can also be used to reduce nightmares and daytime anxiety.
- Propanolol, a centrally acting noradrenergic β blocker, can reduce autonomic hyperarousal.
- Most antipsychotic medications are not used to treat PTSD, especially in patients with comorbid TBI because these agents can interfere with neurological recovery.
- Atypical antipsychotics (e.g., Zyprexa and Risperdal) may be helpful for control of psychotic symptoms of PTSD (e.g., hallucinations), possibly due to serotonergic effects.
- Sedative-hypnotics (e.g., benzodiazepines) provide temporary relief of symptoms but because of rebound and dependence, they are not recommended in PTSD.

Ongoing Care

- Cognitive-behavioral treatment that includes exposure therapy can be introduced early for patients with mild TBI and later in the course of recovery for moderate-to-severe TBI patients. Memory deficits are a substantial obstacle to efficacy; in fact, such impairment may never resolve to the point that psychotherapy is possible.
- Referral to PTSD specialists can be particularly helpful. Centralized referral databases are now offered (listed under "Electronic References").

Treatment Controversies

Eye Movement Desensitization and Reprocessing

An ongoing debate continues about the efficacy of eye movement desensitization and reprocessing (EMDR). Although outcome studies support the use of this technique, many clinicians argue that it is effective because it includes elements of exposure therapy, and that there are no advantages to EMDR over traditional exposure therapy [17].

Additional Considerations

Disability Evaluations

In veterans, a diagnosis of PTSD may be used to support claims of disability. Disabled veterans can receive disability income if they can substantiate these claims. Secondary monetary gain may result in many false disability claims.

Personal Injury Cases

Individuals who file personal injury lawsuits may argue that their injury resulted in PTSD. Again, secondary gain may influence symptom reporting. Consider referral for evaluation by a PTSD specialist and/or neuropsychologist who can determine the extent to which this influence may result in symptom magnification or malingering.

ADDITIONAL READING

Electronic References

VA/DoD Clinical Practice Guideline. http://www.healthquality.va.gov/ptsd/ptsd_poc2.pdf

To find a therapist: http://www.abct.org/Members/?m=FindTherapist&fa=FT_Form&nolm=1

Treatment Options: http://www.dcoe.health.mil/ForHealthPros/PTSDTreatmentOptions.aspx

Textbooks

Foa E, Keane TM, Friedman MJ, Cohen, JA. *Effective Treatments for PTSD: Practice Guidelines from the International Society for Traumatic Stress Studies.* 2nd ed. New York: Guilford Press; 2008.

Rosen GM, Frueh C. *Clinician's Guide to Posttraumatic Stress Disorder.* Hoboken, NJ: Wiley; 2010.

Journal Articles

McAllister TW. Psychopharmacological issues in the treatment of TBI and PTSD. *Clin Neuropsychol.* 2009;23(8):1338–1367.

Van Boven RW, Harington GS, Hackney DB, et al. Advances in neuroimaging of traumatic brain injury and posttraumatic stress disorder. *J Rehabil Res Dev.* 2009;46(6):717–757.

Vanderploeg RD, Belanger HG, Curtiss G. Mild traumatic brain injury and posttraumatic stress disorder and their associations with health symptoms. *Arch Phys Med Rehabil.* 2009;90(7):1084–1093.

REFERENCES

1. American Psychiatric Association. *Diagnostic and Statistical Manual of Mental Disorders, Fourth Ed.* Washington, DC: American Psychiatric Association; 1994.

2. Kim E, Lauterbach EC, Reeve A, et al.; ANPA Committee on Research. Neuropsychiatric complications of traumatic brain injury: a critical review of the literature (a report by the ANPA Committee on Research). *J Neuropsychiatry Clin Neurosci.* 2007;19(2):106–127.

3. Sumpter RE, McMillan TM. Misdiagnosis of post-traumatic stress disorder following severe traumatic brain injury. *Br J Psychiatry.* 2005;186:423–426.

4. Ehlers A, Clark DM. A cognitive model of posttraumatic stress disorder. *Behav Res Ther.* 2000;38(4):319–345.

5. LeDoux JE. Emotion circuits in the brain. *Annu Rev Neurosci.* 2000;23:155–184.

6. Gilbertson MW, Shenton ME, Ciszewski A, et al. Smaller hippocampal volume predicts pathologic vulnerability to psychological trauma. *Nat Neurosci.* 2002;5(11):1242–1247.

7. Kessler RC, Sonnega A, Bromet E, Hughes M, Nelson CB. Posttraumatic stress disorder in the National Comorbidity Survey. *Arch Gen Psychiatry.* 1995;52(12):1048–1060.

8. Brewin CR, Andrews B, Valentine JD. Meta-analysis of risk factors for posttraumatic stress disorder in trauma-exposed adults. *J Consult Clin Psychol.* 2000;68(5):748–766.

9. Parslow RA, Jorm AF. Pretrauma and posttrauma neurocognitive functioning and PTSD symptoms in a community sample of young adults. *Am J Psychiatry.* 2007;164(3):509–515.

10. Gil S, Caspi Y, Ben-Ari IZ, Koren D, Klein E. Does memory of a traumatic event increase the risk for posttraumatic stress disorder in patients with traumatic brain injury? A prospective study. *Am J Psychiatry.* 2005;162(5):963–969.

11. Weathers FW, Litz BT, Herman DS, Huska JA, Keane TM. The PTSD Checklist (PCL): reliability, validity, and diagnostic utility. In: Proceedings of the Annual Conference of the International Society for Traumatic Stress Studies; October 25, 1993; San Antonio, TX.

12. Blake DD, Weathers FW, Nagy LM, et al. *Clinician-Administered PTSD Scale (CAPS), Form 1: Current and Lifetime Diagnosis Version.* West Haven, CT: National Center for Posttraumatic Stress Disorder; 1990.

13. First MB, Spitzer RL, Gibbon M, Williams JBW. Structured Clinical Interview for DSM-IV Axis I Disorders—Non Patient Edition (SCID-I/NP), version 2.0. New York: New York State Psychiatric Institute, Biometrics Research; 1997.

14. Brenner LA, Ladley-O'Brien SE, Harwood JE, et al. An exploratory study of neuroimaging, neurologic, and neuropsychological findings in veterans with traumatic brain injury and/or posttraumatic stress disorder. *Mil Med.* 2009;174(4):347–352.

15. Sbordone RJ, Liter JC. Mild traumatic brain injury does not produce posttraumatic stress disorder. *Brain Inj.* 1995;9(4):405–412.

16. Mayou RA, Black J, Bryant B. Unconsciousness, amnesia and psychiatric symptoms following road traffic accident injury. *Br J Psychiatry.* 2000;177:540–545.
17. Lohr JM, Tolin DF, Lilienfeld SO. Efficacy of eye movement desensitization and reprocessing: implications for behavior therapy. *Behav Ther.* 1998;29:123–156.

21

Factors Suggesting a Need for Referral to Mental Health Providers in Postconcussive Disorder

Matthew R. Powell and Michael McCrea

GENERAL PRINCIPLES

Postconcussive disorder (PCD) has emerged as one of the more controversial and challenging conditions in the neurosciences. PCD is appropriately diagnosed when neurologic, cognitive, behavioral, or somatic symptoms following mild traumatic brain injury (MTBI) persist beyond 3 months [1,2].

Patients with PCD frequently present to the outpatient clinics of primary care physicians, physiatrists, or neurologists seeking relief for lingering symptoms. Although some patients will have already received an initial medical work-up to rule out a more devastating brain injury during the acute phase, many patients will have had no prior contact with health care specialists [3]. Outpatient medical work-ups for PCD-related complaints are typically unremarkable for any identifiable neurologic pathology. Furthermore, there exists no "standard of care" treatment regimen that physicians can rely on to comprehensively address the various symptoms reported. Complicating treatment decision-making even more is the fact that it is not at all uncommon for two MTBI patients with very similar injuries (e.g., based on acute injury characteristics) to report very different symptom profiles following injury.

TREATMENT

Background

A multitude of factors have been shown to contribute to and maintain diverse PCD-related symptoms [3,4]. PCD is not a unidimensional brain-based condition but rather an outcome influenced by cognitive, emotional, medical, psychosocial, and motivational factors [3,5,6], now referred to as the biopsychosocial model of PCD [7].

Because of this complexity, treatments targeting PCD-related symptoms should follow an integrated model of care. In this context, referral to behavioral health providers such as neuropsychologists, rehabilitation psychologists, health psychologists, and/or psychiatrists should be considered, but particularly when patients experience cognitive, emotional, or behavioral changes. If a patient reports the following signs or symptoms, one should consider referal to a mental health provider with experience in managing TBI to assist with evaluation and treatment.

- Cognitive symptoms
- Emotional/behavioral symptoms (e.g., psychiatric disorder or difficulty coping)
- Excessive symptoms or worsening symptoms (without underlying medical cause)
- Persisting pain (e.g., headache, neck or back pain)
- Substance abuse/dependence
- Reported functional impairment (e.g., inability to return to work or school)
- Patients involved in litigation, pursuing or receiving disability and/or workman's compensation benefits

Management Approaches

Behavioral health intervention is not a unitary construct and can be conceptualized in three distinct ways: (1) symptom management (e.g., symptom reduction), (2) cognitive restructuring, and (3) preventative treatment.

Symptom Management

Physicians frequently refer their patients for *behavioral intervention* when it is apparent that their patient's symptoms are medically intractable. Behavioral health specialists help patients develop a behavioral program to facilitate symptom management (e.g., reduction of pain, improving sleep hygiene, using moderation during daily activities). The symptoms targeted under a symptom management approach may or may not be psychiatric symptoms. For example, patients with chronic daily headache or neck pain may benefit from learning progressive muscle relaxation or biofeedback procedures from a qualified health psychologist. Patients with mood disorders (e.g., depression), anxiety disorders (e.g., posttraumatic stress disorder), or adjustment reactions may benefit from time-limited psychotherapy such as cognitive behavioral treatments. Moreover, psychotherapy may increase patients' awareness of factors contributing to psychiatric difficulties, reduce their symptoms, or help them develop appropriate short- and long-term goals post injury.

Cognitive Behavioral Health Treatments

These treatments focus on *cognitive restructuring*. Patients with well-established PCD frequently develop inaccurate or distorted perceptions of their injury, their recovery, their preserved abilities, and their outcome [7,8]. Psychotherapies focusing on cognitive restructuring work toward dismantling the distorted self-perceptions that frequently accompany PCD and replace them with accurate beliefs and appraisals related to one's injury, recovery, preserved ability, and outcome post injury [8,9]. Ferguson and Mittenberg [8] developed a six-session structured cognitive behavioral therapy program that helps patients understand how psychological factors can intensify and maintain PCD-related symptoms and teach PCD patients cognitive behavioral techniques to manage stress and cope more effectively with PCD symptoms.

Prevention

Although symptom management and cognitive restructuring approaches are very important for patient health and quality of life, treatment approaches focusing on *prevention* of PCD are ideal. Because psychological and social factors of disease, including PCD, are clearly modifiable variables (e.g., the patient, the provider, and the patient's environment can influence outcome), it should not be surprising that MTBI patients who receive brief cognitive behavioral health treatments in the acute or subacute phase of recovery report fewer and less severe PCD-related symptoms months later compared to patients with MTBI who do not receive these early behavioral interventions [10–18]. Brief psychoeducational interventions administered during early recovery following MTBI, with or without concomitant cognitive behavioral teaching, also decrease the risk for PCD. For example, education provided to MTBI patients prior to hospital discharge resulted in significantly shorter symptom duration, decreased frequency of symptoms, fewer symptomatic days per week, and a lower severity of symptoms [10]. Further, because the symptoms of PCD are nonspecific, and because they are so prevalent in normal, healthy non–brain injured persons, symptoms may be misattributed to the injury. For example, attention and memory concerns post injury may be related to side effects from certain medications (e.g., narcotic pain medications or tricyclic antidepressants) a patient received to treat PCD symptoms rather than from a MTBI. Similarly, attention or memory complaints may be better explained by a posttraumatic stress reaction associated with a motor vehicle collision than a MTBI. Encouraging patients to consider alternative explanations for their symptoms may be an appropriate means of remediating this tendency.

SUMMARY

Behavioral health and neuropsychological interventions can be useful for preventing the development of PCD, for symptom management, and/or for reducing disability associated with MTBI. Recognition that there are factors beyond the neurobiological abnormalities associated with MTBI that cause or maintain PCD-related symptoms may have a key impact on overall outcome.

ADDITIONAL READING

Electronic Reference

Psychological approaches to treatment of postconcussion syndrome: a systematic review. http://jnnp.bmj.com/content/81/10/1128.full

Textbook/Chapters

Iverson GL, Zasler ND, Lange RT. Post-concussive disorder. In: Zasler ND, Katz DI, Zafonte RD, eds. *Brain Injury Medicine: Principles and Practice.* New York: Demos Medical Publishing; 2007:373–405.

McCrea MA. *Mild Traumatic Brain Injury and Postconcussion Syndrome: The New Evidence Base for Diagnosis and Treatment.* New York: Oxford University Press; 2008.

Journal Articles

Borg J, Holm L, Peloso PM, et al. Non-surgical intervention and cost for mild traumatic brain injury: results of the WHO Collaborating Centre Task Force on Mild Traumatic Brain Injury. *J Rehabil Med.* 2004;(43 suppl):76–83.

Comper P, Bisschop SM, Carnide N, Tricco A. A systematic review of treatments for mild traumatic brain injury. *Brain Inj.* 2005;19(11):863–880.

Iverson GL. Outcome from mild traumatic brain injury. *Curr Opin Psychiatry.* 2005;18(3):301–317.

Mittenberg W, Canyock EM, Condit D, Patton C. Treatment of post-concussion syndrome following mild head injury. *J Clin Exp Neuropsychol.* 2001;23(6):829–836.

Mittenberg W, Tremont G, Zielinski RE, Fichera S, Rayls KR. Cognitive-behavioral prevention of postconcussion syndrome. *Arch Clin Neuropsychol.* 1996;11(2):139–145.

Ruff RM, Camenzuli L, Mueller J. Miserable minority: emotional risk factors that influence the outcome of a mild traumatic brain injury. *Brain Inj.* 1996;10(8):551–565.

REFERENCES

1. American Psychiatric Association. *Diagnostic and Statistical Manual of Mental Disorders, Fourth Edition.* Washington, DC: American Psychiatric Association; 1994.

2. World Health Organization. *International Statistical Classification of Diseases and Related Health Problems—10th Edition.* Geneva, Switzerland: World Health Organization; 1992.

3. McCrea MA. *Mild Traumatic Brain Injury and Postconcussion Syndrome: The New Evidence Base for Diagnosis and Treatment.* New York: Oxford University Press; 2008.

4. Iverson GL. Outcome from mild traumatic brain injury. *Curr Opin Psychiatry.* 2005;18(3):301–317.

5. Ruff RM, Camenzuli L, Mueller J. Miserable minority: emotional risk factors that influence the outcome of a mild traumatic brain injury. *Brain Inj.* 1996;10(8):551–565.

6. Ruff RM, Richardson AM. Mild traumatic brain injury. In: Sweet JJ, ed. *Forensic Neuropsychology: Fundamentals and Practice. Studies on Neuropsychology, Development and Cognition.* Bristol, UK: Swets & Seitinger; 1999:315–338.

7. Iverson GL, Zasler ND, Lange RT. Post-concussive disorder. In: Zasler ND, Katz DI, Zafonte RD, eds. *Brain Injury Medicine: Principles and Practice.* New York: Demos Medical Publishing; 2007:373–405.

8. Ferguson RJ, Mittenberg W. Cognitive-behavioral treatment of postconcussion syndrome. In: Van Hasselt VB, Hersen M, eds. *Sourcebook of Psychological Treatment Manuals for Adult Disorders.* New York: Plenum Press; 1996:615–655.

9. Miller LJ, Mittenberg W. Brief cognitive behavioral interventions in mild traumatic brain injury. *Appl Neuropsychol.* 1998;5(4):172–183.

10. Mittenberg W, Tremont G, Zielinski RE, Fichera S, Rayls KR. Cognitive-behavioral prevention of postconcussion syndrome. *Arch Clin Neuropsychol.* 1996;11(2):139–145.

11. Ponsford J, Willmott C, Rothwell A, et al. Impact of early intervention on outcome after mild traumatic brain injury in children. *Pediatrics.* 2001;108(6):1297–1303.

12. Ponsford J, Willmott C, Rothwell A, et al. Cognitive and behavioral outcome following mild traumatic head injury in children. *J Head Trauma Rehabil.* 1999;14(4):360–372.

13. Ponsford J, Willmott C, Rothwell A, et al. Impact of early intervention on outcome following mild head injury in adults. *J Neurol Neurosurg Psychiatry.* 2002;73(3):330–332.

14. Ponsford J, Willmott C, Rothwell A, et al. Factors influencing outcome following mild traumatic brain injury in adults. *J Int Neuropsychol Soc.* 2000;6(5):568–579.

15. Paniak C, Toller-Lobe G, Durand A, Nagy J. A randomized trial of two treatments for mild traumatic brain injury. *Brain Inj.* 1998;12(12):1011–1023.

16. Paniak C, Toller-Lobe G, Reynolds S, Melnyk A, Nagy J. A randomized trial of two treatments for mild traumatic brain injury: 1 year follow-up. *Brain Inj.* 2000;14(3):219–226.

17. Borg J, Holm L, Peloso PM, et al. Non-surgical intervention and cost for mild traumatic brain injury: results of the WHO Collaborating Centre Task Force on Mild Traumatic Brain Injury. *J Rehabil Med.* 2004(43 suppl):76–83.

18. Comper P, Bisschop SM, Carnide N, Tricco A. A systematic review of treatments for mild traumatic brain injury. *Brain Inj.* 2005;19(11):863–880.

PART 4

Moderate to Severe Traumatic Brain Injury

22

Field Management
Prehospital Care

Clare L. Hammell

GENERAL PRINCIPLES

Prehospital management is increasingly recognized as influencing outcome in moderate to severe traumatic brain injury (TBI). One-third of patients with severe TBI have a documented secondary brain insult on hospital admission [1].

Aims of Prehospital (Field) Care

It includes rapid scene and patient assessment, necessary interventions only, prevention of secondary brain injury, short scene time (ideally <10 to 15 minutes), rapid transfer to appropriate secondary care facility.

ASSESSMENT

- **Scene assessment**—the initial priority. Is the area safe for you to work in? Common prehospital hazards—motor vehicle instability, traffic, risk of fire/explosions from fuel, hazardous materials, and firearms risk. Assessing and managing the patient may occasionally have to wait until emergency services personnel make the scene safe.
- **Patient assessment**—limited patient access and space in which to work common. Initial assessment focused on identifying and managing life threatening injuries. Structured assessment required:
  - **Airway** (and cervical spine control)
  - **Breathing** (respiratory rate, pattern, obvious external chest injury, chest expansion, percussion, and auscultation often unhelpful because of surrounding noise)
  - **Circulation** (obvious external hemorrhage, peripheral pulses present, capillary refill time, blood pressure recording often not possible/unreliable)

- **Disability** (Glasgow Coma Score [GCS], pupil size and reactivity, seizures)

Work together with other rescue personnel to formulate extrication plan if patient is trapped in a vehicle. Time is of essence; outcome is improved with a shorter injury-definitive care time.

- **Common problems identified during patient assessment**—airway obstruction, hypoventilation, hypoxemia, hypo- or hypertension, and reduced conscious level. Extracranial-associated injuries are common; their management may take preference. Spinal injury should be assumed in all patients with moderate to severe head injury.

PATIENT MANAGEMENT

Airway Management

- Basic airway opening maneuvers including oropharyngeal airways. Supraglottic airways (e.g., laryngeal mask airways) are easy to insert if patient access is difficult and will free up rescuers hands. Such devices achieve faster time to ventilation than endotracheal tubes in models of restricted airway access [2].
- **Prehospital endotracheal intubation (ETI):** Indications (from International Brain Trauma Foundation [BTF])—TBI patients with a GCS < 8, the inability to maintain an adequate airway, hypoxemia not corrected by supplemental oxygen. Adequate skills and expertise must be available. Evidence for its benefit is conflicting; some studies have shown increased mortality with prehospital ETI [3,4], others have shown survival benefit [5]. All current published studies are retrospective, often with unmatched controls and most ETIs in the studies are performed without sedative drugs. This approach leads to raised intracranial pressure (ICP) with laryngoscopy and increased incidence of adverse events. Use of sedative agents and muscle relaxants (rapid sequence induction) improves success rates and may reduce complications. Expect a difficult airway (suboptimal patient positioning, blood/debris in mouth, difficult environment).
- **Checklist prior to prehospital ETI**—suitably experienced personnel, airway equipment working (+ spare laryngoscope), alternative airways, for example, supraglottic/oropharyngeal, cricothyroidotomy kit, self inflating bag and mask, monitoring including pulse oximetry/capnography, drugs (sedatives, muscle relaxants, vasopressors, anticholinergics).
- **Complications of prehospital ETI**—failure (must have back up plan), esophageal intubation (fatal if unrecognized), hypoxemia, aspiration of gastric contents, hypo- or hypertension. Ensure adequate sedation and muscle relaxation postintubation to avoid coughing and rises in ICP.

Ventilation

- Hypoxemia increases mortality and the chance of a poorer neurological outcome following TBI [6]. It may result from hypoventilation but significant chest injuries often coexist, for example, hemopneumothorax/pulmonary contusions.
- All self ventilating patients should receive oxygen via facemask with a reservoir bag.
- Assisted ventilation is required in all patients post-ETI; it may also be required in unintubated patients with respiratory depression. Normal ventilation rate in adults is 12 breaths per minute. Inadvertent hyperventilation and hypocapnia is common in intubated patients; this is associated with a poorer neurological outcome and should be avoided. End tidal carbon dioxide monitoring helps prevent this.

Circulatory Management

- One single episode of hypotension doubles the risk of mortality in severe TBI patients [6].
- Assume that hypotension is due to hypovolemia from coexisting injuries initially.
- Cerebral perfusion pressure (CPP) = mean arterial pressure (MAP) – ICP. So if ICP is increased (common in moderate/severe TBI), MAP must be increased to maintain CPP.
- In-hospital management usually aims for CPP 60 to 70 mm Hg; there is no evidence to suggest what level to aim for in prehospital environment. Impractical to calculate MAP and blood pressure measurement may also be difficult and unreliable outdoors or in moving vehicle.
- In isolated TBI, BTF recommend a minimum systolic blood pressure of 90 mm Hg. Higher values are desirable if ICP is raised in order to maintain CPP.
- Small boluses (e.g., 250 mL) of isotonic crystalloid fluid should be administered to maintain target systolic blood pressure. Use of vasopressors are impractical in the field.
- There is increasing interest in use of hypertonic fluids in this group for fluid resuscitation. Subgroup analysis of a TBI group receiving hypertonic saline (HTS) for volume restoration showed a mortality benefit [7].

Neurological assessment should be brief and reproducible. GCS, pupil size, and reactivity are used. It is often poorly recorded at scene but is useful (and prognostic) to compare on-scene and admission GCS.

Raised ICP

- Assess periodically for signs of raised ICP at scene and during transfer (reducing GCS, pupil dilatation and reduced reactivity, increasing systemic hypertension with reflex bradycardia). Possible treatments at scene or during transport include:

- Addressing hypoxemia, hypotension, hypercapnia, and inadequate sedation (in intubated patients) first
- 30-degree head up tilt of spinal board
- Pharmacological strategies—include osmotic diuretics (mannitol) and hypertonic crystalloid solutions
- **Mannitol**—previously the first line osmotic drug for management of raised ICP (HTS largely replacing; see following section). There exists little data regarding prehospital administration. Produces a dieresis that may provoke hypotension if patient is hypovolemic
- **HTS**—reduces ICP reliably in animal and human studies. Also survival benefit in bleeding head-injured patients has been demonstrated [7]. The largest randomized study of the use of HTS (HTS vs. Ringer's lactate) prehospitally [8] failed to repeat this survival finding although the HTS group had lower ICP and higher CPP measurements on hospital admission. In hypovolemic patients, it augments volume resuscitation by increasing circulating blood volume, MAP, and CPP. Usual solutions are 3% to 7.5% sodium chloride. Initial dose of 3 to 4 mL/kg; repeat dose is occasionally needed. Reported side effects (hypernatremia, increased osmolality) of no importance in prehospital environment.

Spinal Immobilization

All head-injured patients require spinal immobilization except if very combative. Hard cervical collar and long spinal board usually. Beware of cervical collars obstructing cerebral venous return and raising ICP. If signs of raised ICP are present, tilt the head of the board to 30° to facilitate venous drainage. Aim for early removal of long boards and cervical collars in the emergency department.

Transfer to Secondary Care Facility

Must have neuroimaging and ideally neurosurgery on site. A recent retrospective analysis of patients with severe TBI showed reduced mortality if they were managed in centers with onsite neurosurgical expertise [9]. Air transport may be required if there are long transfer distances.

ADDITIONAL READING

Electronic Reference

Brain Trauma Foundation website. http://tbiguidelines.org/glHome.aspx?gl=2

Journal Articles

Badjadata M, Carney, Crocooc TJ, et al. Guidelines for prehospital management of traumatic brain injury, 2nd edition (Brain Trauma Foundation). *Prehosp Emerg Care.* 2008;12 suppl:S1–S5.

Hammell CL, Henning JD. Prehospital management of severe traumatic brain injury: a clinical review. *BMJ.* 2009;338:b1683.

Parr M. Prehospital airway management for severe brain injury. *Resuscitation.* 2008;76(3):321–322.

Stahil PF, Smith WR, Moore EE. Hypoxia and hypotension, the 'lethal duo' in traumatic brain injury: implications for prehospital care. *Intensive Care Med.* 2008;34(3):402–404.

REFERENCES

1. Myburgh JA, Cooper DJ, Finfer SR, et al. Epidemiology and 12-month outcomes from traumatic brain injury in Australia and New Zealand. *J Trauma.* 2008;64(4):854–862.

2. Hoyle JD Jr, Jones JS, Deibel M, Lock DT, Reischman D. Comparative study of airway management techniques with restricted access to patient airway. *Prehosp Emerg Care.* 2007;11(3):330–336.

3. Davis DP, Peay J, Sise MJ, et al. The impact of prehospital endotracheal intubation on outcome in moderate to severe traumatic brain injury. *J Trauma.* 2005;58(5):933–939.

4. Wang HE, Peitzman AB, Cassidy LD, Adelson PD, Yealy DM. Out-of-hospital endotracheal intubation and outcome after traumatic brain injury. *Ann Emerg Med.* 2004;44(5):439–450.

5. Winchell RJ, Hoyt DB. Endotracheal intubation in the field improves survival in patients with severe head injury. Trauma Research and Education Foundation of San Diego. *Arch Surg.* 1997;132(6):592–597.

6. Chesnut RM, Marshall LF, Klauber MR, et al. The role of secondary brain injury in determining outcome from severe head injury. *J Trauma.* 1993;34(2):216–222.

7. Vassar MJ, Perry CA, Gannaway WL, Holcroft JW. 7.5% sodium chloride/dextran for resuscitation of trauma patients undergoing helicopter transport. *Arch Surg.* 1991;126(9):1065–1072.

8. Cooper DJ, Myles PS, McDermott FT, et al. Prehospital hypertonic saline resuscitation of patients with hypotension and severe traumatic brain injury: a randomized controlled trial. *JAMA.* 2004;291(11):1350–1357.

9. Patcl HC, Bouamra O, Woodford M, King AT, Yates DW, Lecky FE. Trends in head injury outcome from 1989 to 2003 and the effect of neurosurgical care: an observational study. *Lancet.* 2005;366(9496):1538–1544.

23

Emergency Department Management and Initial Trauma Care Considerations

Stephen V. Cantrill

GENERAL PRINCIPLES

Classification

Traumatic brain injury (TBI) is usually initially classified as to severity (mild, moderate, severe) based on Glasgow Coma Scale (GCS) score, mechanism (blunt, penetrating), and whether it is isolated head trauma, or one of multiple injuries the trauma patient has sustained (multiple trauma patient; see also Chapter 1).

Pathophysiology (see also Chapters 2, 25, and 26)

The following aspects of potential secondary injury must be identified rapidly in the emergency department, and appropriate interventions should be initiated.

- Elevated intracranial pressure (ICP) is often seen in severe head injury and, if untreated, can cause significant secondary brain injury through reduction of cerebral perfusion pressure (CPP). Elevation in the ICP can be due to mass lesions (e.g., hemorrhage) or cerebral edema. Sudden severe increases in the ICP can result in the Cushing reflex—widened pulse pressure (systolic blood pressure minus diastolic), irregular respirations, and bradycardia.
- Brain swelling can be the result of brain hyperemia or an increase in brain intracellular water, that is, cerebral edema.
- Cerebral herniation may occur because of brain swelling or an expanding mass lesion. This requires immediate action if the patient is to survive.

INITIAL EVALUATION AND TREATMENT

Guiding Principles

- The initial resuscitation of the moderate to severely head-injured patient represents one of the most significant challenges in medicine. Very frequently these patients suffer from multiple injuries requiring the concerted efforts of the entire trauma team—the emergency physician, the neurosurgeon, the trauma surgeon, and the orthopedist, as well as nursing and ancillary staff. This is truly a team effort, with evaluation, diagnosis, and treatment being performed simultaneously in a very tight feedback loop.

- Any head trauma patient must have their initial resuscitation guided by the principles of advanced trauma life support (ATLS) [1]. This will include, if necessary, immediate endotracheal intubation, fluid resuscitation, oxygenation, and sedation. The goal is to stabilize the patient to the point that a head computed tomography (CT) scan may be performed to

  - diagnose the nature of the head trauma and
  - identify any neurosurgically correctable lesions [2,3]

Clinical Presentation

The mechanism of the patient's injury should be obtained from the patient (if possible) or from bystanders or prehospital care providers. In patients with blunt trauma, a cervical spine injury must be assumed until disproved.

Symptoms

Mental status is of major concern. Any change in mental status, including the duration of any loss of consciousness, should be identified. Symptoms of headache, vertigo, nausea, vomiting, weakness, ataxia, or other neurological symptoms should be sought. History of recent drug or alcohol use should be obtained in addition to past medical history and current medications (with special attention to any anticoagulation medications).

Physical Examination

- The cornerstone of the physical examination is the GCS (see Table 1.1), although the initial values can be influenced by non–head injury issues (such as alcohol intoxication, which in extreme conditions can result in a GCS of 3). The use of the GCS may be problematic in non–English speaking patients and in children. Orthopedic and spinal cord injuries may also interfere with its application.

- Pupil size, symmetry, and responsiveness should be assessed.
- A motor examination should be performed with evaluation of strength and symmetry of the major muscle groups. Any abnormal movements should be noted, especially decorticate or decerebrate posturing.
- Cranial nerve function (II-XII) should be evaluated, to the extent possible. In the severe head-injured patient, this may be limited.
- Deep tendon reflexes should be assessed with any asymmetry noted.
- The head and neck should be carefully inspected for any evidence of trauma with special attention to the ears (hemotympanum or otorrhea), the nose (rhinorrhea), Battle's sign (retroauricular hematoma), or raccoon's eyes (periorbital ecchymoses), all indicators of a potential basilar skull fracture.
- The remainder of the physical examination should be performed based upon the mechanism of injury and any other findings.
- Any decrease in a patient's mental status or GCS after arrival must be assumed to indicate a worsening of their head injury and must drive an immediate therapeutic response.

Diagnostic Evaluation

The gold standard for initial diagnostic evaluation of the moderate to severely head-injured patient is a rapid noncontrast CT scan of the head. If the history is unclear in the comatose patient, it is prudent to quickly evaluate the patient for hypoglycemia (via point-of-care glucometer) before obtaining the CT.

Laboratory Studies

In the severe TBI patient, an ethanol level, toxicology screen, complete blood count, basic metabolic panel (electrolytes, glucose), and coagulation studies are indicated.

Initial Management

- In the severely brain-injured patient, airway protection via rapid sequence intubation should be given serious consideration. This not only serves to protect the airway, but avoids hypoxia [4]. If at all possible, the neurologic examination should be performed prior to the administration of drugs for intubation.
- Any presence of systemic hypotension is cause for concern in the TBI patient. This mandates a search for the cause of the hypotension and treatment of the hypotension with crystalloid or blood products

(if indicated). Untreated hypotension portends a worse neurological outcome for any TBI patient [4].

- In patients who deteriorate after their initial evaluation, their worsening condition may be temporarily stabilized by hyperventilation [5]. Decreasing the patient's Pco_2 to 30 mm Hg will cause a temporary decrease in the (elevated) ICP through cerebral vasoconstriction with subsequent decrease in cerebral blood flow. This should be done only for a brief period of time, because an undesirable side-effect of this action is further cerebral ischemia with increased secondary brain injury.

- In the most severe TBI patients, or in those who are deteriorating, treatment with an osmotic diuretic, usually mannitol 0.25 to 1 g/kg IV may improve the patient's condition through the reduction of cerebral edema [6]. These patients may also benefit from the induction of a barbiturate coma to reduce the metabolic demands of the brain [7].

- Severely brain-injured patients may benefit from treatment with antiseizure medication such as phenytoin or fosphenytoin. This decreases the incidence of seizures in the immediate postinjury period [8].

Treatment Controversies

- The use of hypertonic saline solution to assist in the treatment of cerebral edema has been studied and does show some initial promise, but further studies are necessary to determine optimal administration dosage and concentration [6].

- Prophylactic hypothermia has undergone some study with pooled data showing decreased mortality, but many of these studies have serious flaws including small sample sizes. Further work is needed in this area [9].

ADDITIONAL READING

Electronic References

Brain Trauma Foundation. http://tbiguidelines.org/glHome.aspx
Review of use of hypothermia. http://www.medscape.com/viewarticle/585192

Textbook/Chapter

Heegard WG, Biros MH. System injuries: head. In: Marx J, Hockberger R, Walls R, eds. *Rosen's Emergency Medicine: Concepts and Clinical Practice.* 7th ed. St Louis, MO: Mosby; 2009:349–382.

Journal Articles

Brain Trauma Foundation. Guidelines for the management of severe traumatic brain injury, 3rd edition. *J Neurotrauma.* 2007;24(suppl 1).

Muizelaar JP, Marmarou A, Ward JD, et al. Adverse effects of prolonged hyperventilation in patients with severe head injury: a randomized clinical trial. *J Neurosurg*. 1991;75(5):731–739.

REFERENCES

1. American Medical Association. *Advanced Trauma Life Support*. 8th ed. Chicago, IL; 2008.
2. Jagoda AS, Bazarian JJ, Bruns JJ Jr, et al.; American College of Emergency Physicians; Centers for Disease Control and Prevention. Clinical policy: neuroimaging and decisionmaking in adult mild traumatic brain injury in the acute setting. *Ann Emerg Med*. 2008;52(6):714–748.
3. Shackford SR, Wald SL, Ross SE, et al. The clinical utility of computed tomographic scanning and neurologic examination in the management of patients with minor head injuries. *J Trauma*. 1992;33(3):385–394.
4. Brain Trauma Foundation. Guidelines for the management of severe traumatic brain injury. I. Blood pressure and oxygenation, 3rd edition. *J Neurotrauma*. 2007;24(suppl 1):S7–S13.
5. Brain Trauma Foundation. Guidelines for the management of severe traumatic brain injury. XIV. Hyperventilation, 3rd edition. *J Neurotrauma*. 2007;24(suppl 1):S87–S90.
6. Brain Trauma Foundation. Guidelines for the management of severe traumatic brain injury. II. Hyperosmolar therapy, 3rd edition. *J Neurotrauma*. 2007;24(suppl 1):S14–S20.
7. Brain Trauma Foundation. Guidelines for the management of severe traumatic brain injury. XI. Anesthetics, analgesics and sedatives, 3rd edition. *J Neurotrauma*. 2007;24(suppl 1):S71–S76.
8. Brain Trauma Foundation. Guidelines for the management of severe traumatic brain injury. XIII. Antiseizure prophylaxis, 3rd edition. *J Neurotrauma*. 2007;24(suppl 1):S83–S86.
9. Brain Trauma Foundation. Guidelines for the management of severe traumatic brain injury. III. Prophylactic hypothermia, 3rd edition. *J Neurotrauma*. 2007;24(suppl 1):S21–S25.

24

Imaging in Moderate to Severe Traumatic Brain Injury

David N. Alexander

BACKGROUND: IMAGING TECHNIQUES

The two most commonly used imaging procedures in traumatic brain injury (TBI) are computerized tomography (CT) of the brain and magnetic resonance imaging (MRI or MR) of the brain. Less commonly used imaging procedures that are helpful in selected patients with brain injury for specific purposes include lateral and AP (anteroposterior) skull x-rays (SXRs), cerebral angiography, CT angiography (CTa), magnetic resonance angiography (MRA), magnetic resonance venography (MRV), single photon emission computerized tomography (SPECT) and positron emission tomography (PET), diffusion tensor imaging (DTI), and functional MR imaging (fMRI). Each of these techniques has its own principles, benefits, and limitations. They have been employed in some settings and will be briefly described; however, the primary focus of this chapter is CT and MR.

Computerized Tomography

CT measures the density of structures in the brain displayed in two-dimensional slices that vary in thickness from 2 mm to 1 cm. CT is the initial imaging procedure of choice in acute moderate to severe TBI. CT is readily available, with rapid scanning time, and has excellent imaging of acute blood, fractures, foreign bodies, and hemorrhagic contusion.

High-density structures, such as bone and acute blood, appear white on CT, whereas low-density structures, such as air or cerebrospinal fluid (CSF), appear dark. The white matter of the brain is slightly less dense than gray matter; so white matter is darker than gray matter on CT imaging. Edema reduces the density of the brain, making it appear darker. So density, and therefore whiteness on the scan, is as follows: bone > acute blood > gray matter > white matter > CSF > air. One can choose to view a specific range or a subset of the data obtained; so it is called "windowing." Generally, the CT scan is windowed to visualize brain matter best; a second set of images are windowed to highlight bone densities ("bone windows") to allow better visualization of fractures.

Magnetic Resonance Imaging

MRI is the best single test for assessing injury to the brain in moderate and severe TBI in the subacute or chronic phase after TBI. Its advantages over CT in the subacute phase include excellent imaging of the posterior fossa, assessment of axonal injury, and visualization of cortical and subcortical nonhemorrhagic contusions and edema. The signal characteristics of hematomas on MRI are highly variable. The appearance is greatly influenced by the state of hemoglobin (ferrous vs. ferric), the field strength of the magnet, the pulse sequence used, the status of the RBCs (intact vs. lysed), the age of the clot, the hematocrit, state of oxygenation, and size of the clot.

MR requires a longer scan time than CT, and becomes less useful for agitated patients or patients who cannot remain still during the test. MR is not useful for bone imaging or for fractures. MR cannot be used in patients with pacemakers, or a variety of other metallic implants. When there is concern for venous sinus injury, MRV provides excellent imaging of the sinuses.

MR is an imaging procedure without ionizing radiation. The basic principle of MRI is the imaging of proton magnetism. Protons, a component of water, are ubiquitous in the body and brain. The magnetic field lines up the charged protons like little magnets, then the magnetic field is removed or perturbed. Sequences of perturbation and data acquisition determine imaging characteristics:

- T1-weighted images show the general structure of the brain.
- T2-weighted and FLAIR (fluid attenuation inversion recovery) images show white matter changes.
- DWI (diffusion weighted imaging) is sensitive to early swelling of cells in ischemic infarction, and may show injured neurons and glia in TBI.
- GRE (gradient recalled echo) sequences are very sensitive to blood products, which show up as dark areas.

Skull X-Rays

Historically, SXRs were the initial neuroradiologic procedures. Conventional radiographs were used as early as the Spanish-American War to evaluate the cranial vault for depressed fractures and for localizing radiopaque materials. SXRs have been supplanted by CT scan, although a modified lateral SXR is generally obtained as a "scout film" in preparation for the CT.

Angiography

Angiography defines the intra- and extracranial circulation to the brain. Catheter cerebral angiogram is the definitive test for visualization of the vasculature, but is invasive and uncommonly used in TBI unless an underlying aneurysm or arteriovenous malformation (AVM) is suspected. Noninvasive tests such as CTa are very good for visualizing these same structures. If venous thrombosis is suspected, MRV is a useful and sensitive test.

Single Photon Emission Computerized Tomography

SPECT is a nuclear medicine tomographic imaging technique using γ rays and a γ camera. A common γ-emitting isotope used in SPECT, 99mTc-HMPAO (technetium 99m-hexamethylpropylene amine oxime), is useful in the detection of regional cerebral blood flow. SPECT is uncommonly used in TBI and its clinical value is limited.

Positron Emission Tomography

PET utilizes positron-emitting radiopharmaceuticals to map the physiology, biochemistry, and hemodynamics of the brain. 2-Deoxy-2-[18F]fluoro-D-Glucose (FDG) is the most common radiopharmaceutical used in PET to measure regional glucose metabolism in the brain. A variety of other substrates and radiolabeled compounds can be injected and a cross-sectional map of the brain shows the quantitative distribution, utilization, or binding of these substrates in the brain. The radiation exposure from a PET scan is about the same as a CT. The clinical value of PET in TBI is under investigation.

Diffusion Tensor Weighted Imaging

DTI measures the diffusion of water molecules and their vectors/direction along white matter tracts, using MR techniques. Disruption of white matter tracts, as is typically seen in the context of diffuse axonal injury (DAI), is more dramatically visualized with DTI. Further research is needed to establish the clinical utility of this test [1].

Functional MR Imaging

fMRI measures changes in blood oxygenation levels in specific volumes (voxels) of the brain. The brain rapidly changes its blood flow/oxygen delivery to parts of the brain as they become metabolically more or less active. Recent reports in a small minority of patients with severe brain injury and in a minimally conscious state or vegetative state have shown metabolic patterns that indicate consciousness using fMRI to measure response to questions/commands [2].

PATHOLOGY: IMAGING APPEARANCE OF TBI

The pathologic changes typically associated with moderate to severe closed head injury include DAI, intra- and extra-axial hemorrhages, focal cortical contusions (FCC), and hypoxic-ischemic injury (HII). Open or penetrating head injury leads to direct disruption of brain parenchyma. Other phenomena include skull fractures and diffuse brain swelling. The main mechanical phenomena causing brain damage are that of contact and acceleration.

Extracerebral Hemorrhagic Lesions

Subdural Hematoma
Subdural hematomas (SDHs) are common in severe head injury, occurring in 20% of cases in one large series [3]. SDHs are generally seen unilaterally over the frontal and parietal convexities. They appear as crescent-shaped, high-density extra-axial fluid collections. They can be isodense during the subacute phase, generally at 3 weeks. At that time, they are seen on CT as a displacement of the gray and white matter interface or displacement of surface veins during contrast administration.

MRI easily identifies the isodense subacute phase of SDHs: they are bright on T1, particularly on coronal images. MRI also improves visualization of SDHs that are bilateral, small, interhemispheric, subtemporal, subfrontal, or tentorial (Figure 24.1).

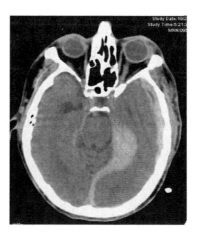

Figure 24.1 Patient with TBI and a left temporal and left tentorial subdural hematoma.

Epidural Hematoma

Epidural hematomas (EDHs) occur as a result of an injury to the middle meningeal artery or, occasionally, the dural venous sinuses. The arterial bleeding strips away the dura, which is normally tightly adherent to the inner table of the skull. EDHs are generally small, biconvex or lens-shaped, high-density extra-axial masses with sharp anterior and posterior margins because of their firm dural attachments (Figure 24.2). Two-thirds of the time they occur over the temporal or parietal region. Less commonly, they occur in the frontal or occipital region. Any extra-axial high-density mass lesion crossing the midline and depressing the superior sagittal sinus is an EDH; SDHs would not cross the midline but will track along the falx or tentorium.

The vascular origin of EDH is (1) middle meningeal artery (50%); (2) meningeal vein (30%); and (3) laceration of dural venous sinuses, diploic veins, and internal carotid artery (20%).

Subarachnoid Hemorrhage

Traumatic subarachnoid hemorrhage (SAH) is a common finding in TBI, occurring in up to 40% of patients [3]. Traumatic SAH can be seen as a subtle increased density along the falx, a feathery appearance due to blood in the sulci over the convexity or in the interpeduncular fossa, particularly with the patient lying supine during scanning procedures. Intraventricular hemorrhage can also occur (the subarachnoid and intraventricular space are contiguous), and may be seen as an accumulation of blood in the occipital horns of the lateral ventricles.

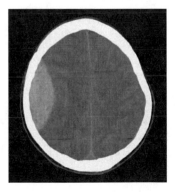

Figure 24.2 Epidural hematoma. This midconvexity, high-density biconvex lens–shaped appearance indicates an acute extradural hemorrhage, possibly because of laceration of the middle meningeal artery.

Intracerebral Nonhemorrhagic Lesions

Parenchymal Contusions
(see also "Intracerebral Hemorrhagic Lesions")

Parenchymal contusion is focal bruising that occurs most commonly along the inferior, lateral, and anterior aspects of the frontal and temporal lobes (Figure 24.3). The irregular bony contours of the floor of the anterior and middle cranial fossae predispose to this focal injury. Both CT and MR visualize hemorrhagic contusion well; however, MR imaging is superior to CT in visualizing nonhemorrhagic contusion.

Edema

Brain edema is divided into vasogenic edema and cytotoxic edema; both mechanisms are seen in TBI. Vasogenic edema is best visualized on MR, with fingers of edema following white matter tracts. Cytotoxic edema, protypically caused by dying neurons and glia because of hypoxic or ischemic injury, can result in generalized brain edema and herniation (Figure 24.4).

Hypoxic-Ischemic Injury

TBI is often associated with hypoperfusion of the brain. Areas of the brain particularly sensitive to hypoxic injury include the hippocampus CA1 pyramidal cells (crucial for memory acquisition), layers 3, 5, and 6 of the cerebral cortex, and Purkinje cells in the cerebellum and striatal neurons. Hypoperfusion may affect watershed areas in the cortex. HII recovers less well than traumatic axonal injury because of the necrosis of large numbers of cortical neurons. CT is insensitive to hypoxic injury, but

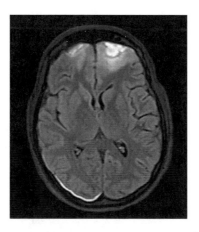

Figure 24.3 T1-weighted MR image of bifrontal contusions and a right posterior thin subdural hematoma in a 31-year-old woman who fell off a skateboard 4 months prior to this scan, now presenting with seizures.

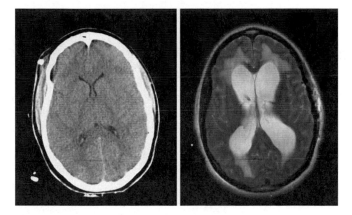

Figure 24.4 TBI in a teenager because of an MVA, initially presenting with mild cerebral edema and small ventricles. Three months post injury, this same patient has ventricular dilatation due to shunt failure combined with atrophy from neuronal and glial loss.

may show watershed infarctions. MR is relatively insensitive to HII but may show subtle changes including bright cortical signal on T1 (indicating cortical laminar necrosis) [4].

Intracerebral Hemorrhagic Lesions

Parenchymal Contusions
Hemorrhagic focal cortical contusion is seen on CT scan as a mottled area of high density, reflecting the petechial bleeding associated with capillary rupture. Contusions appear as inhomogeneous areas of high and low density because of the mixture of blood and edema, varying from minimal focal edema to scattered high-density foci with massive edema. Over time, these gradually resolve to become areas of low density.

Tissue Tear Hemorrhages
TTHs frequently are associated with DAI, and also called "microhemorrhages." These tend to occur in the periventricular white matter, the corpus callosum, and the brainstem [5]. They can be seen most sensitively on higher field strength magnets using GRE (T2*-weighted) or susceptibility weighted imaging (SWI) [6].

Intraparenchymal Hematomas
Traumatic intraparenchymal hematomas can occur in any region of the brain, including the basal ganglia and the internal capsule.

Diffuse Axonal Injury

DAI is a frequent underlying pathology in TBI. The initial pathology of DAI consists of retraction balls with severed, broken, and swollen axons. The axonal or white matter shearing injuries are better evaluated on MR imaging than CT. Nevertheless, the shearing may cause tissue tear hemorrhages (TTH), which can be seen on CT scan. DAI can occur from the level of the gray-white matter junction down to the deep white matter and brainstem structures (Figure 24.5). With more severe injuries, the force tends to be transmitted to the deep middle portion of the brain, with particular involvement of the corpus callosum, dorsal lateral midbrain, white matter at the gray-white junction, and cerebellar white matter near the dentate nucleus.

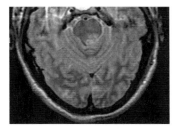

Figure 24.5 Dorsolateral pontomesencephalic axonal injury in a TBI patient with DAI and right frontal contusion.

Extracerebral Lesions

Skull Fractures

CT scanning with bone windowing is needed for an evaluation of suspected fracture. MRI is insensitive and does not visualize fracture. Basilar skull fractures are not well visualized unless the CT is viewed with bone windows. If the clinical situation suggests a basilar skull fracture, with hemotympanum (blood behind the ear drum), Battle's sign (purplish bruising and ecchymosis in the mastoid region), or leakage from the ear, then a CT scan with bone windows is needed despite a negative SXR.

Cervical Spine Injury

Cervical spine films at the onset of head injury are important because of the 6% co-occurrence of cervical spine injury in TBI patients. The digital lateral skull radiograph obtained during CT scan of the head as a scout film should be reviewed, because it may include a portion of the cervical spine to look for cervical spine pathology.

SUMMARY

CT and MR are the mainstays of imaging in TBI. Newer procedures, in addition to identifying anatomic lesions, show changes in metabolism and white matter tract dysfunction in TBI, although they are not in routine clinical use.

ADDITIONAL READING

Electronic References

Chesnut RM, Carney N, Maynard H, et al. Rehabilitation for traumatic brain injury: evidence report/technology assessment no. 2. Rockville, MD: Agency for Health Care Policy and Research; 1999. Available at http://www.ncbi. nlm.nih.gov/bookshelf/br.fcgi?book=hserta&part=A1280#A2176

Imaging of TBI: A Review of Recent Medical Literature: http://www.ncbi.nlm. nih.gov/bookshelf/br.fcgi?book=hserta&part=A1280#A2176

Textbook/Chapter

Robert D. CT and MRI. In: Lewis PR, Pedley TA, eds. *Merritt's Neurology*. 12th ed. Philadelphia, PA: Lippincott Williams & Wilkins; 2010:62–73.

Journal Articles

Le TH, Gean AD. Neuroimaging of traumatic brain injury. *Mt Sinai J Med.* 2009;76(2):145–162.

Park HK, Joo WI, Choung CK, et al. The clinical efficacy of repeat brain computed tomography in patients with traumatic intracranial haemorrhage within 24 hours after blunt head injury. *Br J Neurosurg.*2009;23(6):617–621.

Suskauer SJ, Huisman TM. Neuroimaging in pediatric traumatic brain injury: current and future predictors of functional outcome. *Dev Disabil Res Rev.* 2009;15(2):117–123.

REFERENCES

1. Sidaros A, Engberg AW, Sidaros K, et al. Diffusion tensor imaging during recovery from severe traumatic brain injury and relation to clinical outcome: a longitudinal study. *Brain*. 2008;131(Pt 2):559–572.

2. Monti MM, Vanhaudenhuyse A, Coleman MR, et al. Willful modulation of brain activity in disorders of consciousness. *N Engl J Med.* 2010;362(7):579–589.

3. Eisenberg HM, Gary HE Jr, Aldrich EF, et al. Initial CT findings in 753 patients with severe head injury. A report from the NIH Traumatic Coma Data Bank. *J Neurosurg.* 1990;73(5):688–698.

4. Siskas N, Lefkopoulos A, Ioannidis I, Charitandi A, Dimitriadis AS. Cortical laminar necrosis in brain infarcts: serial MRI. *Neuroradiology.* 2003;45(5):283–288.

5. Wilberger JE Jr, Rothfus WE, Tabas J, Goldberg AL, Deeb ZL. Acute tissue tear hemorrhages of the brain: computed tomography and clinicopathological correlations. *Neurosurgery.* 1990;27(2):208–213.

6. Provenzale JM. Imaging of traumatic brain injury: a review of the recent medical literature. *AJR Am J Roentgenol.* 2010;194(1):16–19.

25

Neurosurgical Management of Skull Fractures and Intracranial Hemorrhage

Joshua M. Rosenow

SKULL FRACTURES

Epidemiology

- There are more than 1.5 million head injuries in the United States annually, with approximately one-third sustaining a skull fracture from the injury [1].

Characteristics Used to Describe Skull Fractures

- Pattern
  - Linear—a simple, straight single fracture line
  - Complex or comminuted—multiple intersecting or radiating fracture lines
  - Nondisplaced—the fractured sections of skull are separated by the fracture line but still aligned
  - Displaced—the fractured sections of skull are misaligned by a variable distance
- Scalp integrity
  - Closed—there is no connection between the fracture and the atmosphere
  - Open—the scalp overlying the fracture has been lacerated to such an extent as to expose the fracture to the atmosphere
- Diastatic—the fracture traverses and separates one of the cranial sutures
- Skull base fracture—involves the bones of the skull base, rather than the cranial vault. These bones include the sphenoid, temporal, and occipital bones, as well as the clivus and orbital roof
- Open depressed fractures expose the patient to an increased risk of intracranial infection and cerebrospinal fluid (CSF) leak due to the

chance of a dural tear caused by the depressed fragment. This results in a communication between the intradural space and the atmosphere

Etiology and Pathophysiology

- Blunt trauma is the most common etiology. The topography of the fracture is dependent on the force of the injury and the surface against which the skull strikes. Striking the skull against a smaller surface increases the force per unit area, thus increasing the chance of a complex and/or depressed skull fracture.

Evaluation

Clinical Presentation

- Asymptomatic—This is the most common presentation of a skull fracture, especially closed, linear, nondisplaced fractures.
- Arterial epidural hemorrhage—Fracture lines may cross the paths of major dural arteries such as the middle meningeal artery (MMA). This causes epidural arterial hemorrhage that may rapidly expand and cause significant neurologic deficit. Evacuation of the hemorrhage and coagulation of the bleeding point is often indicated.
- Venous epidural hemorrhage—Fracture lines may cross the paths of major venous sinuses, such as the transverse sinus or superior sagittal sinus. These are high-flow dural spaces; sinus lacerations can result in substantial hemorrhage. Occipital fractures that cross the transverse sinus can result in epidural hemorrhage in the posterior fossa.
- Carotid injury—The energy from trauma that causes fractures can also lead to injury of intracranial vessels. For example, fractures of the temporal bone that extend across the carotid canal or clival fractures involving the cavernous sinus may lead to carotid dissection and pseudoaneurysm formation [2]. Carotid-cavernous fistulas may also be formed.
- Cranial nerve (CN) deficits—Basal skull fractures crossing the course of cranial nerves may lead to specific deficits as follows:
  - Olfactory nerve (CN I) injury—Although the olfactory nerve may be injured simply by shear injury without a concomitant skull fracture, disruption of the cribriform plate will also result in loss of olfaction because of shearing off of the olfactory processes that extend through the anterior skull base into the upper nasal cavity
  - Optic nerve (CN II) injury—anterior skull base and orbital fractures. Clival fractures may result in midline optic chiasm injury causing bitemporal hemianopia
  - Oculomotor nerve (CN III) injury—skull base fractures across the cavernous sinus

- Abducens nerve (CN VI) injury—clival fractures
- Facial nerve (CN VII), auditory nerve (CN VIII)—peripheral-pattern facial weakness, dry eye, and hearing loss—temporal bone fractures
- CSF leak
  - CSF rhinorrhea—anterior skull base pathology such as fractures of the cribriform plate or frontal sinus with associated dural tear
  - CSF otorrhea—temporal bone fracture and overlying dural tear leading to CSF egress via ear or eustachian tube
  - CSF leakage may lead to the development of meningitis [3]
- Open fractures may present with obvious signs of displaced/protruding skull pieces with or without CSF leakage.
- Encephalocele—If the fracture defect is large enough and there is an adjacent or associated dural tear, a portion of the brain may herniate through the defects. This may be associated with CSF leakage.
  - Anterior skull base—encephaloceles may involve the orbit or ethmoid sinuses
  - Temporal bone—brain may protrude into the mastoid air cells
- External signs of hemorrhage
  - Battle's sign (ecchymosis in the mastoid region) or hemotympanum because of temporal bone fracture
  - Raccoon eyes—periorbital ecchymosis due to anterior skull base fracture

Radiographic Evaluation
- X-rays—These identify fractures very well, but have been largely replaced by computed tomography (CT) scan [4].
- CT scan—Best, most rapid study to define the morphology of a skull fracture, its relationship to the underlying brain and venous sinuses, and to evaluate for associated hemorrhage.

Specific Circumstances Requiring Special Evaluation
- Fractures across venous sinuses—CT venography may be considered if concern for sinus occlusion is present.
- Fractures through the carotid canal or midline sphenoid bone (cavernous carotid)—CT angiography is useful for identifying vascular dissection.
- "Growing skull fractures" in children [5–7]—Otherwise known as posttraumatic leptomeningeal cysts. These are seen in fewer than 1% of pediatric skull fractures and present as an enlarging scalp mass. They result from a dural tear that allows the arachnoid to progressively herniate through the fracture defect. Secure dural closure is required.

Management

- Simple linear fractures—These are managed conservatively.
- Indications for surgery—open depressed and depressed fractures:
  - Depression greater than the thickness of the skull
  - Open depressed fracture
  - Obvious CSF leakage
  - Neurologic deficit due to cerebral compression from fractured segment
  - Frontal sinus fractures with displacement of the inner table and/or fractures of both the inner and outer tables may be considered for cranialization of the sinus with exenteration of sinus contents and packing of the frontonasal ducts. This is done to prevent the development of a mucocele with epidural extension and resulting abscess.
- Special cases
  - Fractures across venous sinuses—Bleeding from venous sinus lacerations can be especially significant and difficult to control. Unless there is a critical reason to intervene, such as open fracture with CSF leakage, neurologic deficit from sinus obstruction or brain compression, or active sinus hemorrhage, consideration may be given to deferring elevation of the fracture segment.
  - Tension pneumocephalus—Increasing pneumocephalus due to progressive air trapping (often from anterior skull base fractures extending into the nasal sinuses) may cause increased intracranial pressure (ICP) requiring operative intervention.
  - Anterior skull base fractures—Avoid passing nasogastric tubes in these patients because of the risk that the tube will pass intracranially through a fractured skull base.

INTRACRANIAL HEMORRHAGE

Epidemiology

- In a survey of 90,250 hospitalized patients with brain injury [8], 30.6% had traumatic intracranial hemorrhage.
- Types of hemorrhage included: subarachnoid—47.9%, subdural—40.6%, epidural—17.5%, intracerebral—14.0%, and intraventricular—4.3%.

Specific Hemorrhage—Locations and Management

Epidural hematoma (EDH)
  - See the section on "Skull Fractures" for etiologies of EDH.

- Presentation—Classically described brief loss of consciousness followed by a lucid interval before neurologic decline occurs in fewer than 30% of patients [9].
- CT scan is the best study for diagnosis and monitoring of EDH. The typical appearance is a biconvex, lenticular lesion caused by the stripping of the dura away from the skull by the hematoma. Lateral spread may stop at the sutures where the dura is most tightly adherent. This then leads to increase in hematoma thickness. Acute blood is typically hyperdense to the brain parenchyma, but in certain circumstances, such as rapid hemorrhage or low hematocrit, it may be iso- or hypodense.
- Hemorrhage causing significant mass effect or neurologic deficit requires emergent evacuation. Very thin EDH (<5 mm) may not require evacuation. However, if the decision is made to observe, these lesions require very close clinical and imaging monitoring as patients (especially children) may deteriorate rapidly. In general, there should be a low threshold for surgical intervention.
- Surgical treatment involves evacuation of the hemorrhage, coagulation of the bleeding point, and tacking up the dura to eliminate the epidural space and prevent reaccumulation. The craniotomy should be large enough to encompass the hematoma.

Intracerebral hemorrhage (cerebral contusion)

- It typically occurs in areas where the polar aspects of the lobes (frontal, temporal, occipital) strike the skull, or where the surface of the brain rubs on the irregular surface of the skull base (inferior frontal, temporal lobes). Shearing of white matter tracts may cause small deep contusions.
    - Coup contusions—occur on the same side of the impact
    - Contrecoup contusions—occur contralateral to the side of impact
- Contusions may initially be caused by impact resulting in hemorrhage, but may expand over time because of necrosis, infarction, further hemorrhage, and cerebral edema.
- The clinical presentation is dependent on size and location; contusions may cause focal deficits if they are located in eloquent cortex.
- Contusions are at high risk for expansion in the first several days following injury due to both expansion of the hemorrhage and increasing surrounding edema. This may lead to an increase in ICP, causing neurologic decline and the need for further treatment. Because of this, CT scans should be intermittently repeated.
- Contusions in the temporal lobe may be especially dangerous because of their location adjacent to the brainstem. Expansion may lead to precipitous neurologic decline and uncal herniation. Substantial temporal lobe contusions need to be monitored especially closely and surgeons should have a lower threshold for evacuation.

- Traumatic brain injury may be associated with coagulopathy due to systemic fibrinolysis [10–12]. For this reason, coagulation parameters should be monitored closely and corrected as needed to prevent expansion of contusions.
- Surgical evacuation of contusions may be indicated in the setting of neurologic deterioration or significant ICP increase.

Subdural hematoma (SDH)

- It is caused by impact that shifts the brain while other structures remain fixed, resulting in tearing of the veins that bridge from the cerebral cortex to the dura and dural venous sinuses.
- Patients with substantial acute SDHs are often severely neurologically ill owing to the significant impact forces involved in these injuries. These patients often have poor neurologic outcomes, even with the most aggressive and rapid treatment.
- CT scan remains the most rapid method of diagnosing SDH. Because there are few barriers to the spread of hemorrhage along the hemispheric surface, these are often crescentic, holohemispheric lesions. Acute blood is typically hyperdense to the brain parenchyma, but in certain circumstances, such as rapid hemorrhage or low hematocrit, it may be iso- or hypodense.
- Hemorrhage causing significant mass effect or neurologic deficit requires emergent evacuation. Small SDHs in patients with good neurologic examinations may sometimes be observed. However, if decision is made to observe, these lesions require very close clinical and imaging monitoring.
- Surgical treatment involves craniotomy for evacuation of the hemorrhage with coagulation of the bleeding point. Burr holes are not adequate for treatment of acute SDH because the clot is often too solid and extensive to be sufficiently treated through such a small exposure. The craniotomy should be large enough to allow sufficient access to the thickest part of the hematoma and to allow visualization of the majority of the subdural space.
- If the brain is significantly swollen at the time of surgery, a decompressive craniectomy may be of use in alleviating the increased ICP. Many of these patients may also require ICP monitoring. A decompressive craniectomy must be generous enough to allow the brain to herniate through the defect without strangulating the herniated portion, thus leading to ischemia and further cerebral edema. The dura must be patched open to allow for this expansion.

Intraventricular hemorrhage (IVH)

- IVH may be caused by tearing of the deep venous system that lines the walls of the lateral and third ventricle, as well as by damage to the vascularized choroid plexus.

- Substantial IVH often obstructs the flow of CSF through the ventricles and cerebral aqueduct, leading to obstructive hydrocephalus and increased ICP.
- Treatment—ventricular drainage. In cases of massive IVH, it may be difficult to keep the drain from becoming repeatedly clogged.

ADDITIONAL READING

Electronic References

AANS/CNS Joint Section on Neurotrauma and Critical Care. http://www.neurotraumasection.org/

Brain Trauma Foundation. www.braintrauma.org

Guidelines for the management of severe traumatic brain injury. http://tbiguidelines.org/glHome.aspx?gl=1

Textbooks/Chapters

Loftus CM. *Neurosurgical Emergencies.* 2nd ed. New York: Thieme; 2007.

Marion DW. *Traumatic Brain Injury.* New York: Thieme; 1999.

Narayan RK, Wilberger JE, Povlishock JT. *Neurotrauma.* New York: McGraw-Hill; 1996.

Journal Articles

Brain Trauma Foundation, American Association of Neurological Surgeons, Congress of Neurological Surgeons. Guidelines for the management of severe traumatic brain injury. Steroids. *J Neurotrauma.* 2007;24(suppl 1):S91–S95.

Edwards P, Arango M, Balica L, et al. CRASH trial collaborators. Final results of MRC CRASH, a randomised placebo-controlled trial of intravenous corticosteroid in adults with head injury-outcomes at 6 months. *Lancet.* 2005;365(9475):1957–1959.

REFERENCES

1. Langlois JA, Rutland-Brown W, Thomas KE. *Traumatic Brain Injury in the United States: Emergency Department Visits, Hospitalizations, and Deaths.* Atlanta, GA: Centers for Disease Control and Prevention NcfIPaC; 2006.
2. Resnick DK, Subach BR, Marion DW. The significance of carotid canal involvement in basilar cranial fracture. *Neurosurgery.* 1997;40(6):1177–1181.
3. Dagi TF, Meyer FB, Poletti CA. The incidence and prevention of meningitis after basilar skull fracture. *Am J Emerg Med.* 1983;1(3):295–298.
4. Cooper PR, Ho V. Role of emergency skull x-ray films in the evaluation of the head-injured patient: a retrospective study. *Neurosurgery.* 1983;13(2):136–140.
5. Rothman L, Rose JS, Laster DW, Quencer R, Tenner M. The spectrum of growing skull fracture in children. *Pediatrics.* 1976;57(1):26–31.
6. Roy S, Sarkar C, Tandon PN, Banerji AK. Cranio-cerebral erosion (growing fracture of the skull in children). Part I. Pathology. *Acta Neurochir (Wien).* 1987;87(3–4):112–118.

7. Tandon PN, Banerji AK, Bhatia R, Goulatia RK. Cranio-cerebral erosion (growing fracture of the skull in children). Part II. Clinical and radiological observations. *Acta Neurochir (Wien)*. 1987;88(1–2):1–9.

8. Lin JW, Tsai SH, Tsai WC, et al. Survey of traumatic intracranial hemorrhage in Taiwan. *Surg Neurol*. 2006;66 (suppl 2):S20–S25.

9. Greenberg MS. *Handbook of Neurosurgery*. New York: Thieme; 2006.

10. Keimowitz RM, Annis BL. Disseminated intravascular coagulation associated with massive brain injury. *J Neurosurg*. 1973;39(2):178–180.

11. Pondaag W. Disseminated intravascular coagulation related to outcome in head injury. *Acta Neurochir Suppl (Wien)*. 1979;28(1):98–102.

12. Preston FE, Malia RG, Sworn MJ, Timperley WR, Blackburn EK. Disseminated intravascular coagulation as a consequence of cerebral damage. *J Neurol Neurosurg Psychiatr*. 1974;37(3):241–248.

26

The Neurointensive Care Unit

Intracranial Pressure and Cerebral Oxygenation

Sarice L. Bassin

GENERAL PRINCIPLES

Pathophysiology

The intracranial compartment is composed of the following components: blood, cerebrospinal fluid (CSF), and brain. The Monro-Kellie hypothesis states that the volume inside the skull is fixed, so that if there is an increase in the volume of any of the components, there must be a decrease in volume of another component. For example, CSF may be shunted into the spinal canal in the setting of a brain mass. This is a compensatory mechanism to keep intracranial pressure (ICP) constant. Once the compensatory abilities are overwhelmed, pressure in the intracranial cavity will rise rapidly.

When ICP is high, herniation can occur. During herniation, brain tissue and blood vessels are compressed causing irreversible damage. If the brainstem is involved, vegetative functions, including respiration, may cease and brain death can ensue.

Cerebral perfusion pressure (CPP; CPP = mean arterial pressure [MAP] – ICP) is the pressure gradient driving blood into the brain. If CPP is too low, the brain can become ischemic. When cerebral autoregulation is intact, blood vessels will constrict or dilate in order to keep cerebral blood flow constant. After traumatic brain injury (TBI), cerebral autoregulation is often dysfunctional, and CPP must be closely monitored and controlled. Therefore, in the setting of severe TBI, ICP measurement is necessary to accurately determine CPP and prevent cerebral ischemia.

Frequent causes of elevated ICP in TBI are impaired autoregulation, diffuse cerebral edema, focal brain contusions, intracerebral hemorrhage, epidural hematoma or subdural hematoma, hydrocephalus, and venous sinus thrombosis.

DIAGNOSIS

Clinical Presentation

- Initial presentation is variable but can include agitation, somnolence, confusion, vomiting, unilaterally or bilaterally dilated pupils, sluggish or absent reaction of pupil to light, and motor posturing.
- Blood pressure may be elevated in the body's effort to maintain CPP.
- Papilledema may develop, although it would not likely be present hyperacutely.

Radiographic Assessment

CT scan to evaluate for:

- Intra- and extra-axial hemorrhages
- Cerebral edema
- Hydrocephalus or compression of ventricles
- Midline shift
- Effacement of the suprasellar or quadrigeminal plate cisterns
- Effacement of sulci and gyri

TREATMENT

Guiding Principles

- Brain Trauma Foundation (BTF) Guidelines [1] recommend ICP monitoring in the following patients:
  - Glasgow Coma Scale (GCS) 3 to 8 with abnormal head CT
  - GCS 3 to 8 with normal head CT, and age > 40, SBP < 90 mm Hg, or motor posturing
- ICP monitors typically used in the intensive care unit are either intraventricular or intraparenchymal
  - An external ventricular drain, a catheter placed into the ventricular system to both monitor ICP and drain CSF, is still considered the gold standard for measurement of ICP. The system is fluid coupled and can be rezeroed after insertion.
  - An intraparenchymal monitor consists of either a miniature strain gauge pressure sensor or a fiberoptic catheter. These devices can neither be rezeroed after insertion, nor drain CSF.
  - ICP goal is less than 20 mm Hg.
  - CPP goal is 50 to 70 mm Hg.

Initial Management of Elevated ICP

- Position—to improve venous drainage from the head:

- Raise the head of bed to at least 30°.
- Keep the head midline.
- Make sure that cervical collar is not too tight.

- Access
  - All patients undergoing ICP management should have a central venous catheter placed for the administration of medications and monitoring of central venous pressure (CVP).
  - Arterial catheters are helpful in closely monitoring MAP and CPP.

- Respiration
  - Patients with inability to protect the airway because of altered sensorium should be intubated and mechanically ventilated.
  - Hyperventilation (arterial partial pressure of carbon dioxide [$PaCO_2$] < 35 mm Hg) decreases ICP by causing cerebral vasoconstriction, therefore decreasing cerebral blood volume. Hyperventilation is associated with diminished cerebral perfusion and it should be avoided, especially in the first 48 hours after TBI.
  - The exact arterial partial pressure of oxygen (Pao_2) goal is unknown for this patient population, but oxyhemoglobin saturation less than 90% correlates with worse outcome. Some data suggests that a minimum Pao_2 of 100 mm Hg should be maintained to prevent cerebral hypoxia [2].

- Blood pressure
  - Systolic blood pressure < 90 mm Hg should be avoided.
  - MAP goal is > 80 mm Hg until CPP can be measured.
  - CPP goal is 50 to 70 mm Hg.
  - One study showed that routinely treating patients with a CPP goal of 70 mm Hg was associated with an increased risk of acute respiratory distress syndrome (ARDS) [3,4], but in individual patients, a higher goal may be indicated (see also the section on Cerebral Oxygenation).
  - If fluid resuscitation does not meet CPP goals, vasopressors should be started.

- CSF drainage
  - If an EVD is in place, CSF can be drained to reduce ICP.
  - If an EVD is not in place, consideration should be given to placing one.

- Osmotic agents
  - Mannitol 0.25 to 1 g/kg every 4 hours
    - Check serum osmolarity (osm) every 6 hours and hold mannitol for serum osm > 320 mOsm/L.
    - Mannitol will cause diuresis and may cause hypovolemia; fluids must be managed to keep patient euvolemic (CVP 5–10).

- Hypertonic saline—must be given through a central line
  - 3% NaCl—Give 250 cc over 30 minutes every 4 hours, or
  - 23.4% NaCl—Give 30 cc over 10 minutes every 4 hours. Note that 23.4% NaCl can cause profound hypotension if infused too rapidly; it must be infused over *no less* than 10 minutes
  - Check serum sodium every 6 hours and hold hypertonic saline for serum sodium > 155 mEq/L
- Sedation and analgesia
  - Adequate sedation and analgesia decrease cerebral metabolism and therefore decrease cerebral blood volume. Sedation options are listed in the following section.
    - Benzodiazepines
      - Lorazepam 2 to 10 mg/hour infusion
      - Midazelam 2 to 10 mg/hour infusion
    - Narcotics
      - Morphine sulfate 4 to 20 mg/hour infusion
      - Fentanyl 25 to 150 µg/hour infusion
    - Anesthetics
      - Propofol 30 to 100 µg/kg/minute. Propofol infusion syndrome (PRIS) is an adverse drug reaction associated with high dose (>65 µg/kg/minute) and long-term (>48 hours) use of propofol. PRIS is almost uniformly fatal. Patients with PRIS develop severe metabolic acidosis, rhabdomyolysis, renal failure, and cardiovascular collapse. If using propofol for long term or at high doses, check creatinine kinase and lactic acid every 6 hours. If either value is rising, or PRIS is otherwise suspected, propofol should be discontinued immediately and an alternative sedative started. Treatment for PRIS is supportive.
    - Barbiturates—These are often reserved for management of elevated ICP that is refractory to other medical treatment. Barbiturates are usually used with continuous electroencephalogram monitoring to determine the depth of pharmacologic coma. Titrating the medication to burst suppression is a common goal. Barbiturate infusions usually cause hypotension. Vasopressors and hemodynamic monitoring must be available to ensure that an adequate blood pressure is maintained.
      - Pentobarbital 10 to 15 mg/kg over 1 to 2 hours loading dose, followed by 1 mg/kg/hour infusion. Infusion may be increased to 2 to 4 mg/kg/hour as needed for goals
- Craniectomy
  - Surgical removal of Part of the skull with a duraplasty can reduce ICP by Decompressive and allowing the brain to expand.
    - Evacuation of blood clots or lobectomy may be indicated.

- Temperature control
  - Fever control helps lower ICP. Normothermia should be a therapeutic goal. Cooling measures include acetaminophen 650 mg every 6 hours, intravenous cooled saline, cooling blankets, and intravascular cooling catheters.
  - Prophylactic hypothermia may be beneficial in special circumstances, but may be associated with an increased risk of pneumonia [1].
- Chemical paralysis
  - In patients with shivering or dyssynchrony with the ventilator, chemical paralysis with neuromuscular blockade may decrease metabolic rate and lower intrathroracic pressure, thereby reducing intracranial blood volume.
  - Daily holidays from chemical paralysis are advised, and adequate sedation must be used in all patients who are chemically paralyzed.
  - Train-of-four monitoring peripheral nerve stimulation should be employed for a goal of 1 to 2 of 4 twitches during the use of neuromuscular blocking agents.

Cerebral Oxygenation

- There are multiple known methods to measure cerebral perfusion. Some measure cerebral blood flow directly, but the more commonly used technologies measure delivery of oxygen to the brain. Although there is evidence linking treatment algorithms that utilize these technologies to improved outcomes, the usage remains controversial.
- Brain tissue oxygen monitors are intraparenchymal probes inserted via a burr hole into the white matter of the brain. A treatment threshold of <15 mm Hg is supported by the latest BTF Guidelines [1]. Treatment options include:
  - Lowering ICP
  - Optimizing CPP (Some patients require CPP values above 70 mm Hg for adequate perfusion.)
  - Increasing Pa_{CO_2}
  - Increasing Pa_{O_2}
  - Increasing hemoglobin
- Jugular venous saturation monitoring requires a fiberoptic catheter to be placed in the internal jugular vein. Per BTF guidelines [1], a reading of <50% is associated with worse outcomes and merits treatment in accordance with the treatment options described earlier

ADDITIONAL READING

Electronic Reference

https://tbiguidelines.org/glHome.aspx?gl=1

Textbook/Chapter

Reilly P, Bullock R, eds. *Head Injury: Pathophysiology and Management.* 2nd ed. London: Hodder Arnold Publication; 2005.

REFERENCES

1. Brain Trauma Foundation, American Association of Neurological Surgeons, Congress of Neurological Surgeons. Guidelines for the management of severe brain injury. *J Neurotrauma.* 2007;24 (suppl 1):S1–S106.
2. Gracias VH, Guillamondegui OD, Stiefel MF, et al. Cerebral cortical oxygenation: a pilot study. *J Trauma.* 2004;56(3):469–72; discussion 472.
3. Robertson CS, Valadka AB, Hannay HJ, et al. Prevention of secondary ischemic insults after severe head injury. *Crit Care Med.* 1999;27(10):2086–2095.
4. Contant CF, Valadka AB, Gopinath SP, Hannay HJ, Robertson CS. Adult respiratory distress syndrome: a complication of induced hypertension after severe head injury. *J Neurosurg.* 2001;95(4):560–568.

27

The Role of Neuroprotective Interventions in Traumatic Brain Injury

David M. Panczykowski and David O. Okonkwo

BACKGROUND

Definitions

- Primary (1°) injury—neuronal death or dysfunction as a consequence of initial impact
- Secondary (2°) injury—progressive ischemic, inflammatory, and cytotoxic processes initiated or potentiated by systemic and/or intracranial insults

  - Systemic insults—hypoxia, hypotension, hyperthermia, hyperglycemia
  - Intracranial insults—intracranial hypertension, cerebral edema, mass lesion, cerebral vasospasm

- Neuroprotective intervention—treatment initiated prior to and/or at the onset of 2° injury with the aim of minimizing its intensity or immediate effects

General Principles

- Prophylaxis and early treatment of secondary insults may mitigate 2° injury and improve outcome following traumatic brain injury (TBI).
- Vast research has been conducted delineating the cascade of factors responsible for 2° injury following TBI, with a subsequent focus on a host of potential agents directed at ameliorating these insults.

  - N-methyl-D-aspartic acid (NMDA) and a-amino-3-hydroxy-methyl-4-isoxazolyl-propionic acid (AMPA) receptor antagonists—suppression of the excitotoxic response that follows TBI
  - Cyclosporine A analogues and caspase and inhibitors—target mitochondrial dysfunction and its interplay with apoptosis

- Progesterone—exerts an effect through neuroprotective hormone receptors
- Despite promising experimental results, all phase III randomized clinical trials (RCTs) evaluating neuroprotection via pharmacological interventions have failed to show an improvement in outcome following TBI.
- Various reasons have been postulated for the lack of efficacy, including:
  - Complexity and poor understanding of the pathophysiologic mechanisms at play in TBI
  - Heterogeneity of the condition and population
  - Flaws in trial design and outcome assessment
- Given the plurality of mechanisms responsible for cellular injury, it remains unlikely that any single-agent treatment can address all aspects of TBI pathophysiology.
- The only widely accepted neuroprotective strategies for 2° injury at present target proven systemic and intracranial insults readily amenable to common therapeutic interventions (e.g., hypoxemia, hypotension, hyperthermia, and hyperglycemia).

HYPOXEMIA

Guiding Principles

- The brain accounts for 20% of the body's oxygen consumption. Blood oxygen content exceeds the brain's utilization by only a factor of 2 or 3, leaving the brain vulnerable to small changes in oxygen supply.
- Primary damage stresses the tenuous balance between supply and demand, making the brain more susceptible to secondary ischemic insults.
- The detrimental effect of secondary ischemic damage is well documented; both depth and duration of hypoxemia are significantly associated with increased morbidity and mortality.
- Cerebral oxygen delivery is a function of cerebral blood flow (CBF) and arterial oxygen content.

Diagnosis and Treatment

- Although no treatment threshold exists per se, studies have found severe morbidity and mortality to be associated with $Pao_2 < 60$ mmHg and O_2 saturation < 90% [1]. Hyperventilation, except as a brief temporizing maneuver in the setting of elevated intracranial pressure (ICP), should be avoided [2].
- Multiple therapies directed at increasing oxygen delivery and utilization have been investigated (e.g., normo- and hyperbaric

hyperoxia, Pbo_2 directed therapy), but have produced only equivocal results [3].

- Direct measures of the cerebral metabolic rate of oxygen consumption (CMRO2) have shown no increase in brain O_2 utilization with normobaric hyperoxia. Hyperbaric treatment has been shown to increase CMRO2; however, a clear clinical benefit has yet to be demonstrated.
- Although studies have shown poor outcome with hypoxic brain oxygen tension (Pbo_2 < 15 mm Hg), no randomized controlled trial currently exists proving Pbo_2 monitoring to be beneficial [4].

- Potential toxicity of hyperoxia

  - Prolonged high fraction of inspired oxygen (Fio_2) has been associated with injury to the lens of the eye, lungs, heart, brain, and gastrointestinal tract and may also lead to cerebral vasoconstriction.
  - High positive end expiratory pressure (PEEP > 15–20 mm Hg) should be avoided; PEEP is transmitted through lungs to thoracic vessels leading to cerebral venous congestion and increased ICP.
  - The potential risks in combination with no clear benefit should preclude the use of hyperoxia until RCTs demonstrate a clear advantage.

- Goals of ventilator management should be eucapnic ventilation ($Paco_2$ 35–40 mm Hg) with sufficient oxygen delivery to avoid hypoxemia or brain hypoxia.

HYPOTENSION

Guiding Principles

- Hypotension is one of the most powerful predictors of outcome—a relationship that is independent of Glasgow Coma Scale (GCS) score, age, or intracranial lesion [1].
- Changes in CBF following TBI generally occur in three phases:
  - Hypoperfusion and ischemia—6 to 12 hours post injury
  - Hyperemia and concomitant ICP increases—24 to 48 hours
  - Vasospasm with decreased perfusion—>72 hours
- Major influences on cerebral circulation include adequate blood pressure, flow-metabolism coupling, $Paco_2$, and cerebral autoregulation; dysfunction in any or all post-TBI puts patients at risk for hyperemia and/or ischemia.
- Mean arterial pressure (MAP) or cerebral perfusion pressure (CPP) are used as surrogates for estimating cerebral perfusion.

Diagnosis and Treatment

For a detailed discussion of this topic, please see Chapter 26.

HYPERTHERMIA

Guiding Principles

- Hyperthermia in the acute postinjury phase is associated with longer ICU stay and worsened neurologic outcome [5].
- Temperature surges occur in up to 67% of TBI patients within the first 72 hours after admission, and may result from multiple causes (hypothalamic disruption, inflammation, medications, surgery, etc.).

Diagnosis and Treatment

- Core temperature should be monitored (preferably by brain temperature probe or rectal thermometer) and temperature spikes $\geq 38°C$ should be avoided and aggressively treated [6].
- Inconsistent research results preclude recommendation of hypothermia as a standard of care intervention in TBI.
- In addition to the common methods of identifying causative factors accompanying fever (e.g., infection), one should also consider central causes of temperature dysregulation.
- Antipyretics, extracorporeal cooling, gastric lavage, and intravascular cooling catheters have all been investigated as means to prophylactically control temperature in TBI patients. Intravascular cooling catheters have shown the most consistency in induced normothermia, without increases in rates of infection, antibiotic, or sedation usage [6,7].

HYPOCAPNIA

Guiding Principles

- Hypocapnia ($Paco_2 \approx 30$–35 mm Hg) is generally caused by intended or accidental hyperventilation (e.g., with therapeutic hyperventilation in managing increased ICP) [1].
- The ability of hyperventilation (and hypocapnia) to reduce cerebral blood volume (CBV) is achieved at a disproportionate cost to CBF, which may be especially harmful in the first 24 hours post injury [8].
- The effects of hypocapnia on vascular smooth muscle are pH mediated; cerebral and renal buffering returns pH to normal within 4 to 6 hours eliminating this effect and precluding the use of sustained hypocapnia. In addition, this buffering leads to pH-overshoot and subsequent rebound hyperemia or increased ICP.

Diagnosis and Treatment

- Prophylactic hyperventilation should not be used, as it has been associated with worsened ICP control and poor neurologic outcome.
- Brief (e.g., 20 minutes) moderate hyperventilation for ICP reduction should be undertaken cautiously and only until a pathology-specific intervention is instituted.

HYPERGLYCEMIA

Guiding Principles

- The massive stress response following TBI results in elevated circulating catecholamine levels with subsequent increases in serum glucose.
- Hyperglycemia, which leads to intracellular acidosis, is associated with the development of reactive oxygen species, especially during the acute ischemic phase of TBI, exacerbating 2° brain injury.
- Admission and early postoperative hyperglycemia (serum glucose ≥ 200 mg/dL) has been associated with worse neurologic and mortality outcomes [9].

Diagnosis and Treatment

- A target serum glucose < 180 to 200 mg/dL decreases episodes of hyperglycemia and has been associated with decreased mortality [9].
- Note that intensive insulin therapy (target glucose 80–110 mg/dL) results in an increased risk of hypoglycemic episodes without conferring mortality benefits. Conservative treatment of glucose levels > 180 mg/dL is generally accepted as striking the best balance.

POSTTRAUMATIC SEIZURES

Guiding Principles

- Posttraumatic seizures (PTS) may occur in 20% to 25% of all patients suffering TBI and the incidence ratio of PTS for mild, moderate, and severe TBI has been shown to be 1.5, 2.9, and 17.0, respectively [10]. PTS can be classified by time of onset—immediate (first few hours), early (occurring during first week), and late (>1 week post insult).
- Late posttraumatic epilepsy is associated with severity and type of injury (subdural and intracerebral hemorrhage, skull fractures, neurologic dysfunction) [11]; biochemical and structural alterations have been the main pathophysiologic mechanisms proposed.

Diagnosis and Treatment

- Studies to date have not addressed effects of PTS on secondary injury. However, early prophylactic treatment with antiepileptic drugs (AEDs; i.e., for the first week post injury) has been shown to decrease the relative risk of early PTS although this is without a concordant decrease in development of late seizures (i.e., posttraumatic epilepsy), morbidity, or mortality [12].

ADDITIONAL READING

Electronic Reference
Stein DG. Progesterone exerts neuroprotective effects after brain injury. Available at http://www.ncbi.nlm.nih.gov/pmc/articles/PMC2699575/

Textbook/Chapter
Cernak I, Lea PM, Faden AI. Neurotrauma. In: Bahr M, ed. *Neuroprotection: Models, Mechanisms, and Therapies.* Weinheim, Germany: Wiley-VCH; 2004:95–115.

Journal Articles
Diringer MN. Hyperoxia: good or bad for the injured brain? *Curr Opin Crit Care.* 2008;14(2):167–171.

Griesdale DE, Tremblay MH, McEwen J, Chittock DR. Glucose control and mortality in patients with severe traumatic brain injury. *Neurocrit Care.* 2009;11(3):311–316.

Guidelines for the management of severe traumatic brain injury. *J Neurotrauma.* 2007;24(suppl 1):S1–S106.

Wang KK, Larner SF, Robinson G, Hayes RL. Neuroprotection targets after traumatic brain injury. *Curr Opin Neurol.* 2006;19(6):514–519.

REFERENCES

1. Guidelines for the management of severe traumatic brain injury. *J Neurotrauma.* 2007;24(suppl 1):S1–106.
2. Robertson CS, Valadka AB, Hannay HJ, et al. Prevention of secondary ischemic insults after severe head injury. *Crit Care Med.* 1999;27(10):2086–2095.
3. Diringer MN. Hyperoxia: good or bad for the injured brain? *Curr Opin Crit Care.* 2008;14(2):167–171.
4. Martini RP, Deem S, Yanez ND, et al. Management guided by brain tissue oxygen monitoring and outcome following severe traumatic brain injury. *J Neurosurg.* 2009;111(4):644–649.
5. Geffroy A, Bronchard R, Merckx P, et al. Severe traumatic head injury in adults: which patients are at risk of early hyperthermia? *Intensive Care Med.* 2004;30(5):785–790.
6. Puccio AM, Fischer MR, Jankowitz BT, Yonas H, Darby JM, Okonkwo DO. Induced normothermia attenuates intracranial hypertension and

reduces fever burden after severe traumatic brain injury. *Neurocrit Care.* 2009;11(1):82–87.

7. Diringer MN, Videen TO, Yundt K, et al. Regional cerebrovascular and metabolic effects of hyperventilation after severe traumatic brain injury. *J Neurosurg.* 2002;96(1):103–108.

8. Curley G, Kavanagh BP, Laffey JG. Hypocapnia and the injured brain: more harm than benefit. *Crit Care Med.* 2010;38(5):1348–1359.

9. Griesdale DE, Tremblay MH, McEwen J, Chittock DR. Glucose Control and Mortality in Patients with Severe Traumatic Brain Injury. *Neurocrit Care.* 2009;11(3):311–316.

10. Annegers JF, Hauser WA, Coan SP, Rocca WA. A population-based study of seizures after traumatic brain injuries. *N Engl J Med.* 1998;338(1):20–24.

11. Kharatishvili I, Pitkänen A. Posttraumatic epilepsy. *Curr Opin Neurol.* 2010;23(2):183–188.

12. Schierhout G, Roberts I. Anti-epileptic drugs for preventing seizures following acute traumatic brain injury. *Cochrane Database Syst Rev.* 2001(4):CD000173.

28

Nutritional Considerations

Aaron M. Cook

GENERAL PRINCIPLES

- Moderate to severe traumatic brain injury (TBI) patients often require the use of parenteral nutrition (PN) or enteral nutrition (EN) because of feeding difficulty.
- Nasogastric EN in TBI patients typically leads to considerable feeding intolerance and ultimately relative malnutrition and immunosuppression; duodenal or jejunal feedings are preferred when providing EN [1,2].
- The Brain Trauma Foundation Guidelines recommend that moderate to severe TBI patients receive full caloric replacement by day 7 after injury (with no specification of route) and suggest initiating feeding within 72 hours after injury and targeting 100% to 140% of estimated resting metabolism expenditure (15%–20% of those calories being protein) [3].

DIAGNOSIS

Clinical Presentation

- Frequently reassess ability to swallow or the need for temporary feeding access.
- Gastrostomy tubes are often more convenient for patients who are unable to swallow for a prolonged period of time (i.e., weeks to months). TBI patients are more likely to tolerate gastric feedings as the acute phase of illness subsides. Typically by week 2 or 3 after TBI, gastric feedings are safe and able to provide adequate calories.
- PN may be considered in patients with early feeding difficulty who do not tolerate EN within the first few days after injury. The benefits of early nutrition must be balanced with the risks of PN.

Monitoring

- Anthropomorphic basal energy expenditure equations may be useful to estimate initial metabolic needs. Assessment and development of a nutritional goal and initiation of nutrition should not be delayed.

- Measurement of metabolic needs by indirect calorimetry is likely more accurate, although less convenient and more time consuming, than estimation using common basal energy expenditure equations.
- Other caloric sources such as lipid emulsion solvents seen with propofol and clevidipine should be included in total calories provided in order to avoid overfeeding when patients receive one of these IV infusions plus full EN or PN.
- Electrolyte abnormalities (particularly hyponatremia), hyperglycemia, and visceral/skeletal protein wasting are commonly problematic and should be addressed with the nutrition plan.

TREATMENT

Guiding Principles

- Despite comatose appearance, TBI patients have increased metabolic needs (~120%–140% of resting metabolic expenditure) because of hypercatabolic response.
- Estimates may be as high as 160% in pediatric patients and adults with multitrauma.
- Conversely, needs may be as low as 80% in pharmacologically induced coma.

Initial Management

- Place postpyloric feeding access as soon as possible.
- Use a calorically dense EN product as early as possible (preferably within 48 hours after injury).
- Provide at least 15% to 20% of calories as protein to account for protein catabolism.
- Some studies suggest success in starting EN near goal rate; common practice tends to focus on slowly increasing EN rate to goal over 12 to 48 hours, depending on patient tolerance [4,5].
- Frequently reevaluate metabolic needs as patient convalesces and clinically improves.
- Large volumes of salt-free water and other hypotonic fluids should be avoided to prevent exacerbation of cerebral edema or hyponatremia.

Glycemic Control

- The optimal range of glucose values is an often debated topic in critically ill individuals.
- Admission hyperglycemia and occurrences of hyperglycemia (>200 to 225 mg/dL) may be associated with morbidity and mortality in TBI patients [6,7].

- The rate of infectious complications, immune dysfunction, and other noninfectious complications such as polyneuropathy are closely associated with elevated glucose concentrations [8].
- Hypoglycemia also appears to be associated with an increased mortality in critically ill individuals [9].
- TBI patients exhibit some differences in brain glucose metabolism and likely require slightly higher glucose values to ensure appropriate brain metabolism; maintenance of serum glucose values between 80 and 110 mg/dL ("intensive insulin") may result in cerebrospinal fluid (CSF) glucose values below the normal threshold [10].
- Serum glucose values of 100 to 180 mg/dL should result in improved CSF glucose values and reduce the risk of hypoglycemia.

Treatment Controversies

- Timing—If early is best, is "settling" for PN in first few days after injury when EN is not feasible likely to confer the same benefit as early EN? If PN is used in this situation, clinicians should be vigilant to avoid permissive delays in EN initiation while providing early PN (i.e., should still be aggressive in attempting to start EN as soon as possible) and caution should be used in patients with intracranial hypertension or the potential for cerebral edema.
- Management of hyperglycemia—Optimal glycemic thresholds are often debated and may be different in TBI patients than in other critically ill populations.
- Immunonutrition—Role of immunonutrients such as glutamine, arginine, and omega-3 fatty acids in the inflammatory response of TBI patients is ill-defined. Theoretical suppositions can be made based on the pathophysiology of TBI and the mechanism of action of these immunonutrients, but clinical data is lacking.
  - No published studies evaluating immunonutrients in TBI patients are available.
  - Based on the current understanding of the mechanism of action of each individual nutrient, caution should be exercised when evaluating the use of immunonutrients.
  - Glutamine, although potentially beneficial in PN patients and those with infections, may be deleterious because of the potential conversion to glutamate, an excitatory neurotransmitter known to be a major factor in the pathology of secondary brain injury.
  - Arginine, although potentially beneficial in trauma patients by increasing nitric oxide–mediated perfusion, may be harmful in TBI patients by increasing nitric oxide in cerebral circulation, thereby increasing cerebral blood volume and intracranial pressure.
  - In contrast, omega-3 fatty acids may be able to mitigate the central inflammatory response and propagation of lipid peroxidation due

to the ischemia and metabolic dysfunction seen after severe TBI by shunting prostaglandin production away from arachidonic acid and associated metabolites.

■ Continued assessment of nutritional needs—Optimal timing of reductions in calories and protein is not well defined as the TBI patient improves clinically. Clinicians should continue to monitor caloric needs, nutrition tolerance, and caloric intake, even after the acute illness subsides.

ADDITIONAL READING

Electronic Reference
http://www.guideline.gov/summary/summary.aspx?doc_id=11000

Journal Articles

Brain Trauma Foundation Guidelines. Management of severe traumatic brain injury. *J Neurotrauma.* 2007;24:S1–S95.

Cook AM, Peppard A, Magnuson B. Nutrition considerations in traumatic brain injury. *Nutr Clin Pract.* 2008;23:608–620.

Marik PE, Zaloga GP. Immunonutrition in critically ill patients: a systematic review and analysis of the literature. *Intensive Care Med.* 2008;34:1980–1990.

Rhoney DH, Parker D Jr. Considerations in fluids and electrolytes after traumatic brain injury. *Nutr Clin Pract.* 2006;21:462–478.

Taylor SJ, Fettes SB, Jewkes C, et al. Prospective, randomized, controlled trial to determine the effect of early enhanced enteral nutrition on clinical outcome in mechanically ventilated patients suffering head injury. *Crit Care Med.* 1999;27:2525–2531.

REFERENCES

1. Ott L, Young B, Phillips R, et al. Altered gastric emptying in the head-injured patient: relationship to feeding intolerance. *J Neurosurg.* 1991;74(5):738–742.
2. Grahm TW, Zadrozny DB, Harrington T. The benefits of early jejunal hyperalimentation in the head-injured patient. *Neurosurgery.* 1989;25(5):729–735.
3. Brain Trauma Foundation. Management of severe traumatic brain injury. *J Neurotrauma.* 2007;24:S1–S95.
4. Taylor SJ, Fettes SB, Jewkes C, Nelson RJ. Prospective, randomized, controlled trial to determine the effect of early enhanced enteral nutrition on clinical outcome in mechanically ventilated patients suffering head injury. *Crit Care Med.* 1999;27(11):2525–2531.
5. Zarbock SD, Steinke D, Hatton J, Magnuson B, Smith KM, Cook AM. Successful enteral nutritional support in the neurocritical care unit. *Neurocrit Care.* 2008;9(2):210–216.
6. Young B, Ott L, Dempsey R, Haack D, Tibbs P. Relationship between admission hyperglycemia and neurologic outcome of severely brain-injured patients. *Ann Surg.* 1989;210(4):466–72; discussion 472.

7. Liu-DeRyke X, Collingridge DS, Orme J, Roller D, Zurasky J, Rhoney DH. Clinical impact of early hyperglycemia during acute phase of traumatic brain injury. *Neurocrit Care.* 2009;11(2):151–157.

8. van den Berghe G, Wouters P, Weekers F, et al. Intensive insulin therapy in the critically ill patients. *N Engl J Med.* 2001;345(19):1359–1367.

9. The NICE-SUGAR Study Investigators. Intensive versus conventional glucose control in critically ill patients. *N Engl J Med.* 2009;360(13):1283–1297.

10. Vespa P, Boonyaputthikul R, McArthur DL, et al. Intensive insulin therapy reduces microdialysis glucose values without altering glucose utilization or improving the lactate/pyruvate ratio after traumatic brain injury. *Crit Care Med.* 2006;34(3):850–856.

Initial Rehabilitation Interventions in the Acute Hospital Setting and Transitioning to the Next Level of Care

Kemesha Delisser and Brian Greenwald

INTRODUCTION

Moderate to severe traumatic brain injury (TBI) carries an overall mortality of 20% to 50% with 85% of those mortalities occurring within the first 2 weeks of injury [1,2]. For those who survive, significant risk of disability remains. Initial TBI treatment goals are focused on decreasing its significant mortality and prevention of negative sequelae and disability. Initial rehabilitation interventions in the acute hospital setting is to begin to shift focus from life-saving measures and medical stabilization to optimization of the medical milieu in the context of CNS recovery and preservation or restoration of function. Early rehabilitation or physiatry consultation and formal intervention programs are associated with decreased acute hospital length of stay and improved functional outcomes [3]. The following topic areas represent commonly encountered acute hospital considerations for patients with TBI.

AGITATION

- Agitation occurs in up to 33% to 50% of moderate to severe TBI patients sometime during the acute course [4,5].
- Search for the cause of agitation which may include seizures, pain, hypoxia, recent medication changes, or infection.
- Implement environmental modifications—lower lights, turn off TV and radio, decrease visitations and/or number of visitors in the room.
- Minimize use of restraints because they can increase agitation and cause harm.

- Pharmacological treatment should be kept to a minimum; use the lowest dose possible to address symptoms, and taper as tolerated (see also Chapters 38 and 39).

  - For restlessness, consider trazodone, carbamazepine, or valproate.
  - For aggression, consider β-blockers (metoprolol and other β selective agents are preferred) or valproate.
  - For emotional lability, consider selective serotonin reuptake inhibitors or valproate.
  - To manage psychotic features, consider risperidone, olanzapine, or other atypical antipsychotics. Typical neuroleptics should be avoided owing to dopamine blockade.
  - Use of Ativan or other benzodiazepines should be discouraged to the extent possible, because they may cause sedation and amnesia and are associated with risk of paradoxical agitation as well as adverse effects on neuroplasticity.

CONTRACTURES AND SPASTICITY[1]

- The first stage of treatment involves aggressive range of motion, stretching, and exercise [6]. Initial interventions should be initiated in the intensive care unit. Repeatedly reassess and modify approach as warranted based on evolving clinical condition.
- Treatment should be geared toward functional improvement and pain relief.
- Splinting or serial casting of extremities should be considered whenever appropriate.
- Pharmacological therapies (e.g., dantrolene, baclofen) may be considered. Close patient monitoring is required, because tone-lowering medications can have negative effects on cognition.

NUTRITION/SWALLOWING STATUS

- TBI results in catecholamine excess acutely, leading to hypermetabolism, increased energy expenditure, and increased protein loss; as a result, TBI patients have increased caloric requirements [6–9].
- Early nutritional support decreases morbidity and mortality, shortens hospital length of stay, and may decrease disability [7].
- Brain Trauma Foundation (BTF) Guidelines for the Management of Severe Traumatic Brain Injury recommend that patient's feeding requirements be met by the first week after TBI [7] (see Chapter 28 for a detailed discussion of nutritional considerations in TBI).

---

[1] See Chapter 52 for a detailed discussion of spasticity.

- Swallow mechanism may be impaired in up to 82% of TBI patients [10]. Note that 12% of patients with swallowing disorders may have normal gag reflex and 77% have good voluntary cough reflex [11].
- TBI patients may have impaired gastric emptying secondary to vagus nerve damage, elevated levels of endogenous opioids, or use of medications such as narcotics.
  - If using enteral nutrition, check feeding residuals periodically.
  - Promotility agents such as erythromycin may be considered.
  - Metoclopramide should be used sparingly if at all because of its dopamine antagonist activity.

BOWEL AND BLADDER[2]

- Injury to frontal lobes can cause loss of cortical control over bowel and bladder.
- Incidence of urinary incontinence is 62% [12] and that of urinary retention is 9% [6].
  - Note associated increased risk of urinary tract infection and skin ulcer development.
- Urinary incontinence treatment options include timed voiding programs and use of anticholinergic agents. Urinary retention treatment may include intermittent catheterization or Foley catheter placement.
- Constipation can also be present secondary to immobility and medications.
- Bowel treatment options include use of a timed bowel program, fiber supplementation, maintenance of adequate hydration, and selected medication use (e.g., stool softeners, stimulant suppositories).

PAIN[3]

Pain is a common cause of agitation; evaluating for etiology may be difficult due to patient confusion or decreased consciousness.

- Management guidelines
  - Use long-acting or around-the-clock dosing for patients unable to effectively communicate pain medication needs.
  - Minimize use of sedatives and opiates.
    - Scheduled acetaminophen and nonsteroidal anti-inflammatory drugs are highly effective in many instances.

---

[2] See Chapter 32 for a further discussion of management of bowel and bladder issues in TBI.

[3] See also Chapter 40 for a detailed discussion of pain management in TBI.

- Whenever possible, use mechanical interventions to prevent exacerbation of pain (e.g., positioning, splinting).

SEIZURE PROPHYLAXIS[4]

- Posttraumatic seizures are classified as immediate (first 24 hours), early (≤7 days after TBI), or late (>7 days after TBI) [7,13].
- BTF Guidelines suggest the use of phenytoin as prophylaxis to prevent early seizures in high-risk patients, defined as those with GCS < 10, cortical contusion, depressed skull fracture, hematoma, penetrating head wound, or seizure within 24 hours of head injury [7].
- Phenytoin trials demonstrate efficacy in preventing early seizures but no impact on incidence of long-term seizures [14].
- Anticonvulsants have been associated with adverse side effects, including hematologic abnormalities, ataxia, and neurobehavioral side effects; they may also impair neural plasticity. Therefore, prophylaxis is not recommended beyond 7 days post injury [14–19].
- Monitor use of anticonvulsants, and discontinue after the first week whenever possible.

DEEP VEIN THROMBOSIS PROPHYLAXIS

- There is a reported 20% incidence of deep vein thrombosis (DVTs) first detected in TBI patients upon admission to inpatient rehab [6].
- High-risk patients are those with advanced age, severe injury, clotting disorders, prolonged immobilization, and multiple transfusions [7].
- General guidelines for DVT prophylaxis
  - Pharmacological intervention has been shown to be efficacious. Early use must be weighed against the risk of expansion of hemorrhage. Subcutaneous heparin (or a low-molecular-weight heparinoid [LMWH]) can generally be started 36 hours after trauma [17].
  - Mechanical compression stockings, aspirin, and lose-dose warfarin may reduce risk, but data does not suggest equivalent efficacy.
  - Discuss timing of initiation with primary service.
- Very high-risk patients with contraindications for other methods of prophylaxis can be considered for inferior vena cava filter placement.
  - Consider use of a retrievable filter with removal soon after clinical indication for placement resolves.
- DVT prophylaxis should be continued until the patient is ambulatory, or sufficient time has passed, given the comorbidities and clinical status.

---

[4] See also Chapter 47 for a detailed discussion of posttraumatic seizure management.

ENDOCRINE ABNORMALITIES[5]

The signs and symptoms of hypothalamopituitarism may be subtle and may overlap with the neurologic and psychiatric sequelae of TBI [18,19]. Maintain a low threshold for suggesting or initiating an endocrine work-up when clinically indicated, as described in the following section.

- Acute corticosteroid deficiency—adrenal crisis
  - Symptoms—weakness, nausea, vomiting, abdominal or flank pain, hyperthermia or hypothermia, and hypovolemic shock
  - Clinical and laboratory findings—hypotension, hypoglycemia, hyponatremia, myopathy, anemia, eosinophilia, QT prolongation, or deep T waves on electrocardiogram
  - Adrenal crisis is life-threatening and should be treated immediately with glucocorticoid replacement.
- Syndrome of Inappropriate Antidiuretic Hormone Secretion (SIADH)
  - Symptoms—anorexia, vomiting, worsening cognitive function, agitation, headache, and seizures
  - Clinical and laboratory findings—hyponatremia; fractional excretion of sodium is greater than 1%
  - May be precipitated by medications such as amitriptyline, carbamazepine, and phenobarbital
  - Treatment—fluid restriction, saline infusion. Correct no more than 12 mEq/L in first 24 hours and no more than 6 mEq/L on subsequent days.
- Neurogenic diabetes insipidus
  - Associated with basalar skull fractures
  - Treat with increased oral fluid intake, IV hypotonic fluid, and/or vasopressin.

MEDICATIONS TO BE AVOIDED

Regardless of clinical condition, certain medications should be avoided in TBI because of the risk of increased sedation, worsening cognitive, behavioral, or affective impairments, and/or adverse effect on neural plasticity. Some common examples are as follows:

- Anticholinergics (e.g., Benadryl, some tricyclic antidepressants)—can cause delirium and worsen sedation
- Dopamine blockers (e.g., metoclopramide, typical antipsychotics such as haloperidol)
  - Dopamine blockade is associated with worse motor recovery in animal studies and prolonged posttraumatic confusion in human trials

---

[5] See also Chapter 49 for a detailed discussion of this topic.

- Central-acting α-1 antagonists (prazosin) and α-2 agonists (clonidine)—can increase sedation
- H2 Blockers (e.g., famotidine)—can increase confusion and sedation

ADDITIONAL READING

Electronic References

CHEST—recommendations for DVT prophylaxis: http://chestjournal.chestpubs. org/content/126/3_suppl/338S.full.pdf+html

http://www.biausa.org/_literature_49033/Early_vs_Late_Treatment_ Position_Paper

Textbook/Chapter

Mysiw WJ, Fugate LP, Clinchot DM. Assessment, early rehabilitation intervention, and tertiary prevention. In: Zasler N, Katz D, Zafonte R, eds. *Brain Injury Medicine: Principles and Practice*. New York, NY: Demos Medical Publishing; 2007:283–301.

Journal Article

Yablon SA, Rock WA Jr, Nick TG, Sherer M, McGrath CM, Goodson KH. Deep vein thrombosis: prevalence and risk factors in rehabilitation admissions with brain injury. *Neurology*. 2004;63:485–491.

REFERENCES

1. Moppett IK. Traumatic brain injury: assessment, resuscitation and early management. *Br J Anaesth*. 2007;99(1):18–31.
2. Roberts I, Yates D, Sandercock P, et al. Effect of intravenous corticosteroids on death within 14 days in 10008 adults with clinically significant head injury (MRC CRASH trial): randomised placebo-controlled trial. *Lancet*. 2004;364(9442):1321–1328.
3. Mackay LE. Benefits of a formalized traumatic brain injury program within a trauma center. *J Head Trauma Rehabil*. 1994;9:11–19.
4. Tateno A, Jorge RE, Robinson RG. Clinical correlates of aggressive behavior after traumatic brain injury. *J Neuropsychiatry Clin Neurosci*. 2003;15(2):155–160.
5. Silver JM, Yudofsky SC. Aggressive disorder. In: Silver JM, Yudofsky SC, Hales RE, eds. *Neuropsychiatry of Traumatic Brain Injury*. Washington, DC: American Psychiatric Press; 1994:313–353.
6. Mysiw WJ, Fugate LP, Clinchot DM. Assessment, early rehabilitation intervention, and tertiary prevention. In: Zasler N, Katz D, Zafonte R, eds. *Brain Injury Medicine: Principles and Practice*. New York, NY: Demos Medical Publishing; 2007:283–301.
7. Brain Trauma Foundation; American Association of Neurological Surgeons; Congress of Neurological Surgeons; et al. Guidelines for the management of severe traumatic brain injury. XIII. *J Neurotrauma*. 2007;24(suppl 1):S1–106.
8. Härtl R, Gerber LM, Ni Q, Ghajar J. Effect of early nutrition on deaths due to severe traumatic brain injury. *J Neurosurg*. 2008;109(1):50–56.

9. Krakau K, Omne-Pontén M, Karlsson T, Borg J. Metabolism and nutrition in patients with moderate and severe traumatic brain injury: A systematic review. *Brain Inj.* 2006;20(4):345–367.

10. Logemann JA, Pepe J, Mackay LE. Disorders of nutrition and swallowing: intervention strategies in the trauma center. *J Head Trauma Rehabil.* 1994;9:43–56.

11. Winstein CJ. Neurogenic dysphagia. Frequency, progression, and outcome in adults following head injury. *Phys Ther.* 1983;63(12):1992–1997.

12. Chua K, Chuo A, Kong KH. Urinary incontinence after traumatic brain injury: incidence, outcomes and correlates. *Brain Inj.* 2003;17(6):469–478.

13. Yablon SA, Dostrow VG. Post-traumatic seizures and epilepsy. In: Zasler N, Katz D, Zafonte R, eds. *Brain Injury Medicine: Principles and Practice.* New York, NY: Demos Medical Publishing; 2007:443–468.

14. Temkin NR, Dikmen SS, Wilensky AJ, Keihm J, Chabal S, Winn HR. A randomized, double-blind study of phenytoin for the prevention of post-traumatic seizures. *N Engl J Med.* 1990;323(8):497–502.

15. Dikmen SS, Temkin NR, Miller B, Machamer J, Winn HR. Neurobehavioral effects of phenytoin prophylaxis of posttraumatic seizures. *JAMA.* 1991;265(10):1271–1277.

16. Cifu DX, Kaelin DL, Wall BE. Deep venous thrombosis: incidence on admission to a brain injury rehabilitation program. *Arch Phys Med Rehabil.* 1996;77(11):1182–1185.

17. Clagett GP, Anderson FA Jr, Geerts W, et al. Prevention of venous thromboembolism. *Chest.* 1998;114(5 suppl):531S–560S.

18. Kelly DF, Gonzalo IT, Cohan P, Berman N, Swerdloff R, Wang C. Hypopituitarism following traumatic brain injury and aneurysmal subarachnoid hemorrhage: a preliminary report. *J Neurosurg.* 2000;93(5):743–752.

19. Lieberman SA, Oberoi AL, Gilkison CR, Masel BE, Urban RJ. Prevalence of neuroendocrine dysfunction in patients recovering from traumatic brain injury. *J Clin Endocrinol Metab.* 2001;86(6):2752–2756.

30

Disorders of Consciousness

Brian Greenwald and Phalgun Nori

BACKGROUND

Definition

States of altered consciousness, referred to as disorders of consciousness (DOC), can be categorized as follows: coma, vegetative state (VS), and minimally conscious state (MCS). This classification is based on the recommendations of Aspen neurobehavioral conference workgroup in 1995 [1,2].

Pathophysiology

The etiology of DOC can be broadly categorized into traumatic versus nontraumatic brain injuries. Coma results from severe diffuse dysfunction of cerebral cortices, underlying white matter, or brainstem structures. The most common acute causes of VS are head trauma and hypoxic-ischemic encephalopathy. After an initial severe head injury, a patient may enter the comatose stage, which can last from several days to weeks. Thereafter, the brainstem and lower diencephalon resume function and the patient enters the VS. In a minority of patients, the VS occurs immediately after the insult, without an initial period of coma. The two most common neuropathologic changes noted in patients in VS are diffuse laminar cortical necrosis and diffuse axonal injury (DAI).

Differential Diagnosis

Other causes of altered mental status, including subclinical seizures, toxic, metabolic, and infectious encephalopathies, and structural changes such as hydrocephalus should be considered and ruled out.

Evaluation of the Patient

A thorough bedside neurologic examination should be performed to evaluate a patient with altered consciousness. The examination must be repeated to avoid misdiagnosis. The neurologic examination should evaluate the integrity of the brainstem and presence of higher cortical level functions.

COMA

Coma is a state of pathologic unconsciousness in which eyes remain closed and patient cannot be aroused. Defining feature is absence of sleep-wake cycles.

Evaluation

- Glasgow Coma Scale (GCS)—measures the best eye, motor, and verbal responses, and is a widely used and accepted severity score for traumatic brain injury (TBI). A score of 13 to 15 is considered mild TBI, whereas a score of 9 to 12 is considered moderate TBI and a score of 3 to 8 is classified as severe TBI. The lowest total score (i.e., 3 out of 15) indicates likely fatal damage, especially if both pupils fail to respond to light and oculovestibular responses are absent. Higher initial scores tend to predict better recovery [3]. By convention, the severity of head injury is initially defined by the GCS.
- JFK Coma Recovery Scale-Revised (CRS-R)—CRS-R is considered the most accurate objective clinical evaluation measure of DOC [4]. CRS-R was developed to help characterize and monitor patients with DOC, and has been used widely in both clinical and research settings within the United States and Europe. The CRS-R assesses auditory, visual, verbal, and motor functions as well as communication and arousal level.

VEGETATIVE STATE

VS is characterized by the absence of behavioral evidence of self or the environment in the context of evidence of functional restoration of the reticular system (e.g., eye opening or wakefulness). This diagnosis is made when there is no evidence of sustained or reproducible purposeful behavioral response to visual, auditory, tactile, or noxious stimuli, and no evidence of language comprehension or expression. VS is usually preceded by a period of coma.

- The terms Persistent VS (PVS) and Permanent VS (PNS) have been used by some, but these terms are discouraged because they imply not only level of consciousness but also prognosis, and may be misleading. The Aspen group recommends simply using the term VS accompanied by the cause of injury along with the specific length of time since onset.
- Prognosis—The Multi-Society Task Force on PVS concluded that patients in VS due to a TBI for greater than 1 year had a low probability of recovering awareness [5]. Based on a recent study by Estraneo [6], however,

33% of patients who were in a VS > 12 months from onset of injury either progressed to the MCS or regained consciousness with severe to extremely severe disability. Outcome is generally more favorable in younger patients. For patients who remain in the VS, the Task Force summarized the duration of survival time as follows: "Life expectancy ranges from 2 to 5 years, survival after 10 years is unusual" [5].

- Neuroimaging—Functional neuroimaging has been shown to aid in identification of covert cognitive function in patients in the VS. Activation studies have the potential to demonstrate distinct and specific physiological responses to environmental stimuli, such as changes in regional blood flow or changes in regional cerebral hemodynamics [6,7]. This approach presently remains largely experimental, although broader routine clinical application may develop in time.

MINIMALLY CONSCIOUS STATE

MCS is a condition of severely altered consciousness in which minimal but definite behavioral evidence of self or environmental awareness is demonstrated. In MCS, cognitively mediated behavior occurs inconsistently, but is reproducible or sustained long enough to be differentiated from reflexive behavior. A patient must demonstrate awareness of self and environment on a sustained basis by one or more of the following: following simple commands, gestural or verbal yes/no responses, intelligible verbalization, or purposeful behavior.

Emergence From MCS

Emergence from MCS to a higher state of consciousness is characterized by *reliable and consistent* demonstration of functional interactive communication and/or functional use of two different objects [2].

- Functional interactive communication may occur through verbalization, writing, yes/no signals, use of augmentative communication devices, or following commands. Six out of six correct responses to basic orientation or situational questions marks the transition from MCS to recovery of full consciousness [2].
- Functional use of objects requires that the patient demonstrate behavioral evidence of object discrimination; the patient should be able to use two different objects on two consecutive evaluations [2].

Avoiding Misdiagnosis

MCS can be differentiated from coma and VS by documenting the presence of specific behavioral features not found in either of these conditions. Patients in MCS demonstrate some capacity for cognitive processing and perception of pain; patients in VS do not experience pain. Overall prognosis of patients in MCS is more favorable relative to those in VS. Misdiagnosis can be minimized by structured clinical evaluation.

Prognosis for Recovery Following MCS

When comparing patients in MCS to those in VS, functional outcome appears to be better for the group of patients in MCS. Individuals in MCS showed more rapid improvement, a longer period of recovery, and significantly less functional disability at 12 months [8].

In a recent study by Luaute [10] which sought to characterize outcomes of a etiologically heterogeneous population of patients in VS and MCS for greater than one year, 30% of patients in MCS regained consciousness between one and five years after injury, though all were severely disabled.

TREATMENT

Pharmacological

- The mainstay of pharmacological management in DOC is minimization of use of medication that may exacerbate central nervous system depression or sedation (e.g., opiates, benzodiazepines, β-blockers, and anticonvulsants).
- Amantadine—There is paucity of data on the effects of medications on recovery from prolonged impairments of consciousness. Amantadine is a tricyclic water-soluble amine salt that affects the synthesis, accumulation, release, and reuptake of catecholamines in the central nervous system. Amantadine has been hypothesized to facilitate brain recovery through effects on dopamine and N-methyl-D-aspartate (NMDA) receptors. In a small randomized controlled trial [9], amantadine was shown to improve rate of recovery in patients with DAI-associated TBI, but was not specific for patients with impaired consciousness. Stimulants such as amphetamine and methylphenidate have been used to facilitate arousal and recovery as well, but at present there is insufficient data to promote routine use of these agents to promote recovery from DOC in TBI.

Nonpharmacological

- Supportive care is key in management of DOC. Maintaining skin integrity, preventing or treating infections, assessing or providing for adequate splinting and equipment needs, and educating family or caregivers about the nature of this condition are core components of management for these patients.

Table 30.1 Comparison of Clinical Features Associated With Coma, Vegetative State, and Minimally Conscious State

Condition	Consciousness	Sleep/Wake	Motor Function	Auditory Function	Visual Fixation	Communication	Emotion
Coma	None	Absent	Reflex and postural responses only	None	None	None	None
Vegetative state	None	Present	Postures or withdraws to noxious stimuli	Startle	Startle	None	None
			Occasional nonpurposeful movement	Brief orienting to sound	Brief visual fixation		Reflexive crying or smiling
Minimally conscious state	Partial	Present	Localizes noxious stimuli	Localizes sound location	Sustained visual fixation	Contingent vocalization	Contingent smiling or crying
			Reaches for objects	Inconsistent command following	Sustained visual pursuit	Inconsistent but intelligible verbalization or gesture	
			Holds or touches objects in a manner that accommodates size and shape				
			Automatic movements (e.g., scratching)				

From Ref. [2].

- Deep brain stimulation (DBS)—In a recent study by Schiff [10], DBS was undertaken in a patient who remained in MCS 6 years after TBI. At baseline, the patient was nonverbal and had inconsistent command following. The DBS electrodes were implanted targeting the anterior intralaminar thalamic nuclei and adjacent paralaminar regions of both thalami. After DBS implantation, changes were noted in the behavior of the patient, including longer periods of eye opening, increased responsiveness to commands, and intelligible verbalization. The observed improvements in arousal level, motor control, and behavioral persistence might be due to direct activation of frontal cortical and basal ganglia systems, which play a key role in the brainstem arousal systems. This single case report suggests that further study may be warranted to determine whether the implantation of central DBS might benefit patients who are in MCS. DBS was not shown to have any effect on patients in either coma or VS [11].

ADDITIONAL READING

Electronic References
JFK Coma Recovery Scale. http://www.tbims.org/combi/crs/index.html
Schiff ND. Measurements and models of cerebral function in the severely injured
    brain. http://www-users.med.cornell.edu/~jdvicto/pdfs/schi06a.pdf

Textbook/Chapter
Giacino JT, Katz DI, Schiff N. Assessment and rehabilitative management of
    individuals with disorders of consciousness. In: Zasler ND, Katz DI, Zafonte
    RD, eds. *Brain Injury Medicine: Principles and Practice.* New York, NY:
    Demos Medical Publishing; 2007:423–439.

Journal Articles
Giacino JT, Ashwal S, Childs N. The minimally conscious state definition and
    diagnostic criteria. *Neurology.* 2002;58:349–353.
Monti MM, Vanhaudenhuyse A, Coleman MR. Willful modulation of brain activ-
    ity in disorders of consciousness. *New Engl J Med.* 2010;362:579–589.

REFERENCES

1. American Congress of Rehabilitation Medicine. Recommendations for use
   of uniform nomenclature pertinent to patients with severe alterations in
   consciousness. *Arch Phys Med Rehabil.* 1995;76:205–209.
2. Giacino JT, Ashwal S, Childs N, et al. The minimally conscious state: definition and diagnostic criteria. *Neurology.* 2002;58(3):349–353.
3. Jennett B, Teasdale G, Braakman R, Minderhoud J, Heiden J, Kurze T. Prognosis
   of patients with severe head injury. *Neurosurgery.* 1979;4(4):283–289.
4. Giacino JT, Kalmar K, Whyte J. The JFK Coma Recovery Scale-Revised:
   measurement characteristics and diagnostic utility. *Arch Phys Med Rehabil.*
   2004;85(12):2020–2029.

5. The Multi-Society Task Force on PVS. Medical aspects of the persistent vegetative state. *N Engl J Med.* 1994;330:1499–1508, 1572. [Erratum, *N Engl J Med.* 1995;333:130.]

6. Estraneo A, Moretta P, Loreto V, et al. Late recovery after traumatic, anoxic, or hemorrhagic long-lasting vegetative state. *Neurology.* 2010;75(3):239–245.

7. Coleman MR, Davis MH, Rodd JM, et al. Towards the routine use of brain imaging to aid the clinical diagnosis of disorders of consciousness. *Brain.* 2009;132(Pt 9):2541–2552.

8. Monti MM, Vanhaudenhuyse A, Coleman MR, et al. Willful modulation of brain activity in disorders of consciousness. *N Engl J Med.* 2010;362(7):579–589.

9. Whyte J, Katz D, Long D, et al. Predictors of outcome in prolonged post-traumatic disorders of consciousness and assessment of medication effects: A multicenter study. *Arch Phys Med Rehabil.* 2005;86(3):453–462.

10. Luaute J, Maucort-Boulch D, Tell L, et al. Long-term outcomes of chronic minimally conscious and vegetative states. *Neurology.* 2010;75(3):246–252.

11. Giacino JT, Whyte J. Amantadine to improve neurorecovery in traumatic brain injury-associated diffuse axonal injury: a pilot double-blind randomized trial. *J Head Trauma Rehabil.* 2003;18(1):4–5; author reply 5.

12. Schiff ND, Giacino JT, Kalmar K, et al. Behavioural improvements with thalamic stimulation after severe traumatic brain injury. *Nature.* 2007;448(7153):600–603.

13. Yamamoto T, Katayama Y. Deep brain stimulation therapy for the vegetative state. *Neuropsychol Rehabil.* 2005;15:406–413.

31

The Role of Specialized Brain Injury Units in the Rehabilitation Process

Allen W. Brown

LONGITUDINAL CARE

- Consensus exists for providing a continuum of care to individuals and their families or significant others after moderate to severe traumatic brain injury (TBI), from acute hospitalization to outpatient clinical care and community-based services.
- Ideally, inpatient rehabilitation brings into focus the comprehensive rehabilitation plan of care initiated by rehabilitation consultation and services provided during acute hospitalization, medical and surgical treatment, and stabilization.
- Inpatient brain injury rehabilitation provides comprehensive medical rehabilitation services as individuals emerge from trauma-induced alterations of consciousness and families or significant others begin adjusting to these changing circumstances.
- As the link between acute medical care and community-based services, specialized inpatient brain injury rehabilitation units are a crucial source of clinical data, to define baseline injury severity, monitor progress, measure outcome and satisfaction, and to use for benchmarking and practice improvement [1].

PRACTICE MODELS

Centralized Brain Injury Units

- Geographically smaller countries with nationalized health care, and states in the United States with single urban medical centers and large rural populations, often have trauma systems that direct individuals who experience catastrophic and polytraumatic injuries to single trauma centers for definitive care.
- This practice model has been shown to improve outcome compared to usual care [2]. This model of care, providing acute and rehabilitation

services in a single location from admission to the acute hospital through discharge after rehabilitation, is uncommon in the United States, and not as developed in Europe for TBI as it is for stroke [3].

Brain Injury Services in Rehabilitation Units

- Most brain rehabilitation units in the United States exist either within acute hospitals or as free-standing rehabilitation hospitals.
- Clinical services—Consensus exists about what clinical services should be provided during inpatient rehabilitation for TBI [4].
  - Rehabilitation services should be customized to individual needs and refined with clinical change.
  - Services should be comprehensive and interdisciplinary.
  - Cognitive and behavioral assessment should be included.
  - Evaluation of and treatment for substance abuse should be a component of these rehabilitation programs.
  - Persons with TBI, and their families or significant others should be involved in the rehabilitation process. Families and significant others should also be supported through the rehabilitation process.
  - The use of medications for behavioral management and cognitive enhancement should be carefully considered.
  - Specialized programming is necessary for individuals in pediatric and geriatric populations with TBI.
- Admission guidelines—Many rehabilitation units use admission guidelines as set forth by the Centers for Medicare and Medicaid Services, although these guidelines may not apply to individuals not covered by government-funded health care.
  - An individual should be able and willing to actively participate in an intensive rehabilitation program (recommended intensity and duration: 3 hours of daily therapy services, 5 out of each 7 days) and should be expected to make measurable improvement in functional capacity or adaptation to impairments.
  - Rehabilitation services should be ordered by a rehabilitation physician with specialized training and experience in rehabilitation services and be administered by an interdisciplinary team.
  - Specialized rehabilitation physician and nursing care is needed.
  - Rehabilitation care should be provided by qualified personnel in rehabilitation nursing, physical therapy, occupational therapy, speech-language pathology, social services, psychological services, and prosthetic and orthotic services.
  - Appropriate care can not be provided in a less intensive medical setting, such as in a skilled care environment.

- Rehabilitation treatment for individuals in coma or a minimally conscious state include the following.

  - Rehabilitation care for individuals who remain in coma or who are minimally conscious after reaching medical stability is provided in specialized hospital-based rehabilitation settings, long-term acute care facilities, or in a skilled care environment.
  - Treatment approaches are generally grouped into three types—sensory stimulation, physical management, and neuromodulation [5].
  - Variations in determining level of consciousness, small sample sizes, and poor study design have limited the application of existing research to develop clinical assessment and treatment guidelines.
  - Many interventions have shown some positive effects on increasing arousal, but more methodologically rigorous study is needed [6].

- Rehabilitation after TBI and polytrauma in the military (see also Chapter 64)

  - The Polytrauma System of Care is an integrated system of specialized care created by the Department of Veterans Affairs.
  - It serves veterans and active duty service members who have TBI and polytrauma injuries through regional centers around the country.
  - Clinical trials in these centers have shown differential positive effects in subpopulations for cognitive and functional treatment approaches [7].

BRAIN INJURY TREATMENT EFFECTIVENESS

- In an evidence-based review of randomized controlled trials, quasi-randomized and quasi-experimental designs—comparing multidisciplinary rehabilitation with either routinely available local services or lower levels of intervention; or trials comparing an intervention in different settings or at different levels of intensity—it was found that [8]:

  - for moderate to severe injury, there was "strong evidence" of benefit from formal intervention;
  - for patients with moderate to severe TBI already in rehabilitation, there was "strong evidence" that more intensive programs are associated with earlier functional gains;
  - there was "limited evidence" that specialized inpatient brain injury rehabilitation units may provide additional functional gains.

- In an assimilation of randomized controlled trials in the literature and a review of TBI rehabilitation trials chosen based on evaluation of research quality irrespective of study design, it was found that [9]:

- early intensive rehabilitation is recommended;
- specialized brain injury programs are recommended for individuals with complex needs;
- vocational programs are recommended for individuals with this potential.

BRAIN INJURY REHABILITATION DATABASES

- A national consortium of 16 academic rehabilitation research centers, the Traumatic Brain Injury Model Systems (funded by the National Institute on Disability and Rehabilitation Research), have contributed data about individuals admitted to specialized brain injury inpatient rehabilitation units to a common database since 1989.
- Data from acute care and inpatient rehabilitation are submitted, and outcome data are collected from subjects at 1, 2, and 5 years after injury and every 5 years thereafter.
- This database is used for longitudinal analysis of data from people with TBI in their communities and supports research toward developing evidence-based TBI rehabilitation interventions [10].
- Other proprietary data sources (such as eRehabData.com and the Uniform Data System for Medical Rehabilitation) allow inpatient brain injury rehabilitation practices to monitor clinical metrics and outcomes for benchmarking and to support practice improvement [11].

ADDITIONAL READING

Electronic References

Model Systems Knowledge Translation Center. http://msktc.washington.edu/
The TBI Model System National Data and Statistical Center at Craig Hospital. http://www.tbindsc.org

Textbook/Chapter

Mysiw WJ, Fugate LP, Clinchot DM. Assessment, early rehabilitation intervention, and tertiary prevention. In: Zasler ND, Katz DI, Zafonte RD, eds. *Brain Injury Medicine: Principles and Practice*. New York, NY: Demos Medical Publishing; 2007:283–301.

Journal Articles

Prvu Bettger JA, Stineman MG. Effectiveness of multidisciplinary rehabilitation services in postacute care: state-of-the-science. A review. *Arch Phys Med Rehabil*. 2007;88(11):1526–1534.
Ragnarsson KT. Traumatic brain injury research since the 1998 NIH consensus conference: accomplishments and unmet goals. *J Head Trauma Rehabil*. 2006;21(5):379–387.

REFERENCES

1. Horn SD, Gassaway J. Practice-based evidence study design for comparative effectiveness research. *Med Care*. 2007;45(10 suppl 2):S50–S57.
2. Engberg AW, Liebach A, Nordenbo A. Centralized rehabilitation after severe traumatic brain injury–a population-based study. *Acta Neurol Scand*. 2006;113(3):178–184.
3. Stroke Unit Trialists' Collaboration: Organised inpatient (stroke unit) care for stroke [Systematic Review]. *Cochrane Database of Syst Rev*. 2007;4:CD000197.
4. Anonymous. Consensus conference. Rehabilitation of persons with traumatic brain injury. NIH Consensus Development Panel on Rehabilitation of Persons With Traumatic Brain Injury. *JAMA*. 1999;282:974–983.
5. Giacino JT, Katz DI, Schiff N. Assessment and rehabilitative management of individuals with disorders of consciousness. In: Zasler ND, Katz DI, Zafonte RD, eds. *Brain Injury Medicine: Principles and Practice*. New York, NY: Demos Medical Publishing; 2007:432–439.
6. Meyer MJ, Megyesi J, Meythaler J, et al. Acute management of acquired brain injury Part III: an evidence-based review of interventions used to promote arousal from coma. *Brain Inj*. 2010;24(5):722–729.
7. Vanderploeg RD, Schwab K, Walker WC, et al. Rehabilitation of traumatic brain injury in active duty military personnel and veterans: Defense and Veterans Brain Injury Center randomized controlled trial of two rehabilitation approaches. *Arch Phys Med Rehabil*. 2008;89(12):2227–2238.
8. Turner-Stokes L, Nair A, Sedki I, Disler PB, Wade DT. 2009 Multi-disciplinary rehabilitation for acquired brain injury in adults of working age. Cochrane Database of Systematic Reviews.
9. Turner-Stokes L. Evidence for the effectiveness of multi-disciplinary rehabilitation following acquired brain injury: a synthesis of two systematic approaches. *J Rehabil Med*. 2008;40(9):691–701.
10. Dijkers MPP, Harrison-Felix CP, Marwitz JHMA. The traumatic brain injury model systems: history and contributions to clinical service and research. *J Head Trauma Rehabil*. 2010;25:1–12.
11. Granger CV, Markello SJ, Graham JE, Deutsch A, Reistetter TA, Ottenbacher KJ. The uniform data system for medical rehabilitation: report of patients with traumatic brain injury discharged from rehabilitation programs in 2000–2007. *Am J Phys Med Rehabil*. 2010;89(4):265–278.

32

Rehabilitation Nursing

Ann S. Bines

DEFINITION

Rehabilitation nursing is a specialty that centers on the diagnosis and treatment of human responses of individuals and/or groups to actual or potential health problems relative to altered function ability and lifestyle [1].

- Major areas of focus with the inpatient traumatic brain injury (TBI) population:
  - Pain assessment and treatment
  - Maintenance/assessment and treatment of skin integrity
  - Promotion of a physiologic sleep/wake pattern
  - Continence of bowel and bladder
  - Assessment/participation in behavior modification
  - Providing for safety/promoting independence restraint reduction
  - Promoting advocacy through education
  - Emotional/psychosocial support

PAIN ASSESSMENT AND TREATMENT

- Incidence of pain significant, etiology variable, and assessment is difficult due to cognitive issues. Consistency of care givers (nurses, unlicensed personnel, and family) is very beneficial in recognizing signs of pain in cognitively impaired patients.
- Assessment is inherently difficult in this patient population. No conventional tools have been validated in the cognitively impaired TBI population. Pain assessment in patients who cannot verbalize their pain should include subjective assessment of pain behaviors [2,3].
- Validated tools (primarily validated in elderly patients with dementia):
  - Checklist of Nonverbal Pain Indicators. Scoring of 6 behaviors—vocalization, grimaces, bracing, rubbing, restlessness, and verbal complaints [4]
  - Critical Care Pain Observation Tool. Facial expression, body movements, muscle tension, vocalization, or compliance with ventilator [5]

- Face, Legs, Activity, Cry, Consolability scale. Facial expression, leg movement, body activity, cry/vocalization, and consolability [6]
- Treatment
  - Use multimodal therapy to provide pain relief with less toxicity.
  - Nonpharmacological therapies include heat, cold, repositioning, diversion, and behavioral management. Maximize use of these modalities.
  - Use analgesics for analgesia, not to control behavior. Taper or discontinue drugs that are not effective.

ASSESSMENT AND PREVENTION OF SKIN BREAKDOWN

- This is a high-risk population for development of pressure ulcers. Risk factors include decreased sensation/movement, agitation/nonpurposeful movement (e.g., spasticity/dystonia), nutritional impairment, and incontinence.
- Extrinsic factors causing pressure ulcers include pressure, shear, friction, moisture, and equipment.
- An estimated 1.6 billion dollars is spent annually on care of pressure ulcers. Cost per hospital stay ranges from $200 up to $7000 (for complex stage IV) [7].
- Most frequently used risk assessment tools are the Braden and Norton scales. Risk for skin breakdown should be initially assessed on admission and then on a routine frequency. Assess skin for breakdown daily.
  - Norton-5 parameters scored/assessed: physical condition, mental state, activity, mobility, and incontinence. Lower scores indicate high risk. Risk onset begins at 12 or less.
  - Braden-6 parameters scored/assessed: sensory perception, skin moisture, physical activity, nutritional status, friction/shear, and ability to change body position. Lower scores indicate high risk. Risk onset begins at 16 or less [8].
- Prevention
  - Reduce/limit moisture: Establish a program to enhance continence. Use pH balanced soaps/cleansers. Use moisture barrier as needed to prevent skin breakdown. Perineal areas open to air when in bed.
  - Optimize nutrition/hydration: Calorie counts, mineral/vitamin supplements.
  - Pressure relief: Bed surfaces, chair cushions, turning frequency/ use of log to track, adequate padding of orthotics, and padding of rigid surfaces in bed and wheel chair. Repositioning program for wheelchair-bound patients who cannot weight shift independently off-load bony prominences.

- Shear/friction prevention: Use of lifting aids/equipment when repositioning. Raise knee gatch of bed when the head of the bed is elevated to decrease shear/friction forces.

PROMOTION OF SLEEP/WAKE PATTERN

- Assessment: Use of log by caregivers due to limited ability of patients to self report information. Document sleep onset and duration of sleep periods. Include patient/family assessment of quality of sleep
- Interventions
  - Use of pharmacological agents. Timing of administration early enough to enhance sleep but not affect ability to participate actively in therapy is important. Use sleep aids to promote sleep—not to control behavior.
  - Control environmental factors such as noise, light. Employ non-pharmacological sleep aids—music, evening showers, or TV. Be aware of patient's premorbid sleep behavior; hours of sleep per night shift work. Do not force sleep. Schedule nursing care so as not to interfere with sleep.

CONTINENCE OF BOWEL AND BLADDER

Continence is a major area of nursing focus. Functional Independence Measure gain/loss in bowel and bladder continence is an externally reported outcome measure/benchmark for rehab programs. Continence is also a primary goal for families/caregivers. Incontinence may present a burden of care that prevents home discharge.

- Bladder incontinence in TBI patients
  - Incontinence is most often due to uninhibited neurogenic bladder-cerebral control decreased, reduced bladder capacity, or frequent uninhibited bladder contractions with voiding as soon as urge is perceived. Sensation and bulbocavernosus reflex are intact. Bladder empties completely
  - Transient, acute functional incontinence, often of precipitous onset, is typically reversible. Related to impaired physical/cognitive/behavioral function
  - Assessment-monitor postvoid residual; review medications, consider presence of age/premorbid incontinence issues, urinary tract infection
  - Interventions to reestablish continence: Prior to initiating any program, assess patient's behavior, core strength, balance, and level of assistance with transfers. Continence can be achieved using bedpans, urinals, commodes, or condom catheters. Consistency of caregivers in adhering to the program outlined is very important.

Regulate fluid intake. Ensure privacy. Provide positive reinforcement [9,10].
- Scheduled/timed voids—assess patients voiding patterns and replicate (usually every 2–4 hours)
- Habit training
- Prompted voiding

- Bowel incontinence
  - Cause—uninhibited neurogenic bowel—reflexes, spinal reflex arc, and bowel and saddle sensation intact. Decreased awareness of need to defecate and decreased control of external sphincter/ability to inhibit defecation. May have a sense of urgency (perceived).
  - Assessment: consider premorbid bowel habits. Identify date of last bowel movement. Review current diet, hydration status.
  - Interventions to promote bowel continence: assess patient's ability to transfer to/use the toilet. Be consistent in administering the bowel program. Promote an upright sitting position, with knees bent for defecation. Avoid use of a bedpan; utilize shower or toileting chair. Consider an abdominal binder to increase abdominal pressure. Adequate hydration/fiber. Initiate program after food intake to activate gastrocolic reflex. Plan bowel program so as not to interfere with participation in therapy. Provide privacy [10].
  - Medications may include.
    - stool softeners (scheduled, not as needed) with or without a laxative component
    - bulk products
    - suppositories to stimulate the defecation reflex

BEHAVIOR MODIFICATION

Use consistent tool(s) to assess behaviors by entire team. Document behaviors, factors that provoke undesirable behaviors and response to interventions. Medications should be used in conjunction with a consistent approach to management of adverse behaviors.

PROVIDING FOR SAFETY/PROMOTING INDEPENDENCE/RESTRAINT REDUCTION

- A restraint is the direct application of physical force to an individual, to restrict his/her freedom of movement. Medications can also be considered a form of restraint. Restraints have not been proven to decrease falls.
- The Joint Commission and other regulating bodies have developed standards for the use of restraints. Overriding premise is to reduce/limit the use of restraints. Institutions must develop policies to govern

the use of restraints. The policy defines what types of restraints can be used, who can apply restraints, how often the patient must be assessed while in a restraint and by whom, the time frame within which an order for restraint must be written, and how often the order must be renewed. There are specific criteria that define why a restraint can be used, and these criteria must be documented and consistent among the caregivers. Also required is documentation of alternatives tried prior to a restraint being initiated. The standards also speak to the patient/family education that must be done when restraints are used. Restraint orders cannot be written as "prn or standing orders" [11].

- Common restraints include limb restraints, side rails (not when used to facilitate repositioning in bed by patient), mittens, wrap around seat belts (any belt that cannot be easily removed by the patient), and bed enclosures.

- Restraint alternatives: Devices that do not restrict movement but either alert staff to egress or "slow down" a patient's ability to engage in an unsafe behavior. Examples of restraint "alternatives" include bed exit alarms systems, wheel chair alarm systems ("talking" seat belts), abdominal binders, wheel chair lap trays, upper limb orthotic devices for functional positioning, Velcro straps for positioning in wheel chairs, video observation areas/rooms, and 1:1 caregivers/sitters [12].

- Most institutions have Continuous Quality Improvement programs that monitor fall rates and restraint usage. At minimum, daily assessment should be made by the entire team of the need to continue use of restraints. Interventions that can be used as alternatives to restraints, to maintain patient safety, should be explored.

ADDITIONAL READING

Electronic References

http://www.jointcommission.org/AccreditationPrograms/Hospitals/
http://www.aacbis.net/downloads.html

Textbooks/Chapters

Hoeman, SP. *Rehabilitation Nursing: Prevention, Intervention and Outcomes.* St Louis, MO: Mosby Inc; 2008.

Mauk KL, ed. *The Specialty Practice of Rehabilitation Nursing: A Core Curriculum.* 5th ed. Skokie, IL: Rehabilitation Nursing Foundation; 2007.

Journal Articles

American Association of Neuroscience Nursing. *Nursing management of adults with severe traumatic brain injury: Clinical Practice Guidelines.* Glenview, IL: Author; 2008.

Lemke, DM. Riding out the storm: sympathetic storming after traumatic brain injury. *J Neurosci Nurs.* 2004;36(1):4–9.

REFERENCES

1. Association of Rehabilitative Nurses. *Standards and Scope of Rehabilitation Practice.* Glenview, IL: Author; 2000.
2. Herr K, Coyne PJ, Key T, et al.; American Society for Pain Management Nursing. Pain assessment in the nonverbal patient: position statement with clinical practice recommendations. *Pain Manag Nurs.* 2006;7(2):44–52.
3. McGrath PJ, Rosmus C, Canfield C, Campbell MA, Hennigar A. Behaviours caregivers use to determine pain in non-verbal, cognitively impaired individuals. *Dev Med Child Neurol.* 1998;40(5):340–343.
4. Feldt KS. The checklist of nonverbal pain indicators (CNPI). *Pain Manag Nurs.* 2000;1(1):13–21.
5. Gélinas C, Fillion L, Puntillo KA, Viens C, Fortier M. Validation of the critical-care pain observation tool in adult patients. *Am J Crit Care.* 2006;15(4):420–427.
6. Voepel-Lewis T, Merkel S, Tait AR, Trzcinka A, Malviya S. The reliability and validity of the Face, Legs, Activity, Cry, Consolability observational tool as a measure of pain in children with cognitive impairment. *Anesth Analg.* 2002;95(5):1224–1229.
7. Arnold MC. Pressure ulcer prevention and management: the current evidence for care. *AACN Clin Issues.* 2003;14(4):411–428.
8. Braden B, Bergstrom S. A conceptual scheme for the study and etiology of pressure sores. *Rehabilitation Nurs.* 1989;14(5):258.
9. Doughty DB, ed. *Urinary and Fecal Incontinence: Nursing Management.* 3rd ed. St Louis, MO: Mosby; 2006.
10. Mauk KL, ed. *The Specialty Practice of Rehabilitation Nursing.* 5th ed. Skokie, IL: Rehabilitation Nursing Foundation.
11. Joint Commission E-Dition http://e-dition.jcrinc.com/Frame.aspx
12. Cohen C, Neufeld R, Dunbar J, Pflug L, Breuer B. Old problem, different approach: alternatives to physical restraints. *J Gerontol Nurs.* 1996;22(2):23–29.

33

Physical Therapy
Mobility, Transfers, and Ambulation

Catherine Burress

EPIDEMIOLOGY

According to the National Institute of Health, traumatic brain injury (TBI) is the leading cause of long-term disability in children and young adults in the United States [1]. TBI patients present with a wide variety of impairments and functional limitations that require physical therapist (PT) intervention. The management of TBI patients can be complex, as they present with a wide range of symptoms that may be further complicated by impairments in cognition, communication, and behavior.

PRESENTATION AND EVALUATION

A major challenge of the TBI population is the heterogeneous presentation without clear patterns of physical impairment. This requires the PT to have a thorough understanding of all systems that require examination. Often the evaluation will be incomplete and observational due to the patient's inability to fully participate in the examination.

- Sensory impairments may include deficits in light touch, temperature sensation, deep pressure, pain sensation, proprioception, and vibratory sensation. Testing may be limited by communication impairments.
- Decreased range of motion (ROM) or contracture may develop secondary to decreased mobility, suboptimal positioning, and spasticity. Evaluation includes the use of goniometry and visual observation.
- Motor control impairments present as weakness, decreased coordination, impaired balance, and movement disorders. Evaluation includes use of manual muscle testing and observation of antigravity movement, assessment of heel to shin and rapid alternating movements, evaluation of static and dynamic balance—including balance reactions—and use of standardized tests such as the Berg Balance Scale [2].
- Changes in tone may present in a hemiparetic pattern, tetraparetic pattern, or may be localized. It may manifest as spasticity, spasms,

or localized dystonias. Objective assessment of spasticity uses the Modified Ashworth Scale [2].

- Thirty percent to 65% of TBI patients will present with some variety of vestibular pathology [3]. Symptoms may include dizziness, vertigo, nausea, disequilibrium, and visual disturbances. Assessment may include use of the Dix-Hallpike test, observation of visual tracking, saccades, and nystagmus, and when appropriate the Dynamic Gait Index or Clinical Test of Sensory Integration in Balance (Foam and Dome) [3]. Location of the lesion, determined through clinical testing, will dictate appropriate treatment.

- Fractures and soft tissue injuries are often comorbid diagnoses that the therapist must consider and that may impact treatment.

- Functional mobility is often the area of greatest focus with TBI patients.

  - Bed mobility assessment should include rolling and supine to-and-from sit transitions. Rolling assessment will provide the PT with information on possible vestibular deficits, trunk ROM and strength. Supine to-and-from sit transitions may provide information on trunk ROM and strength, as well as general upper and lower extremity ROM and strength.

  - Transfer assessment, including assist level, may incorporate use of the Hoyer, squat pivot transfer, lateral or sliding board transfers, and stand pivot or stand step transfers. Choosing the appropriate transfer requires the clinical assessment, observation, and judgment of the PT. This assessment provides the therapist with further insight into strength, ROM, coordination, spasticity, and balance skills.

  - Ambulation assessment is not always appropriate with moderate to severe TBI patients. The PT's clinical judgment will dictate whether to proceed with this activity. Gait assessment is typically initiated in a highly supported environment, such as the parallel bars or a supported ambulation system such as the Lite Gait, and will provide further observational evidence of strength, ROM, balance, spasticity, and coordination.

TREATMENT

A recent systematic review found high-level evidence that more intensive rehabilitation programs for TBI patients lead to greater functional outcomes, and that patients with moderate to severe brain injuries benefit from formal therapeutic intervention [2].

- Sensory stimulation within the context of physical therapy will include weight bearing activities in sitting and standing, change of position— including sidelying, prone, and upright—and proprioceptive input through stretching and ROM.

- ROM and stretching programs are important to prevent or reduce loss of flexibility. Splinting or bracing may be used as an adjunct to more active interventions to maintain and, at times, increase ROM [3].
- Strengthening programs are important to allow progression of functional mobility skills. TBI patients are often not able to participate in traditionally structured progressive resistive strengthening programs. In these instances, patients can benefit from strengthening within the context of functional mobility. When patients present with less than antigravity strength, using slings to suspend the extremity or friction-free surfaces can allow the patient to more effectively activate very weak muscles.
- Balance training will likely start in sitting, initially working on static sitting balance, progressing as appropriate to dynamic standing balance. Therapists may include use of compliant surfaces, perturbations, and distracting environments to progress balance training dependent on patient-specific impairments. Dault and Dugas demonstrated that a balance training program is also beneficial in addressing muscle strengthening in TBI patients [4].
- Coordination training may include object manipulation with extremities, varying speed, and use of weights to manage ataxia and movement disorders.
- Spasticity is often a limiting factor for TBI patients, impacting positioning in bed and wheelchairs, setup and positioning for transfers, and limiting motor control. When left untreated, spasticity leads to muscle and soft tissue shortening and eventual contractures [5]. Physical therapy management will include stretching and ROM programs, strengthening of the antagonist muscles, bracing, and serial casting.
  - Serial casting can improve ROM, reduce muscle tone [2], and reduce plantar flexion contractures [6].
  - PTs should consider how ROM gains will be maintained, determine a strategy for ongoing spasticity management when casting is discontinued, and what functional goals may be achieved with casting.
- Vestibular rehabilitation programs will incorporate the use of habituation exercises, gaze stabilization exercises, corrective maneuvers for benign paroxysmal positional vertigo, compensatory training, and progressing functional mobility as appropriate [3]. TBI patients will often require modifications to the vestibular rehabilitation program, including hand-over-hand assist for cervical rotation when performing gaze stabilization exercises, using modified positioning for the Epley maneuver, or simply utilizing position changes and mobility training for habituation.

- Functional mobility training should include bed mobility, transfers, and sitting, and progress to standing and ambulation as appropriate. Current literature supports the use of task-specific training for improved skill acquisition: A recent systematic review of the literature found high-level evidence to support the use of task-oriented and repetitive training [2]. This would support training patients by performing specific functional mobility skills multiple times sequentially during a session. However, this may be challenging for TBI populations with poor attention or problems with agitation, therefore therapists may need to consider the use of varied practice throughout the session.

  Recovery of ambulation is frequently a high priority for patients and family members. Traditional gait training is often initiated in the parallel bars and progressed to an assistive device such as a walker or cane as patients improve their balance and strength. Body weight–supported treadmill training (BWSTT) has been shown to be highly effective in the stroke population, but research with TBI patients has shown less beneficial results [2,7]. However, in clinical practice, BWSTT may be useful with TBI patients who are not following commands, may have poor attention or initiation for ambulation, impaired safety awareness, poor balance or coordination, or require a significant amount of physical assist. BWSTT can be a safer, more successful and earlier intervention to initiate gait training.

- Orthotics are used by many clinicians to improve ambulation, although others avoid it because of concerns that an orthosis may disrupt normal gait kinematics and lead to disuse atrophy of the muscles that control the joint [8].

  - A systematic review of the literature on the use of ankle foot orthoses (AFO) to improve ambulation concluded that there is good evidence that the AFO increased walking speed, increased stride length, increased cadence, and decreased energy expenditure during ambulation. The review found conflicting evidence on increasing or decreasing muscle activation of the anterior tibialis and gastrocnemius/soleus complex [8].

  - The use of AFOs is often beneficial to facilitate early ambulation in brain injury patients, however timing/appropriateness of prescription must be based on clinical judgment.

- Specialized seating and positioning is often required to prevent skin breakdown, decrease risk of secondary complications, maintain patient safety, optimize positioning, and allow patient mobility when ambulation is not an appropriate goal. Power wheelchair mobility should be considered for TBI patients with very low-level mobility but minimal cognitive deficits.

BEHAVIOR MANAGEMENT

Behavioral impairments occur in 35% to 70% of patients with acquired brain injury [9]. These may include agitation, restlessness, aggression, disinhibition, impulsiveness, distractibility, and inattention. Implementing a structured and comprehensive behavior management plan can minimize or reduce behavioral manifestations. An effective plan will involve all team members, including the PT, and will include direct observation of the behavior, assessment of the environment, identification of the purpose of the behavior, and identification of antecedents to the behavior, and will provide appropriate reinforcement of desired/functional behaviors [9].

CONCLUSION

Effective management of TBI patients requires thorough evaluation, implementation of an effective treatment plan, and development of an individualized behavior management plan. When these elements are appropriately applied, physical therapy interventions can be successful and rewarding for the patient, family, and treatment team.

ADDITIONAL READING

Electronic Reference
American Physical Therapy Association. www.apta.org

Textbooks/Chapters
Herdman SJ. *Vestibular Rehabilitation*. 3rd ed. Philadelphia, PA: FA Davis Company; 2007.

Pierson FM, Fairchild SL. *Principles and Techniques of Patient Care*. 4th ed. WB Saunders & Company; 2008.

O'Sullivan SB, Schmitz, TJ. *Physical Rehabilitation*. 5th ed. Philadelphia, PA: FA Davis Company; 2007.

Umphred, DA. *Neurologic Rehabilitation*. 4th ed. St Louis, MO: Mosby; 2001.

Journal Articles
Leung J, Mosely A. Impact of ankle-foot orthoses on gait and leb muscle activity in adults with hemiplegia: systematic literature review. *Physiotherapy*. 2003;89(1):39–55.

Marshall S, Teasell R, Bayona N, et al. Motor impairment rehabilitation post acquired brain injury. *Brain In*. 2007;21(2):133–160.

Slifer KJ, Amari A. Behavior management for children and adolescents with acquired brain injury. *Dev Disabil Res Rev*. 2009;15:144–151.

Wilson DJ, Powell M, Gorham JL, et al. Ambulation training with and without partial weightbearing after traumatic brain injury. *Am J Phys Med Rehabil*. 2006;85(1):68–74.

REFERENCES

1. Maskell F, Chiarelli P, Isles R. Dizziness after traumatic brain injury: overview and measurement in the clinical setting. *Brain Inj*. 2006;20(3):293–305.

2. Hellweg S, Johannes S. Physiotherapy after traumatic brain injury: a systematic review of the literature. *Brain Inj*. 2008;22(5):365–373.

3. Herdman SJ. *Vestibular Rehabilitation*. 3rd ed. Philadelphia, PA: FA Davis Company; 2007.

4. Marshall S, Teasell R, Bayona N, et al. Motor impairment rehabilitation post acquired brain injury. *Brain Inj*. 2007;21(2):133–160.

5. Ward AB. Spasticity treatment with botulinum toxins. *J Neural Transm*. 2008;115(4):607–616.

6. Wilson DJ, Powell M, Gorham JL, Childers MK. Ambulation training with and without partial weightbearing after traumatic brain injury: results of a randomized, controlled trial. *Am J Phys Med Rehabil*. 2006;85(1):68–74.

7. Leung J, Mosely A. Impact of ankle-foot orthoses on gait and leb muscle activity in adults with hemiplegia: systematic literature review. *Physiotherapy*. 2003;89(1):39–55.

8. Slifer KJ, Amari A. Behavior management for children and adolescents with acquired brain injury. *Dev Disabil Res Rev*. 2009;15(2):144–151.

9. Lombard LA, Zafonte RD. Agitation after traumatic brain injury: considerations and treatment options. *Am J Phys Med Rehabil*. 2005;84(10):797–812.

34

Occupational Therapy
Activities of Daily Living and Community Reintegration

Deirdre R. Dawson

BACKGROUND

Definitions

- Occupation: Activity that gives structure, value, and meaning and encompasses work (paid and unpaid), leisure, and self-care [1]—includes activities of daily living (ADLs).
- Occupational performance: The doing of activities in the environment in which they need to be done, for example, cooking a meal at home for the family.
- Occupational therapist (OT): Per the World Federation of Occupational Therapy, an OT is a therapist trained to enable people to participate in everyday life by enhancing their abilities and/or by modifying the environment to better support participation.
- Activities of daily living: Functional daily activities generally divided into basic (self-care tasks) and instrumental (everyday activities necessary for interacting with the environment, more complex than basic activities of daily living (BADLs), for example, driving, managing personal finances, and home management. Instrumental activities of daily living (IADLs) are generally understood to exclude work-related skills.
- Community integration: "Something to do, somewhere to live, someone to love" [2]. Has three primary constructs: independent living, social support, and productive occupation [3].

Epidemiology

More than 5 million Americans are estimated to have long-term disability posttraumatic brain injury (TBI) [4]. An estimated 60% have not returned to preinjury levels in primary occupations including work, leisure, and recreation; 30% report problems with BADLs; and 8% remain in restricted living situations including group homes, nursing homes, and jails [5]. The estimated prevalence of TBI among offender individuals is 60% and among the homeless is 53% [6,7].

ASSESSMENT AND EVALUATION

Basic Considerations

- Performance versus capacity: Questionnaires typically provide information about capability but not performance; performance-based measures involve direct observation and provide a more comprehensive and accurate picture of strengths and weaknesses [8].
- Performance and environment: Performance is influenced by the environment; determining performance is best achieved in the client's own environment [9] and will provide more ecological validity (i.e., performance on the test corresponds to an everyday situation).

Step 1

Client-centred goal setting: Goal setting is critical to identifying key occupational performance issues for each client [10]. It may be necessary, useful, and/or relevant to involve a family member or other caregiver in this interview process.

Step 2

Assessment of specific areas of occupation: Select assessments based on goal setting process and whether you need an "outcome" measure (for evaluation) or a measure to describe client's abilities. Important considerations: Does informant and/or self-report concur with performance; how does a specific environment affect performance?

- Performance-based measures (see *Measuring Occupational Performance* [8]): Consider The ADL and IADL Profile [11,12], comprehensive measures of ADLs, and the impact of executive dysfunction on everyday life; or the Multiple Errands Test [13], which allows observation of strategies employed while shopping and collecting information.
- Questionnaires:
  - BADL and IADL—many available [8].
  - Community Integration Questionnaires (CIQ): Primarily used for evaluation. CIQ (www.tbims.org/combi) and Reintegration to Normal Living Index are psychometrically sound and clinically useful [14].

Step 3

Special areas for consideration

- Cognition (see also Chapters 35 and 37): OTs assess cognition particularly as it relates to everyday life (e.g., safety with household ADLs, navigating in the community).
- Driving assessment: A comprehensive multidisciplinary assessment, inclusive of visual, cognitive, and an on-road test, is critical [15]. The Association for Driving Rehabilitation Specialists provides information on specialized testing and training services across North America <www.driver-ed.org>. The few studies investigating whether people with TBI who return to driving have more accidents than healthy controls have produced mixed results [16].
- Return to work and school—see Chapter 73.
- Social support, social integration, and sexuality: Reductions in social support, social isolation, and negative changes in perceived sexuality are frequent outcomes [17] and need to be considered in a comprehensive assessment of community integration.

INTERVENTION

Five key areas to consider: regaining functional independence (BADLs and IADLs), social support and integration, housing, transportation, and ongoing community participation. Participation in meaningful life situations is the goal, gains can be achieved many years post injury [18].

- Regaining functional independence:
  - Comprehensive rehabilitation programs focusing on (1) integration of therapies, (2) metacognition, (3) self-regulation, and (4) participating in personally meaningful life activities have better outcomes than neuropsychological rehabilitation alone [18].
  - Electronic portable cueing devices (e.g., personal digital assistants) increase the frequency with which people carry out a variety of target tasks [19]. Those who have severe episodic memory problems can learn the skills needed to operate these devices using an errorless learning approach [20]. Paper memory notebooks or electronic cueing devices are useful only when applied to functional activities [21].
  - Metacognitive strategy instruction is recommended for adults with TBI with executive dysfunction, and should include "acknowledging or generating goals, self-monitoring and self-recording of performance and strategy decisions based on performance-goal comparison" [22, p. 37]. Metacognitive strategy training improves problem solving in personally relevant and/or simulated problem situations [22].

- For severely impaired survivors, improving performance on selected skills may be achieved by specific functional skills training [23] comprising task analysis, written prompts, embedding retrained skills in programming, consistent practice, and fading cues. Independence in any particular skill can take months to achieve, and as benefits are often not generalizable cost-benefit should be evaluated carefully.

- Social support, social integration, and sexuality interventions related to enhancing social support, social integration, and positive expressions of sexuality are very limited.

  - Multifaceted social support groups that focus on education, coping-skills training, and goal setting may reduce hopelessness and engender a greater sense of control [17].
  - Social-skills training, including individualized goal setting, shaping of behaviors, and social perception training, may improve specific aspects of social behavior [24,25].
  - Peer mentoring may improve social participation [17].

- Housing: OTs should provide input to team members regarding level of independence so appropriate housing can be arranged.

- Transportation: Access to transportation is key for community integration. Thus, in addition to careful assessment of return to driving, public transportation should be investigated as it is cognitively complex.

- Community participation: Emerging research evidence and considerable anecdotal data suggests the value of community-based support programs for enhancing community participation even many years post TBI [26,27]. Important components appear to be (1) a long-term approach, (2) individualized goal clarification, and (3) therapy in the person's own environment.

  - Multidisciplinary rehabilitation programs improve overall community integration [26].
  - Participants in community-based day programs report better social participation and quality of life than nonparticipants [28,29].

ADDITIONAL READING

Electronic References

Evidence-Based Review of Moderate to Severe Acquired Brain Injury (ABIEBR).
    http://www.abiebr.com
International Brain Injury Clubhouse Alliance.
    http://www.braininjuryclubhouses.net/

Textbooks/Chapters

FILM: Braindamadj'd...Take II. http://braind.apartment11.tv/index
Gillen G. *Cognitive and Perceptual Rehabilitation: Optimizing Function.* St Louis, MO: Mosby-Elsevier; 2009.
Law M, Baum C, Dunn W. *Measuring Occupational Performance: Supporting Best Practice in Occupational Therapy.* Thorofare, NJ: Slack Incorporated; 2001.

Journal Articles

Dawson DR, Gaya A, Hunt A, et al. (2009). Using the Cognitive Orientation to Occupational Performance with adults with traumatic brain injury. *Can J Occup Ther.* 2009;76:115–127.

McColl M. Post-acute programming for community integration: A scoping review. *Brain Impairment.* 2007;8(3):238–250.

REFERENCES

1. Townsend EA, Polatajko HJ. *Enabling Occupation II: Advancing Occupational Therapy Vision for Health, Well-Being, and Justice through Occupation.* Ottawa, ON: CAOT Publications; 2007.

2. Jacobs HE. *Behaviour Analysis Guidelines and Brain Injury Rehabilitation: People, Principles, and Programs.* Gaithersburg, MD: Aspen Publication; 1993.

3. McColl MA. Postacute programming for community integration: a scoping review. *Brain Impairment.* 2007;8(3):238–250.

4. Thurman DJ, Alverson C, Dunn KA, Guerrero J, Sniezek JE. Traumatic brain injury in the United States: A public health perspective. *J Head Trauma Rehabil.* 1999;14(6):602–615.

5. Dikmen SS, Machamer JE, Powell JM, Temkin NR. Outcome 3 to 5 years after moderate to severe traumatic brain injury. *Arch Phys Med Rehabil.* 2003;84(10):1449–1457.

6. Shiroma EJ, Ferguson PL, Pickelsimer EE. Prevalence of traumatic brain injury in an offender population: a meta-analysis. *J Correct Health Care.* 2010;16(2):147–159.

7. Hwang SW, Colantonio A, Chiu S, et al. The effect of traumatic brain injury on the health of homeless people. *CMAJ.* 2008;179(8):779–784.

8. Law M, Baum C, Dunn W. *Measuring Occupational Performance: Supporting Best Practice in Occupational Therapy.* Thorofare, NJ: Slack Incorporated; 2001.

9. Toneman M, Brayshaw J, Lange B, Trimboli C. Examination of the change in Assessment of Motor and Process Skills performance in patients with acquired brain injury between the hospital and home environment. *Aust Occup Ther J.* 2010;57(4):246–252.

10. Bovend'Eerdt TJ, Botell RE, Wade DT. Writing SMART rehabilitation goals and achieving goal attainment scaling: a practical guide. *Clin Rehabil.* 2009;23(4):352–361.

11. Dutil E, Bottari C, Vanier M, Gaudreault C. *ADL Profile: Description of the Instrument.* 4th ed. Montreal: Les Éditions Émersion; 2005.

12. Bottari CL, Dassa C, Rainville CM, Dutil E. The IADL profile: development, content validity, intra- and interrater agreement. *Can J Occup Ther.* 2010;77(2):90–100.

13. Alderman N, Baker, D. Beyond the shopping centre: using the Multiple Errands Test in the assessment and rehabilitation of multitasking disorders. In: Oddy M, Worthington A, eds. *Rehabilitation of Executive Disorders: A Guide to Theory and Practice.* New York: Oxford University Press; 2009.

14. Salter K, Foley N, Jutai J, Bayley M, Teasell R. Assessment of community integration following traumatic brain injury. *Brain Inj.* 2008;22(11):820–835.

15. Hopewell CA. Driving and traumatic brain injury (c. 5). In: Schultheis MT, DeLuca J, Chute DL. *Handbook for the Assessment of Driving Capacity.* New York: Academic Press; 2009.

16. Schanke AK, Rike PO, Mølmen A, Osten PE. Driving behaviour after brain injury: a follow-up of accident rate and driving patterns 6–9 years post-injury. *J Rehabil Med.* 2008;40(9):733–736.

17. McCabe P, Lippert C, Weiser M, Hilditch M, Hartridge C, Villamere J; Erabi Group. Community reintegration following acquired brain injury. *Brain Inj.* 2007;21(2):231–257.

18. Geurtsen GJ, van Heugten CM, Martina JD, Geurts AC. Comprehensive rehabilitation programmes in the chronic phase after severe brain injury: a systematic review. *J Rehabil Med.* 2010;42(2):97–110.

19. Marshall S, Rees L, Weiser M, et al. Cognition interventions post-ABI. In *Evidence-Based Review of Moderate to Severe Acquired Brain Injury* (ABIEBR). 5th ed. 2009. http://www.abiebr.com/. Accessed January 25, 2010.

20. Svoboda E, Richards B, Polsinelli A, Guger S. A theory-driven training program in the use of emerging commercial technology: application to an adolescent with severe memory impairment. *Neuropsychol Rehabil.* 2010;20(4):562–586.

21. Cicerone KD, Dahlberg C, Malec JF, et al. Evidence-based cognitive rehabilitation: updated review of the literature from 1998 through 2002. *Arch Phys Med Rehabil.* 2005;86(8):1681–1692.

22. Kennedy MR, Coelho C, Turkstra L, et al. Intervention for executive functions after traumatic brain injury: a systematic review, meta-analysis and clinical recommendations. *Neuropsychol Rehabil.* 2008;18(3):257–299.

23. Parish L, Oddy M. Efficacy of rehabilitation for functional skills more than 10 years after extremely severe brain injury. *Neuropsychol Rehabil.* 2007;17(2):230–243.

24. McDonald S, Tate R, Togher L, et al. Social skills treatment for people with severe, chronic acquired brain injuries: a multicenter trial. *Arch Phys Med Rehabil.* 2008;89(9):1648–1659.

25. Dahlberg CA, Cusick CP, Hawley LA, et al. Treatment efficacy of social communication skills training after traumatic brain injury: a randomized treatment and deferred treatment controlled trial. *Arch Phys Med Rehabil.* 2007;88(12):1561–1573.

26. Kim H, Colantonio A. Effectiveness of post-acute rehabilitation in enhancing community integration for people with traumatic brain injury: A systematic review. *Am J Occup Ther.* 2010;64(5):709–719.

27. Sloan S, Callaway L, Winkler D, McKinley K, Ziino C, Anson K. Changes in care and support needs following community-based intervention for individuals with acquired brain injury. *Brain Impair.* 2009;10(3):295–306.

28. Fraas M, Balz M, Degrauw W. Meeting the long-term needs of adults with acquired brain injury through community-based programming. *Brain Inj.* 2007;21(12):1267–1281.

29. McClean A. Social participation, quality of life and attendance in brain injury drop-in centres: An exploratory study. Masters thesis. https://circle.ubc.ca/handle/2429/23485. Accessed April 23, 2010.

35

Speech Therapy
Dysphagia and Cognitive Communication Impairments

Kara Kozub O'Dell

DYSPHAGIA

Background

Definition

Dysphagia is a condition characterized by abnormality in the transfer of a bolus from the mouth to the stomach. Dysphagia results in unsafe or inefficient oral intake, which can cause aspiration, pneumonia, discomfort, and/or poor caloric intake. Behaviors associated with traumatic brain injury (TBI) such as impulsivity and unawareness can affect the safety and efficiency of oral intake [1].

Epidemiology

Incidence is not well documented, although dysphagia is estimated to occur in approximately 33% of all patients with a TBI (includes mild to severe injuries) [2]. Incidence is as high as 61% in patients following severe TBI; there is a relationship between length of coma, presence of a tracheostomy tube and/or mechanical ventilation, and severity of dysphagia [3].

Etiology

A delay in triggering the pharyngeal swallow is the most prevalent cause of dysphagia and aspiration in individuals following TBI. Other problems include structural injuries to the oral cavity, pharynx, and/or esophagus; atrophy/weakness due to prolonged intubation and cognitive deficits; or behaviors that interfere with oral intake [4].

Pathophysiology

Swallowing is typically described in four phases: (1) The oral preparatory phase, when liquid or food (the bolus) is manipulated in the mouth and masticated, if necessary, to ready it for the swallow; (2) The oral phase, when the tongue propels food posteriorly until the pharyngeal swallow is triggered; (3) The pharyngeal phase, when the pharyngeal swallow is triggered and the bolus moves through the pharynx; and (4) The esophageal phase, when peristalsis carries the bolus through the esophagus and into the stomach. Dysphagia results when one or more of these phases is disrupted [4].

Assessment

Risk Factors
Low Glasgow Coma Scale (GCS) scores and low scores on the Ranchos Los Amigos (RLA) scale of cognitive function are associated with aspiration. Additionally, low GCS scores, low RLA levels, the presence of a tracheostomy tube, and increased ventilation time are associated with impairments affecting oral intake [5].

Signs and Symptoms
These include, but are not limited to,

- Poor secretion management and/or need for frequent suctioning
- Inability to recognize food
- Difficulty placing food in the mouth
- Holding or pocketing liquid/food in the mouth
- A delay in swallowing
- Throat clearing, coughing, or choking before, during, or after swallowing
- Wet, gurgly vocal quality or audible respirations
- Pain/discomfort in throat or chest when swallowing
- Sensation of food stuck in the throat or chest [4]

Bedside Swallowing Evaluation
- Preparatory examination
    - Patient chart review
    - Observation of level of alertness and awareness
    - Observation of respiratory status and secretion management
    - Suction patient orally and/or via the tracheostomy tube, if applicable
    - Oral examination
    - Oral motor control examination
    - Laryngeal function examination
- Initial swallowing examination: The clinician determines if trial swallows are safe based on the information obtained from the preparatory examination. If the patient is acutely ill, has significant pulmonary

complications, is not alert, has poor secretion management, and/or an obvious pharyngeal swallowing disorder, trial swallows may not be indicated. The patient is then suctioned orally and through the tracheostomy tube, when applicable, and observations are made during trial swallows that lead to recommendations.

Instrumental Evaluation
The following instrumental swallow studies are commonly used to study various aspects of the swallow. Following the initial swallowing examination, a referral for an instrumental study is appropriate for any patient who is suspected to be aspirating or have a pharyngeal phase dysphagia.

- Fluoroscopic Swallow Study: a radiographic procedure that obtains real time images of the oral, pharyngeal, and esophageal phases of the swallow
- Fiberoptic Endoscopic Swallow Study: an endoscopic procedure in which a flexible scope visualizes the pharyngeal phase of the swallow

Management

Compensatory Treatment Procedures
- Postural techniques
    - Chin tuck—Patient puts chin to chest and pulls up: helpful for patients with a delayed swallow, reduced airway closure, and/or problems with residue in the valleculae
    - Head rotation—Turning the head to the affected side closes the pharynx on that side so that the bolus flows down the unaffected side: helpful for patients with a unilateral vocal fold paralysis or unilateral pharyngeal wall problem
    - Head tilt—Tilting head to the strong side allows food to drain down the strong side: helpful for patients with oral and pharyngeal problems on the same side
- Techniques to improve oral sensory awareness—The following techniques may be utilized with patients with swallow apraxia, tactile agnosia of food, reduced oral sensation, and delayed onset of the oral and/or pharyngeal swallow
    - Thermal tactile stimulation: contacting the tongue or faucial arches with a cold laryngeal mirror or metal spoon
    - Increasing downward pressure of the spoon against the tongue when presenting food
    - Varying taste, volume, and/or texture of bolus (i.e., sour, cold, solid)

- Diet changes: The diet should be changed only if other compensatory or therapy strategies are not effective or feasible given behavior, cognition, physical impairments, or other reasons.

  - Liquids—thin, nectar thick, honey thick, pudding thick; initially thickened liquids are easier for a patient to control and manage, reducing the risk of aspiration
  - National Dysphagia Diets (NDD):

    - NDD Level 1 (pureed): homogenous, very cohesive, pudding-like, require very little chewing ability
    - NDD Level 2 (mechanically altered, mechanical soft, ground): cohesive, moist, semisolid foods that require some chewing
    - NDD Level 3 (advanced, soft): soft foods that require more chewing ability, no hard, sticky, or crunchy items
    - Regular or general diet [6]

Swallowing Therapy

- Direct therapy—involves presenting food or liquid to the patient and asking him or her to swallow while the therapist manipulates the bolus or the patient follows specific instructions
- Indirect therapy—involves exercise programs or swallows of saliva, but no food or liquid is given: typically used with patients who are at high risk of aspiration
- Types of direct and indirect therapy include exercises for oral manipulation, bolus propulsion, tongue base retraction, laryngeal elevation and/or vocal fold adduction, thermal tactile stimulation, and swallow maneuvers. Exercises and swallow maneuvers require good attention and ability to follow complex instructions and are not indicated for patients with significant cognitive or language impairments

Other Modifications

When patients cannot follow instructions due to cognitive or language impairments, the following suggestions can help prevent aspiration and pneumonia in dysphagic patients.

- Frequent and thorough oral care to reduce bacteria
- Elevate the head of the bed to decrease the risk of aspirating saliva and/or tube feeding
- Limit the number of items during meals to increase attention to safe intake
- Encourage individuals to set utensil, food, or cup down and swallow before taking another bite or sip
- Encourage small, single cup sips and avoid straws if signs of aspiration increase with straw use
- Encourage individuals to take a sip of liquid after every 2 to 3 bites

COGNITIVE COMMUNICATION IMPAIRMENTS

Background

Definition

Communication results from a complex interaction between cognition, language, and speech. Cognitive communication impairments result from underlying deficits in cognitive processes such as awareness, attention, memory, organization, and reasoning that impact the efficiency and effectiveness of communication skills [7]. Posttraumatic amnesia (PTA) is a period of confusion, disorientation, impaired attention, and poor memory for day-to-day events resulting from inability to encode, and therefore learn, new information. Individuals who are experiencing PTA exhibit moderate to severe cognitive communication impairments [8].

Epidemiology

Moderate and severe TBIs are typically associated with cognitive deficits 6 months or longer post injury. Factors that modify association include location of injury in the brain, intelligence preinjury, and severity of injury [9]. PTA occurs in all individuals when they emerge from coma [8].

Assessment

Clinical Signs and Symptoms of
Cognitive Communication Impairments

The following signs and symptoms of cognitive communication impairments result in reduced effectiveness and efficiency of communication of wants, needs, and ideas. Perseveration and confabulation are frequently present.

- Poor arousal, alertness, and/or reaction to environmental stimuli
- Increased fatigue, decreased endurance
- Restlessness and/or agitation
- Agnosagnosia: denial or poor awareness of deficits, difficulties, and errors [10]
- Poor concentration in open or closed environments, reduced attention to detail
- Confusion, disorientation
- Perseveration: the repetition of a particular response, such as a word, phrase, or gesture, despite the absence or cessation of a stimulus [7]
- Verbal confabulation: the spontaneous narrative report of events that never happened due to memory impairment [7]
- Poor impulse control resulting in inappropriate comments and/or behavior during social exchanges

- Poor eye contact, inappropriate response length (long or short), poor topic maintenance
- Inability to verbally reason or solve basic problems in the environment

Diagnostic Evaluation

The aforementioned signs and symptoms are best detected during observation of patients during functional task completion. In addition, a number of formal and informal assessment tools will be discussed elsewhere in this book. Every patient who has suffered from a loss of consciousness should be assessed to determine the presence or absence of PTA. Tests sensitive to the detection of PTA typically assess orientation, immediate memory, and/or concentration. One such test, the Galveston Orientation and Amnesia Test (Table 35.1), can be administered daily until a patient scores a 76 or higher on 3 consecutive days. The scale measures orientation to person, place, and time, as well as memory for events preceding and following the injury [11]. Other frequently used assessments evaluate cognitive domains, including memory, attention, awareness, reasoning, auditory processing, and executive functioning. Such assessments may evaluate each domain independently, such as the California Verbal Learning Test [12] does with memory, or a number of domains simultaneously, such as the Cognitive Linguistic Quick Test [13].

Management

Cognitive communication deficits can be managed by changing the patient's environment and/or behavior. Early in recovery, patients in PTA are not consistently able to modify their behavior. Techniques for modifying a patient's environment and/or behavior include

- Eliminating, decreasing, or modifying stimuli and distractions
- Allowing patient sufficient time to respond
- Gently allowing patient to fail in safe environment during functional task to promote deficit awareness
- Providing frequent orientation; write the day and place for individual to see and refer to frequently throughout the day
- Verbally identifying perseveration or confabulation for the patient and educating and/or redirecting as appropriate
- Providing specific, concrete feedback when a communication attempt is not successful or appropriate
- Accepting all communication attempts including facial expression and gesture
- Providing written and gesture cues when necessary.

Table 35.1 The Galveston Orientation and Amnesia Test

Question	Error Score	Notes
What is your name?	–2	Must give both first name and surname.
When were you born?	–4	Must give day, month, and year.
Where do you live?	–4	Town is sufficient.
Where are you now		
(a) City	–5	Must give actual town.
(b) Building	–5	Usually in hospital or rehab center. Actual name necessary.
When were you admitted to this hospital?	–5	Date.
How did you get here?	–5	Mode of transport.
What is the first event you can remember after the injury?	–5	Any plausible event is sufficient (record answer).
Can you give some detail?	–5	Must give relevant detail.
Can you describe the last event you can recall before the accident?	–5	Any plausible event is sufficient (record answer).
What time is it now?	–5	–1 for each half-hour error.
What day of the week is it?	–3	–1 for each day error.
What day of the month is it? (i.e., the date)	–5	–1 for each day error.
What is the month?	–15	–5 for each month error.
What is the year?	–30	–10 for each year error.
Total Error		
Total Actual Score = (100–total error)=100–_____=		Can be a negative number.
76–100 = Normal/66–75 = Borderline/<66 = Impaired		

Instructions: Can be administered daily. Score of 76 or more on three consecutive occasions is considered to indicate that patient is out of posttraumatic amnesia.

From Ref. [11].

ADDITIONAL READING

Electronic Reference

American Speech-Language-Hearing Association website.
   http://www.asha.org/

Textbooks/Chapters

Halper A, Cherney L, Miller T. *A Framework for Clinical Management: Clinical Management of Communication Problems in Adults with Traumatic Brain Injury.* Gaithersburg, MD: Aspen; 1991.

Logemann J. *Evaluation and Treatment of Swallowing Disorders.* Austin, TX: Pro-Ed; 1998.

Sohlberg M, Mateer C. *Cognitive Rehabilitation: An Integrative Neuropsychological Approach.* New York: The Guilford Press; 2001.

Journal Articles

Ward E, Green K, Morton A. Patterns and predictors of swallowing resolution following adult traumatic brain injury. *J Head Trauma Rehab.* 2007;22(3):184–191.

REFERENCES

1. Groher M. *Dysphagia: Diagnosis and Management.* Boston: Butterworth-Heinemann; 1997.
2. Dray T, Hillel AD, Miller RM. Dysphagia caused by neurologic deficits. *Otolaryng Clinics of North America.* 2008;31(3):507–524.
3. Hansen TS, Engberg AW, Larsen K. Functional oral intake and time to reach unrestricted dieting for patients with traumatic brain injury. *Arch Phys Med Rehabil.* 2008;89(8):1556–1562.
4. Logemann J. *Evaluation and Treatment of Swallowing Disorders.* Austin, TX: Pro-Ed; 1998.
5. Mackay LE, Morgan AS, Bernstein BA. Factors affecting oral feeding with severe traumatic brain injury. *J Head Trauma Rehabil.* 1999;14(5):435–447.
6. Quinn B. New Standards: National Dysphagia Diet. *Nutrition News.* Cengage Learning; 2003; Jan 1. Available at http://www.wadsworth.com/nutrition_d/special_features/news/jan03/dysphagia.html. Accessed January 11, 2011.
7. Murray L, Chapey R. Assessment of language disorders in adults. *Language Intervention Strategies in Aphasia and Related Neurogenic Communication Disorders.* Baltimore, MD: Lippincott Williams & Wilkins; 2001.
8. Horn LJ, Zasler ND. *Medical Rehabilitation of Traumatic Brain Injury.* St Louis, MO: Mosby; 1996.
9. Dikmen SS, Corrigan JD, Levin HS, Machamer J, Stiers W, Weisskopf MG. Cognitive outcome following traumatic brain injury. *J Head Trauma Rehabil.* 2009;24(6):430–438.
10. Crosson B, Barco PP, Velozo CA, et al. Awareness of compensation in post acute head injury rehabilitation. *J Head Trauma Rehab.* 1989;4(3):46–54.
11. Levin HS, Vincent M, O'Donnell MA, Grossman RG. The Galveston Orientation and Amnesia Test. A practical scale to assess cognition after head injury. *J Nerv Ment Dis.* 1979;167(11):675–684.
12. Delis D, Kramer J, Kaplan E, Ober B. *California Verbal Learning Test (this is a registered trademark)—Second Edition (CVLT-II).* The Psychological Corporation: A Harcourt Assessment Company; 2000.
13. Helm-Estabrooks N. *Cognitive Linguistic Quick Test (CLQT).* The Psychological Corporation; 2001.

36

Neuro-optometric Rehabilitation for Visual Dysfunction

William V. Padula

BACKGROUND

Definitions

- *Doctors of optometry* are "independent primary health care providers who specialize in the examination, diagnosis, treatment, and management of diseases and disorders of the visual system, the eye, and associated structures as well as the diagnosis of related systemic conditions" [1].
- *Neuro-optometric rehabilitation (NOR)* is "an individualized treatment regimen for patients with visual deficits as a direct result of physical disabilities, traumatic brain injury (TBI), and other neurological insults" [2].
- *Vision therapy* is "a sequence of activities individually prescribed and monitored by a doctor to develop efficient visual skills and processing. Vision therapy is administered in the office under the guidance of a doctor. Activities paralleling in office techniques are typically taught to the patient to be practiced at home to reinforce the developing visual skill" [3].

Symptoms related to visual dysfunction following a TBI may include: headache, diplopia, homonymous hemianopsia, vertigo, asthenopia, and difficulty with focusing the eyes, movement of print when reading, tracking difficulty, photophobia, and blurred vision [4].

- *Diplopia*, typically due to binocular dysfunction, is quite prevalent following TBI [5,6]. Binocular dysfunction may result in difficulties with balance, posture, and spatial orientation [2].
- Visual field defect/visual neglect
  - *Homonymous hemianopsia,* field loss affecting either the entire left or right field, is often seen in the setting of TBI [7,8].

- *Visual neglect,* a lack of spatial conscious awareness in the absence of a homonymous hemianopsia, may also be seen [9].
- Homonymous hemianopsia or visual neglect can induce a shift in concept of visual egocenter, resulting in Visual Midline Shift Syndrome (VMSS) [2,9,10].

Normal Visual Processing

The visual system is composed of two visual processes. The *focal visual process* is oriented toward detail, identification, attention, concentration, and isolation of the figure from the ground, is conscious, and related to function of the occipital cortex and associated cortices. The *ambient or spatial visual process* is oriented toward spatial orientation, balance, posture, and movement, and is preconscious. It is mediated primarily at the level of the midbrain, although the occipital cortex also plays a role [11,12]. The ambient visual process integrates information with the sensorimotor system [13].

Visual Processing Dysfunction

It refers to visual impairments that are due to central (as opposed to ocular or oculomotor) pathology. Two clinical syndromes are recognized:

- Posttrauma Vision Syndrome (PTVS)
  - Following a TBI, centrally mediated visual symptoms and binocular difficulties can be caused by dysfunction between focal and ambient or sensorimotor (bimodal) visual processing producing:
    - diplopia [5];
    - exotropia and exophoria [14,15,16]; and
    - postural changes associated with compensation for vision dysfunction and diplopia [10,17].
  - Although symptoms and characteristics of binocular dysfunction are logically related to occulomotor nerve palsy, the mechanism for the cause of binocular dysfunction in the setting of PTVS appears to be related to trauma affecting the bimodal visual processing systems. Research has documented that changes in visual evoked potential amplitude occurred following treatment through use of prisms and binasal occlusion. Following such treatment, researchers documented a rapid decline in symptoms and syndrome characteristics. This condition has been termed PTVS [18].
- VMSS—Problems with balance and posture are common following a TBI. Vision supports organization of balance and posture through the following processes.

- Developmentally, vision matches information with the sensorimotor systems to organize the concept of visual midline [19].
- Feed forward cooperation occurs between ambient visual process and sensorimotor system to the cortices [11].
- The ambient visual process (preconscious anticipation) supports change in posture, balance, and movement [10].
- The visual concept of egocenter (i.e., one's own midline) is a function of interaction between the ambient visual process and the sensorimotor system [10,17].
- TBI is hypothesized to affect the relationship of bimodal visual processes, thereby shifting the preconscious concept of visual egocenter [10,11,19].

Treatment of Centrally Mediated Visual Dysfunction

Involves the discipline of NOR.

The following comprise the NOR evaluation:

- Thorough review of history, visual acuities (near and far), visual field evaluation, sensorimotor evaluation, complex refraction, and refractive sequence evaluating state of binocular ranges and accommodative amplitudes for distance and near viewing, dynamic accommodation, binocularity, depth perception, color vision, visual midline assessment affecting posture and balance, and visual evoked potentials [14].
- Lenses, prisms (compensatory and noncompensatory), and sectoral occlusion should be utilized to affect dysfunction in the bimodal visual process, and response to that intervention observed or recorded [11,14].

Vision therapy

- Strategies to improve visual function (i.e., yoked prisms, binasal occlusion) should be undertaken with caution, because over-emphasis of fixation, tracking, and so on can imbed the condition of PTVS [14,18].
- Following a NOR evaluation, a treatment plan involving vision therapy to address binocularity, accommodation, and visual function should be undertaken following NOR evaluation [11].

  - Yoked prisms can improve spatial orientation for visual neglect [11,20,21]. Yoked prisms realign visual egocenter (midline) in VMSS, thereby improving posture and balance [10,17].
  - Binasal occlusion refers to a vertical opaque or translucent filter strip attached to the nasal border of each eyeglass lens. Its purpose is to provide a boundary or vertical line to support ambient visual processing.

ADDITIONAL READING

Electronic Reference
Neuro-optometric Rehabilitation Association (NORA). www.nora.cc

Textbooks/Chapters
Kapoor N, Cuiffreda K, Suchoff I. Egocentric localization in patients with visual neglect. In: Suchoff I, Ciuffreda K, Kapoor N, eds. *Visual and Vestibular Consequences of Acquired Brain Injury*. Santa Ana, CA: Optometric Extension Publishers; 2001:131–144.

Liu G, Volpe N, Galetta S. *Neuro-ophthalmology, Diagnosis and Management*. Philadelphia, PA: WB Saunders; 2001.

Padula WV. *Neuro-Optometric Rehabilitation*. Santa Ana, CA: Optometric Extension Publishers; 1996.

Padula WV, Wu L, Vicci V, et al. Evaluating and treating visual dysfunction. In: Zasler N, Katz D, Zafonte R, eds. *Brain Injury Medicine: Principles and Practice*. New York, NY: Demos Medical Publishing; 2007:511–528.

Journal Articles
Cockerham G, Goodrich G, Weichel E, et al. Eye and visual function in traumatic brain injury. *J Rehabil Res Dev*. 2009;6:811–818.

Weed H. Divergence paralysis due to head injury. *Transcript, American Academy of Ophthalmology*. 1989;4:27–34.

Padula W, Argyris S, Ray J. Visual evoked potentials (VEP) evaluating treatment for post trauma vision syndrome in patients with traumatic brain injury. *Brain Inj*. 1994;8:125–133.

Padula W, Argyris S. Post trauma vision syndrome and visual midline shift syndrome. *J Neuro Rehab*. 1996;6:165–171.

Rossetti Y, Rode G, Pisella L, Farne A, Li L. Rightward optical deviation rehabilitates left hemispherical neglect. *Nature*. 1998;395:166–169.

Sarno S, Erasmus G, Lippert M, Lipp B, Schlaegel W. Electrophysiological correlates of visual impairment after traumatic brain injury. *Vision Research*. 2000;40:3029–3038.

REFERENCES

1. AOA Web site. http://www.aoa.org. Accessed 31 July, 2010.
2. Padula W. *Neuro-optometric Rehabilitation*. Santa Ana, CA: Optometric Extension Publishers; 2000.
3. AOA Web site. http://www.aoa.org/x5411.xml1. Accessed 31 July 2010.
4. Sabates NR, Gonce MA, Farris BK. Neuro-ophthalmological findings in closed head trauma. *J Clin Neuroophthalmol*. 1991;11(4):273–277.
5. Gianutsos R, Glosser D, Elbaum J, Vroman GM. Visual imperception in brain-injured adults: multifaceted measures. *Arch Phys Med Rehabil*. 1983;64(10):456–461.
6. Scheiman M, Gallaway M. Vision therapy to treat binocular vision disorders after acquired brain injury. In: Suchoff I, Ciuffreda K, Kapoor N, eds. *Visual and Vestibular Consequences of Acquired Brain Injury*. Santa Ana, CA: Optometric Extension Publishers; 2001:89–113.

7. Silverstone D, Hirsh J. *Automated Visual Field Testing: Techniques of Examination and Interpretation.* Norwalk, CT: Appleton Century-Crofts; 1986.

8. Harrington D. *The Visual Fields.* St Louis, MO: Mosby; 1971.

9. Georgis J. Treatment of carbon monoxide poisoning with yoked prisms. In: Penney DG, ed. *Carbon Monoxide Poisoning.* Lakeland, FL: CRC Press; 2008:619–641.

10. Padula WV, Nelson CA, Padula WV, Benabib R, Yilmaz T, Krevisky S. Modifying postural adaptation following a CVA through prismatic shift of visuo-spatial egocenter. *Brain Inj.* 2009;23(6):566–576.

11. Padula W, Wu L, Vicci V, et al. Evaluating and treating visual dysfunction. In: Zasler N, Zafonte R, Katz D. *Brain Injury Medicine: Principles and Practice.* New York, NY: Demos Publishers; 2006:511–527.

12. Trevarthen CB. Two mechanisms of vision in primates. *Psychol Forsch.* 1968;31(4):299–348.

13. Liebowitz H, Post R. The two modes of visual processing concept and some implications. In: Beck JJ, ed. *Organization and Representation in Perception.* Hillsdale, NJ: Erlbaum; 1982:77–125.

14. Padula W. *Neuro-Visual Processing: An Interdisciplinary Model for Neuro-Rehabilitation.* Santa Ana, CA: Optometric Extension Publishers; 2011.

15. Hart C. Disturbances of fusion following head injury. *Proc R Soc Med.* 1964;62:704–706.

16. Carroll R. Acute loss of fusional convergence following head trauma. *Arch Ophthal.* 1984;4:27–34.

17. Benabib R, Nelson C. Efficiency in visual skills and postural control: dynamic interaction. *Occupational Therapy Practice.* 1991;3:57–68.

18. Padula WV, Argyris S, Ray J. Visual evoked potentials (VEP) evaluating treatment for post-trauma vision syndrome (PTVS) in patients with traumatic brain injuries (TBI). *Brain Inj.* 1994;8(2):125–133.

19. Brooks V. *The Neural Basis of Motor Control.* New York, NY: Oxford University Press; 1986.

20. Milner AD, Dijkerman HC, McIntosh RD, Rossetti Y, Pisella L. Delayed reaching and grasping in patients with optic ataxia. *Prog Brain Res.* 2003;142:225–242.

21. Padula W, Argyris S. Post trauma vision syndrome and visual midline shift syndrome. *NeuroRehabilitation.* 1996;6:165–171.

37

Cognitive Impairment
Characterization and Management

Eric B. Larson

BACKGROUND

Cognitive impairment caused by traumatic brain injury (TBI) can be viewed *dichotomously*. That is, a patient may or may not retain a capacity for thought that is expected of intact individuals (e.g., orientation to person, place and time, ability to follow commands). Impairment can also be defined *continuously*. That is, a patient may demonstrate a greater or lesser degree of thinking ability (e.g., short-term memory) relative to some criterion. This chapter will focus on characterization and management of cognitive impairment in patients with moderate to severe TBI.

Classification of Cognitive Impairment

- This provides a means for describing the extent to which cognitive impairment is manifest and affects different aspects of functioning.
- *Severity of injury* is rated by the Glasgow Coma Scale [1], duration of loss of consciousness, and the duration of posttraumatic amnesia (PTA; reviewed elsewhere in the present text).
- *Stage of recovery* is described using the Rancho Los Amigos Scale of Cognitive Functioning [2] (reviewed elsewhere in the present text).
- Specific cognitive abilities can be reported as percentile ranks relative to a neurologically intact population. It is important to note what population provides the ranges. Usually these ranges refer to individuals who are matched to the patient by age and education.

  - Very superior: >98th percentile
  - Superior: 91st to 97th percentile
  - High average: 75th to 90th percentile
  - Average: 25th to 74th percentile
  - Low average: 9th to 24th percentile
  - Borderline: 2nd to 8th percentile
  - Extremely low: <2nd percentile

- Cognitive abilities can also be rated by percentile ranks relative to a clinical (impaired) population to determine the extent to which a patient resembles those with a particular diagnosis. For example, severity of aphasia in TBI may be characterized with percentiles relative to aphasics. A score corresponding to the 50th percentile relative to aphasics is much worse than a score that corresponds to the 50th percentile relative to a neurologically intact sample.

Etiology of Observed Impairments

- *Mechanism of Injury*—Blunt head trauma can result in diffuse impairment while penetrating wounds may cause circumscribed deficits.
- *Risk Factors*—Factors that predict TBI also predict reduced cognitive performance in individuals both before and after injury. Consequently, they should be considered in interpretation of assessment data and subsequent treatment planning.
  - Low socioeconomic status can result in educational and cultural disadvantages that affect outcome. A high school education in an affluent suburb may be a greater asset than the same number of years of education in a low-income school system.
  - Substance abuse is associated with an increased prevalence of TBI. Resumption of drinking after injury complicates cognitive recovery and increases risk of reinjury.

Role of Neuropsychological Assessment

- Typical time to refer inpatients for formal neuropsychological evaluation is after emergence from PTA
- Typical referral questions. Identify distinct areas of cognitive strengths and weaknesses. Assess severity of cognitive impairment. Determine if patient has independent decision-making ability. Assess need for supervision. Determine if patient is ready to attempt a return to work or school. Assess need for further cognitive rehabilitation. Determine impact of psychiatric factors on independent functioning.

DIAGNOSIS

Most cognitive constructs are complex and consequently the factors that cause a score to fall in the impaired range are very complicated. For example, interpretation of a score on a memory test could take the following into consideration.

- Age and education. This can usually be controlled by selecting the proper norm set (see earlier section). Most memory tests will allow you to compare a patient to others from the same demographic background.

- Premorbid intelligence. This can be estimated through a number of procedures. Demographic variables (e.g., years of education) are sometimes used by clinicians to form a rough estimate of cognitive ability. However, this is subject to substantial error. More precise estimates are provided through a combination of demographic variables and performance on standardized tests such as the Wechsler Test of Adult Reading [3]. The effects of intelligence on memory can then be controlled through analysis of the discrepancy of an actual memory score versus an expected memory score.

- Level of effort. Symptom validity testing can help assess whether patients may be exhibiting symptom magnification.

- Fatigue. Observation of a patient's level of arousal is an essential component of formal evaluation. When a patient shows evidence of somnolence during a particular test, the resulting score should be interpreted with caution.

- Sensory impairment or loss of motor control. Patients who are cognitively intact can appear impaired when physical impairment interferes with testing. For example, patients with intact capacity to learn and retain new information might appear impaired on a visual memory task if they do not wear corrective lenses that they need during assessment.

- Other cognitive abilities. Impairment in one domain often exerts secondary effects in other domains. For example, attention deficits can affect initial encoding of information on memory testing. Language impairment can confound memory assessment when it interferes with comprehension of test items or expression of responses.

- Clinical interpretation of a test score can reliably address the construct it was intended to measure only after all the aforementioned factors have been controlled or taken into consideration.

Clinical Presentation

- Subjective complaints—Moderate and severe TBI are associated with poor recall of diagnosis and limited awareness of disability. Depression or other psychological factors can result in magnification of symptoms and a failure to recognize progress.

- Behavioral observation—The following characteristic behaviors noted in conversation can indicate a need for formal assessment.

  - Attention impairment. A need to have questions repeated or explained
  - Executive dysfunction. Tangential thought or perseveration
  - Language impairment. Word-finding problems, word-substitution errors, irrelevant responses to questions because of poor understanding

- Memory impairment. Inability to recall important personal information (phone number, social security number) or to remember recent events (e.g., circumstances of referral for evaluation or treatment)

Examination

Depending on what stage of recovery the patient has reached, any one of the following assessments are typically conducted at initial contact.

- *Assessment of level of arousal.* Includes eye opening, visual tracking, responsiveness to commands, ability to answer questions. Standardized assessment can be performed with the JFK Coma Recovery Scale [4].
- *Assessment of Posttraumatic Amnesia.* Includes orientation, awareness of medical situation. Standardized assessment can be performed with the Galveston Orientation and Amnesia Test (GOAT) [5]. One accepted convention to establish emergence from PTA is to obtain GOAT scores of 78 and above for 3 consecutive days.
- *Mental status exam.* Includes attention, recall, naming, auditory comprehension, reading, writing, simple construction ability. Standardized assessment can be performed with the Folstein Mini Mental State Examination [6].

Radiographic Assessment

It is important to recognize that localization of a lesion and measurement of its size will not necessarily predict the impact on specific thinking abilities and on related function. Formal cognitive evaluation provides an important complement to imaging studies.

TREATMENT

Guiding Principles

- Assess cost of interventions (not just financial). For example, neurostimulant medication can cause or exacerbate psychosis. Cognitive remediation can cause frustration and fatigue.
- Assess potential benefit of interventions. Treatments that have not undergone randomized clinical trials should be recommended sparingly, if at all. Prescribing experimental interventions may provide false hope or divert patient resources away from validated treatment.
- Assess capacity of patients to participate. For example, psychotherapy may be of limited benefit in patients with marked cognitive impairment unless a neurologically intact family member joins treatment sessions.

Initial Management

In the early stages of recovery, treatment of cognitive impairment can include the following: neurostimulant medications, interaction with family members (verbal or nonverbal), early patient education, and orientation to medical situation. Some recommend withholding distressing news (e.g., recent deaths of loved ones) until the patient has emerged from PTA.

Ongoing Care

Later in recovery, treatment can include cognitive remediation, retraining in independent living skills, training in home exercises that can continue after therapy concludes, and gradual resumption of previously enjoyed activities. Psychotherapy may be beneficial if the family is involved and/ or if the patient has emerged from PTA.

Treatment Controversies

Debate continues about whether significant cognitive recovery can occur after 1 to 2 years post injury [7]. There is also disagreement about the relative merits of direct remediation of cognitive impairment versus training in compensatory strategies to work around permanent deficits [8].

Prognosis

- After 1 month of recovery, severe injury usually results in diffuse impairment (affecting all domains of function). In contrast, at this stage less severe injury results in specific impairments of any of a number of areas, especially memory, cognitive flexibility, and psychomotor speed.
- By 6 years post injury, memory is the most common impairment (observed in more than 50% of TBI survivors) [9].

ADDITIONAL READING

Electronic Reference

National Academy of Neuropsychology. Cognitive rehabilitation: official statement of the national academy of neuropsychology. Retrieved June 22, 2010, from http://www.nanonline.org/NAN/Files/PAIC/PDFs/NANPositionCogRehab.pdf

Textbooks/Chapters

Cicerone K. Cognitive rehabilitation. In: Zasler ND, Katz DI, Zafonte RD, eds. *Brain Injury Medicine: Principles and Practice*. New York, NY: Demos Medical Publishing; 2007:765–777.

Giacino JT, Katz DI, Schiff N. (2007) Assessment and rehabilitative management of individuals with disorders of consciousness. In: Zasler ND, Katz DI, Zafonte RD, eds. *Brain Injury Medicine: Principles and Practice*. New York, NY: Demos Medical Publishing:423–439.

Lezak MD, Howieson DB, Loring DW, Hannay HJ, Fischer JS. *Neuropsychological Assessment*. 4th ed. New York, NY: Oxford University Press; 2004:158–194.

Roebuck-Spencer T, Sherer M. Moderate and severe traumatic brain injury. In: Morgan JE, Ricker JH, eds. *Textbook of Clinical Neuropsychology*. New York, NY: Taylor and Francis; 2008:411–429.

Journal Articles

Dikmen SS, Machamer JE, Powell JM, Temmkin NR. Outcome 3 to 5 years after moderate to severe traumatic brain injury. *Archives of Physical Medicine and Rehabilitation*. 2003;84:1449–1457.

Dreer L, DeVivo M, Novack T, Krzywanski S, Marson D. Cognitive predictors of medical decision making in traumatic brain injury. *Rehabil Psychol*. 2008;53:486–497.

Hanks RA, Millis SR, Ricker JH, et al. The predictive validity of a brief inpatient neuropsychologic battery for persons with traumatic brain injury. *Arch Phys Med Rehabil*. 2008;89:950–957.

REFERENCES

1. Teasdale G, Jennett B. Assessment of coma and impaired consciousness. A practical scale. *Lancet*. 1974;2(7872):81–84.

2. Hagen C, Malkmus D, Durham P. *Levels of Cognitive Functioning. Rehabilitation of the Head Injured Adult: Comprehensive Management*. Downey, CA: Rancho Los Amigos Hospital; 1979.

3. Psychological Corporation. *Manual for the Wechsler Test of Adult Reading (WTAR)*. San Antonio, TX: Author; 2001.

4. Giacino JT, Kalmar K, Whyte J. The JFK Coma Recovery Scale-Revised: measurement characteristics and diagnostic utility. *Arch Phys Med Rehabil*. 2004;85(12):2020–2029.

5. Levin HS, O'Donnell VM, Grossman RG. The Galveston Orientation and Amnesia Test. A practical scale to assess cognition after head injury. *J Nerv Ment Dis*. 1979;167(11):675–684.

6. Folstein MF, Folstein SE, McHugh PR. "Mini-mental state". A practical method for grading the cognitive state of patients for the clinician. *J Psychiatr Res*. 1975;12(3):189–198.

7. Millis SR, Rosenthal M, Novack TA, et al. Long-term neuropsychological outcome after traumatic brain injury. *J Head Trauma Rehabil*. 2001;16(4):343–355.

8. Cicerone KD, Dahlberg C, Kalmar K, et al. Evidence-based cognitive rehabilitation: recommendations for clinical practice. *Arch Phys Med Rehabil*. 2000;81(12):1596–1615.

9. Tate RL, Fenelon B, Manning ML, Hunter M. Patterns of neuropsychological impairment after severe blunt head injury. *J Nerv Ment Dis*. 1991;179(3):117–126.

38

Behavioral Impairment
Recognition and Management

Simon Fleminger

GENERAL PRINCIPLES

Definition

In the early posttraumatic period, in the weeks and months post injury, during recovery from moderate and severe traumatic brain injury (TBI), the most common behavioral problems are: (1) agitation and wandering, (2) lack of insight and psychotic symptoms, and (3) disinhibited behavior.

In the long term, months and years after injury, the most troublesome problems are: (1) self-centered, childish, thoughtless behavior, (2) aggression and violence, and (3) apathy and poor motivation.

Epidemiology

Early after injury about one-third of TBI patients show agitated behavior [1], and many patients show impaired self-awareness [2]. After severe injury as many as 45% may show a complete lack of insight (anosognosia) into their injury [3].

In the longer term, aggressive behavior with irritability and explosive temper is seen in a minority of patients, with severe problems in about 25% [4]. Family members commonly complain of personality change, in particular that the patient is thoughtless, childish, and self-centered [5].

Etiology and Pathophysiology

Frontal lobe injury, particularly medial bifrontal damage, increases the likelihood of early posttraumatic behavioral problems. This may, in part, reflect damage to cholinergic nuclei in the basal forebrain. Pain, systemic illness, hypoxia, medication (particularly if sedative or anticholinergic), and alcohol or other illicit drug withdrawal may be contributory factors.

Later problems with aggression are more common in those with anti-social behavior before the injury and in those with frontal lobe injury [6]. Epilepsy may increase the risk. Depression, anxiety, substance abuse, and psychotic illness may exacerbate symptoms. Apathy and motivational problems are more common in frontal injury or depression [7,8].

DIAGNOSIS

Clinical Presentation

In the days and weeks after injury, patients may show agitation, lack of insight, and/or disinhibited behavior, often concurrently.

Agitation and Wandering

Patients may be restless, and if mobile may wander into other patients' rooms or try to abscond from the ward. They may attempt to pull out an indwelling catheter or intravenous line. Not uncommonly, agitation is first noted on attempting to wean the patient off ventilation. It may be a precursor of aggressive behavior.

Lack of Insight and Psychotic Symptoms

When insight is severely impaired, the patient will deny that he or she has suffered any injury, stating that they are perfectly fit to return to work despite obvious severe problems. Such patients are at risk of confabulation and more overt psychotic states, which usually involve delusional misidentification, for example, believing that they are at work or in a duplicate hospital (reduplicative paramnesia). Persecutory delusions are not uncommon.

Disinhibited Behavior

Sexually disinhibited behavior is particularly challenging for staff, upsetting for family, and a risk to other patients.

These early challenging behaviors tend to remit spontaneously as the patient recovers. They may only last a few days but in some patients persist and limit discharge options.

Late behavioral problems, months and years after injury are more common in those patients with early agitation [1].

History and Assessment

- A precise history of the problem will include detail about specific instances of challenging behavior, and the severity and frequency of the problems. It may be worth doing repeated measurement, for example, with the Overt Aggression Scale [9]. Ask "what is the most dangerous thing that has happened?"

- An assessment of risk will include dangers to self, for example, from wandering and getting lost or because of antisocial behavior leading to assaults on the patient, and dangers to other patients and to staff. Risk is greatest with patients who are mobile, strong, and skilled in combat or fighting, when in the presence of vulnerable patients, and with limited (or insufficient) staffing. For patients who are living at home, remember to assess risks to children.

- Review of the patient's physical health is essential to include secondary complications of the TBI (e.g., hydrocephalus or cerebral infection), systemic illness (e.g., anemia or hypoxia), and causes of pain or discomfort. These conditions may exacerbate behavioral impairment.

- Review of the drug chart will indicate if prescribed medication may be aggravating the behavior; pay particular attention to drugs that are sedative or anticholinergic or enhance dopamine (e.g., methylphenidate). Anticonvulsants should be reduced and stopped unless there is evidence of posttraumatic epilepsy [10].

Physical and Mental State Examination

- Determine if the patient is alert and orientated. Evidence of impaired consciousness will mean that guidelines for management or delirium will be appropriate. Disorientation is common in those with early agitation, poor insight, or disinhibition. Measure cognitive performance using the O-log [11] if severely impaired, otherwise use the Mini Mental State Examination (MMSE) [12] and Frontal Assessment Battery [13]. These assessments will indicate the severity of cognitive impairment, important as a guide to the etiology of the behavioral problem, and can be used to track recovery.

- General physical and neurological examination will allow assessment of secondary and other complications that may aggravate behavioral problems.

- Check for symptoms of withdrawal from alcohol or illicit drugs, or drug cravings.

- Assess the mental state for evidence of depression, mania, anxiety disorder, fear, or psychotic illness.

- Assess the patient's insight into their problems and their capacity to make decisions about their treatment. This may be important if they are going to need to be detained against their will for their own safety.

Laboratory Studies and Radiographic Assessment

- These will need to be reviewed to assess for the presence of infectious or metabolic complications or systemic illness.

TREATMENT—EARLY BEHAVIORAL PROBLEMS

Prevention

- On a medical or surgical ward, behavioral problems are less likely if the patient has plenty of space and the room is not too hot.
- Early rehabilitation minimizes the risk by engaging the patient in activity, thereby reducing boredom and facilitating a positive attitude toward recovery.
- Flexible visiting hours enable family and friends to help support the patient.
- Encourage staff, nursing in particular, to engage with the patient. Ensure that they are confident, that they are properly trained in the management of agitation and aggression, and have the necessary backup, for example, from the hospital security team or access to police.
- Keep medication that can increase delirium to a minimum. Discourage knee-jerk prescription of sedative medication.
- Encourage good liaison with local neuropsychologist or neuropsychiatrist to establish policies for management [14].

Initial Management

- Assess the patient (see earlier sections), and assess and ensure the safety of all concerned. The patient may require one-to-one nursing. Attend to strategies related to prevention.
- Treat any associated mental disorder, for example, depression.
- If possible, use masterly inactivity with careful observation and monitoring of the patient, support for staff, but little in the way of active interventions; most early behavioral problems rapidly improve.
- Small doses of sedation may be needed only if there is evidence of repeated problems. If possible, have a treatment protocol to follow; do not constantly experiment with different drugs.
- Consider behavioral guidelines for management, but these are often difficult to implement on a busy medical or surgical ward.
- Consider onward referral to cognitive behavior unit if available or needed. Do not leave this too late.

Ongoing Management

- If problems persist, ensure that patient is not given frequent as needed doses of short-acting benzodiazepines (e.g., lorazepam) or typical antipsychotics (e.g., haloperidol). Instead, consider regular long-acting benzodiazepine (e.g., diazepam) or regular atypical antipsychotics. There is also evidence supporting the use of β-blockers for the management of agitation and aggression [15].

- Monitor for adverse side effects, in particular increased disinhibition due to benzodiazepine, akathisia due to antipsychotics, and increasing confusion due to sedation.

- Consider antitestosterones or antipsychotics for sexual disinhibition. However, these drugs should only be used as a last resort given that sexual disinhibition early post injury almost always remits spontaneously.

- Set up regular review meetings with staff to check how they are coping and to provide advice.

- Given that the patient almost certainly lacks capacity to consent to treatment, ensure you understand the legal basis on which medication is being offered, and that this is documented. It is wise to negotiate carefully with family and caregivers.

Treatment Uncertainties

- There is no good evidence on which to base guidance as to which drug to use to control agitation and disinhibition after TBI [15]. On the other hand, there is a risk of adversely affecting neural plasticity and functional recovery with the use of benzodiazepines and typical antipsychotics such as haloperidol. Proper medication selection should take all of these issues into consideration.

TREATMENT—LATE BEHAVIORAL PROBLEMS

Aggression is the commonest problem in the long term.

Prevention

- Address any psychosocial factors that may be present, for example, housing, benefits, debt and so on.
- Minimize disability by ensuring good access to rehabilitation.
- Ensure structured activities, for example, vocational activities or day care.
- Provide education for patient and family about brain injury, its sequelae, and management.

Initial Management

- Assess the patient and ensure the safety of all concerned, in particular children.

- Consider late secondary complications, for example, subdural hematoma or posttraumatic epilepsy.
- Treat any associated mental disorder, for example, alcohol or other substance abuse, depression, and anxiety disorder.
- Refer to a psychologist who will undertake an assessment of antecedents, behavior, and consequences (ABC) and may rate the behavior using a standardized rating scale.
- The psychologist will consider behavioral guidelines for management; these may be appropriate for the staff in the nursing home or as guidance to the family or caregiver [16].

Ongoing Management

- Personality change, including problems with irritability and aggression after TBI, is difficult to treat.
- If problems persist, consider mood stabilizer, sedative antidepressant (e.g., trazodone), or atypical antipsychotic (e.g., risperidone).
- Apathy may respond to dopamine agonist (e.g., bromocriptine).
- Consider respite care for caregivers.
- If problems persist and cannot be tolerated, then specialized placement may be needed.

Treatment Uncertainties

- There is no good evidence on which to base guidance as to which drug to use to control aggression after TBI [15].

SUMMARY

Prescribing for behavioral problems:

- no knee-jerk reactions—wait to see if the problem recurs or needs drug treatment
- start low, go slow—initially use at most half of the recommended dose for a patient without brain injury
- beware of "cocktails" of medication
- beware "chasing your tail," for example, by increasing akathisia or confusion
- trial of treatment—if it does not work, stop it
- use drugs with less:
  - potential for drug interactions
  - risk of aggravating epilepsy
  - anticholinergic activity
  - potential to adversely affect neural plasticity

- for the treatment of behavioral problems after TBI drugs are generally being used off label; ensure you negotiate with family and caregivers

ADDITIONAL READING

Electronic Reference
http://www.caregiver.org/caregiver/jsp/content_node.jsp?nodeid=396

Textbook/Chapter
Fleminger S. Head injury. In: David AS, Fleminger S, Kopelman MK, Lovestone S, Mellers J, eds. *Lishman's Organic Psychiatry: A Textbook of Neuropsychiatry.* 4th ed. Oxford: Wiley-Blackwell; 2009:167–280.

Journal Articles
Gordon WA, Zafonte R, Cicerone K, et al. Traumatic brain injury rehabilitation: state of the science. *Am J Phys Med Rehabil.* 2006;85:343–382.

Silver JM, Yudofsky SC, Anderson KE. Aggressive disorders. In: Silver JM, McAllister TW, Yudofsky SC, eds. *Textbook of Traumatic Brain Injury.* Arlington, TX: American Psychiatric Association; 2005:259–278.

REFERENCES

1. van der Naalt J, van Zomeren AH, Sluiter WJ, Minderhoud JM. Acute behavioural disturbances related to imaging studies and outcome in mild-to-moderate head injury. *Brain Inj.* 2000;14(9):781–788.
2. Sherer M, Hart T, Nick TG, Whyte J, Thompson RN, Yablon SA. Early impaired self-awareness after traumatic brain injury. *Arch Phys Med Rehabil.* 2003;84(2):168–176.
3. Weinstein EA, Lyerly OG. Language behavior during recovery from brain injury as predictive of later adjustment. *Trans Am Neurol Assoc.* 1968;93:292–294.
4. Baguley IJ, Cooper J, Felmingham K. Aggressive behavior following traumatic brain injury: how common is common? *J Head Trauma Rehabil.* 2006;21(1):45–56.
5. Lezak MD. Living with the characterologically altered brain injured patient. *J Clin Psychiatry.* 1978;39(7):592–598.
6. Tateno A, Jorge RE, Robinson RG. Clinical correlates of aggressive behavior after traumatic brain injury. *J Neuropsychiatry Clin Neurosci.* 2003;15(2):155–160.
7. Andersson S, Krogstad JM, Finset A. Apathy and depressed mood in acquired brain damage: relationship to lesion localization and psychophysiological reactivity. *Psychol Med.* 1999;29(2):447–456.
8. Kant R, Duffy JD, Pivovarnik A. Prevalence of apathy following head injury. *Brain Inj.* 1998;12(1):87–92.
9. Yudofsky SC, Silver JM, Jackson W, Endicott J, Williams D. The Overt Aggression Scale for the objective rating of verbal and physical aggression. *Am J Psychiatry.* 1986;143(1):35–39.

10. Schierhout G, Roberts I. Prophylactic antiepileptic agents after head injury: a systematic review. *J Neurol Neurosurg Psychiatr.* 1998;64(1):108–112.

11. Jackson WT, Novack TA, Dowler RN. Effective serial measurement of cognitive orientation in rehabilitation: the Orientation Log. *Arch Phys Med Rehabil.* 1998;79(6):718–720.

12. Folstein MF, Folstein SE, McHugh PR. "Mini-mental state". A practical method for grading the cognitive state of patients for the clinician. *J Psychiatr Res.* 1975;12(3):189–198.

13. Dubois B, Slachevsky A, Litvan I, Pillon B. The FAB: a Frontal Assessment Battery at bedside. *Neurology.* 2000;55(11):1621–1626.

14. Fleminger S. The neuropsychiatry of head injury. In: Gelder M, Andreasen N, Lopez-Ibor J, Geddes J, eds. *New Oxford Textbook of Psychiatry.* 2nd ed. Oxford: Oxford University Press; 2009,(1):387–399.

15. Warden DL, Gordon B, McAllister TW, et al.; Neurobehavioral Guidelines Working Group. Guidelines for the pharmacologic treatment of neurobehavioral sequelae of traumatic brain injury. *J Neurotrauma.* 2006;23(10):1468–1501.

16. Ylvisaker M, Turkstra L, Coehlo C. Behavioural interventions for children and adults with behaviour disorders after TBI: a systematic review of the evidence. *Brain Inj.* 2007;21(8):769–805.

39

Rational Neuropharmacology in Traumatic Brain Injury

Cynthia D. Fields and Vani Rao

BACKGROUND

Neuropsychiatric impairments are common after traumatic brain injury (TBI). These include cognitive impairment, mood and anxiety disorders, psychosis, behavioral problems, apathy, and sleep disturbance. Table 39.1 highlights the prevalence, core features, and first-line treatment of post-TBI neuropsychiatric symptoms and syndromes [1,2]. More detailed descriptions of various disorders and their management, including less commonly used medications not mentioned in this chapter, can be found elsewhere (see Additional Reading section). This chapter will provide a brief overview of the pharmacological treatment of common neuropsychiatric sequelae of TBI.

GENERAL GUIDELINES FOR MANAGEMENT

Choose a Medication

In general, pharmacotherapy for post-TBI disorders is similar to that for primary psychiatric disorders. There are few well-designed randomized, placebo controlled trials to guide treatment decisions in this population. Evidence is limited and consists mostly of case reports and case series.

Start Low and Go Slow

Start any agent at the lowest possible dose (usually one-third to one-half the usually recommended dose) and increase the dose slowly. TBI patients are very sensitive to side effects of medications. Medications with known adverse central nervous system (CNS) effects, such as sedatives or anticholinergic drugs, should be avoided whenever possible as they have the potential to impair cognition and impede neural plasticity.

Table 39.1 Prevalence, Core Features, and First-Line Treatment of Post-TBI Neuropsychiatric Syndromes

Syndrome	Prevalence (%)	Core Features	First-Line Treatment
Cognitive deficits	20–80	Disturbances of memory, attention/ processing speed, and/or executive function	Cholinesterase inhibitors, noradrenergic agonists, and/or dopamine agonists
Depression	6–77	Low mood, loss of pleasure, hopelessness, suicidal ideation	SSRIs
Mania	3–9	Elated mood and/or irritability, increased energy, impulsivity	Mood stabilizers
Anxiety	11–70	Persistent worry, tension, dread or apprehension; autonomic arousal	SSRIs
Psychosis	2–20	Hallucinations, delusions, thought disorder	Atypical antipsychotics
Behavioral dyscontrol	11–98	Agitation, aggression, mood lability, disinhibition, impulsivity	β-blockers, SSRIs
Apathy	10	Lack of motivation or drive, loss of initiative (euthymic mood)	Noradrenergic agonists, dopamine agonists
Sleep disorders	30–70	Insomnia (early or middle); hypersomnia and fatigue	Melatonin agonists, tetracyclic antidepressants; noradrenergic agonists

Minimize the Number of Medications

Treat at an adequate dose and for an appropriate length of time with a single agent before switching medications. If there is a partial response, consider augmenting with another agent. Because CNS side effects are additive, use caution when prescribing more than one psychotropic agent. Watch for drug-drug interactions and monitor serum levels of medications if available.

Consider Coexisting Medical Problems

Because seizure disorders are more common in TBI patients than in the general population, drugs that lower the seizure threshold—for example, bupropion, clozapine, and clomipramine—should be avoided, if possible.

Caution

Avoid first generation anticonvulsants such as phenytoin, benzodiazepines, and dopamine agonists such as haloperidol in the acute post-TBI period, because there is strong evidence that they can worsen cognitive functioning [3] and adversely affect neural plasticity [4]. Anticholinergics (e.g., hydroxyzine) and antihistamines (e.g., diphenhydramine) should also be avoided due to their adverse effects on the CNS. Monoamine oxidase inhibitors should be avoided due to their extensive food and drug interactions.

TREATMENT OF SPECIFIC POST-TBI DISORDERS

Cognitive Impairment

- *Cholinesterase inhibitors*—Cholinergic augmentation with cholinesterase inhibitors is a reasonable first-line treatment for memory impairment. In particular, donepezil has been studied for impairments in both memory and attention in moderate to severe TBI [5].
- *Noradrenergic agonists*—Noradrenergic agonist agents, which increase norepinephrine (and to a lesser extent, dopamine) availability, are the mainstay of treatment for impaired attention and processing speed. These agents may also enhance learning and memory. Methylphenidate has been studied extensively in moderate to severe TBI [6].
- *Dopaminergic agents*—Bromocriptine and amantadine [7] can be used to treat executive dysfunction. Amantadine is not only a dopaminergic agent but also a partial N-methyl-D-aspartate (NMDA) antagonist and a noradrenergic agent. These agents also have beneficial effects on

attention and general cognitive functioning. Amantadine is one of the most extensively studied neurostimulant medications in TBI. It is of particular interest because, in addition to its dopaminergic properties, it possesses noradrenergic properties, and therefore has the potential to influence multiple cognitive domains simultaneously.

Depression

- *Selective serotonin reuptake inhibitors (SSRIs)*—SSRIs are the first-line treatment for post-TBI depression because of their safety and tolerability as compared with tricyclic antidepressants (TCAs). Sertraline, the most dopaminergic of the SSRIs, has the best evidence supporting its use [8] and is the authors' preferred SSRI. Other commonly used SSRIs include citalopram and escitalopram.
- *TCAs*—TCAs, which block reuptake of norepinephrine and serotonin, can be quite effective for depression in some TBI patients. Although amitriptyline is recommended by certain groups [8], the authors prefer nortriptyline and desipramine because they are the least anticholinergic. Because of their unfavorable side effect profile, most clinicians use TCAs only if an initial trial of SSRIs has been unsuccessful.
- *Serotonin/norepinephrine reuptake inhibitors (SNRIs)*—SNRIs, dual reuptake inhibitors of both serotonin and norepinephrine (e.g., venlafaxine), may also be effective.
- *Mirtazapine*—Mirtazapine, a presynaptic α-2 adrenergic and serotonin receptor antagonist, can be especially useful when insomnia and/or anorexia are presenting comorbid symptoms.
- *Neuroleptics*—In cases of major depression with psychotic features, or in cases of depression with severe agitation or aggression, atypical antipsychotics (also called second generation antipsychotics; e.g., risperidone, olanzapine) at a standard dose may be used in conjunction with antidepressants. First generation antipsychotics such as haloperidol should be avoided as animal studies reveal that they can increase neuronal toxicity [9] and impede neural plasticity [4].
- *Caution*—Bupropion, which facilitates dopamine transmission and has effects on norepinephrine, is known to lower the seizure threshold. When it must be used, the long-acting XL form is preferred with a daily dosage not to exceed 300 mg.

Mania

- *Anticonvulsants*—Anticonvulsants, such as valproate [10], are the first-line treatment for post-TBI mania and bipolar disorder. Close monitoring of serum levels, liver function, and blood counts is recommended.

- *Lithium*—Anecdotal reports [11] and animal studies [12] suggest the effectiveness of lithium but clinical trials are needed. Because TBI patients are particularly prone to its neurotoxic side effects, lithium should be used with caution and is usually reserved for patients with a prior history of mania. Serum levels should be monitored.
- *Neuroleptics*—Atypical antipsychotics (e.g., risperidone and olanzapine) may be preferred when psychosis, agitation, and/or restlessness are present.

Anxiety

- *SSRIs*—Treatment of persistent anxiety often includes the use of SSRIs, for example, sertraline, at doses that are similar to or sometimes higher than those used for major depression.
- *SNRIs*—SNRIs may also be a good option for anxiety in TBI patients.
- *Buspirone*—Buspirone, a serotonergic and weakly dopaminergic agent, can be used safely as an anxiolytic in patients with TBI. Although it has a slower onset of action than benzodiazepines, buspirone can be considered as a first-line agent because of its benign side effect profile and lack of significant drug-drug interactions.

Psychosis

- *Neuroleptics*—Atypical antipsychotics are the drugs of choice for psychosis following TBI. They are preferred over the older "typical" antipsychotics because of their lower incidence of neurological side effects such as extrapyramidal side effects (EPS) and because they do not inhibit dopamine release to the same degree. Risperidone is a good first-line agent and the one that the authors prefer because of its favorable risk to benefit ratio. Olanzapine is recommended by the Neurobehavioral Guidelines Working Group [8] on the basis of case reports supporting its effectiveness [13,14]; however, metabolic side effects such as weight gain may limit its long-term use. Other atypical antipsychotics may also be reasonable options [15].
- *Anticonvulsants*—If there is no improvement on neuroleptics, anticonvulsants can be tried. Anticonvulsants can be useful for associated agitation.
- *Caution*—Clozapine should be avoided because of its potential to induce seizures.

Behavioral Dyscontrol

- *Antidepressants*—In general, the authors tend to use low-dose SSRIs as a first-line treatment for chronic agitation and aggression, especially if comorbid depressive symptoms exist. Antidepressants have also been shown to be effective in cases of affective lability and syndromes of impulsivity and/or disinhibition related to TBI, such as pathological laughter and crying (formerly referred to as pseudobulbar affect or emotional incontinence).

- *Mood stabilizers*—Mood stabilizers such as anticonvulsants are routinely used in the treatment of post-TBI lability, impulsivity, and/or disinhibition.

- *β-Blockers*—Small randomized controlled trials have demonstrated the efficacy of β-adrenergic receptor blocker agents for the treatment of post-TBI aggression [16] and guidelines have been established for their use [8]. β-Blockers selective for the β-1 subtype (e.g., metoprolol) are generally preferred because they tend to result in less CNS depression.

- *Neuroleptics*—Acutely, if the patient is getting increasingly agitated, low-dose atypical antipsychotics can be used. Note, however, that antipsychotic medications do not help with chronic nonpsychotic aggression.

- *Other*—Noradrenergic agonists and dopaminergics may be useful for impulsivity and disinhibition.

Apathy

Noradrenergic agonists (e.g., methylphenidate) and dopaminergic agents (e.g., amantadine [17]) may be beneficial in the treatment of post-TBI apathy. Cholinesterase inhibitors may also be useful if there is an associated post-TBI dementia. A note of caution: SSRIs, especially in high doses, can worsen apathy and amotivational syndromes [18].

ADDITIONAL READING

Electronic References
http://web.uvic.ca/psyc/skelton/Teaching/415B%20Assignment_Materials/Maythaler_2002.pdf
http://www.liebertonline.com/doi/pdfplus/10.1089/neu.2009.1091

Textbook/Chapter
Silver J, McAllister T, Yudofsky S, eds. *Textbook of Traumatic Brain Injury.* Arlington, TX: American Psychiatric Publishing; 2005.

Journal Articles
Chew E, Zafonte RD. Pharmacological management of neurobehavioral disorders following traumatic brain injury—a state-of-the-art review. *J Rehabil Res Dev.* 2009;46(6):851–879.

Goldstein LB. Neuropharmacology of TBI-induced plasticity. *Brain Inj.* 2003;17(8):685–694.

Kim E, Lauterbach EC, Reeve A, et al. Neuropsychiatric complications of traumatic brain injury: a critical review of the literature (a report by the ANPA committee on research). *J Neuropsychiatry Clin Neurosci.* 2007;19(2):106–127.

Lee HB, Lyketsos CG, Rao V. Pharmacological management of the psychiatric aspects of traumatic brain injury. *Int Rev Psychiatry.* 2003;15(4):359–370.

Vaishnavi S, Rao V, Fann JR. Neuropsychiatric problems after traumatic brain injury: unraveling the silent epidemic. *Psychosomatics.* 2009;50(3):198–205.

Warden DL, Gordon B, McAllister TW, et al. Guidelines for the pharmacologic treatment of neurobehavioral sequelae of traumatic brain injury. *J Neurotrauma.* 2006;23(10):1468–1501.

REFERENCES

1. Rao V, Rollings P, Spiro J. Fatigue and sleep problems. In: Silver JM, McAllister TW, Yudofsky SC, eds. *Textbook of Traumatic Brain Injury.* Arlington, TX: American Psychiatric Publishing; 2005:369–384.

2. Rao V, Lyketsos CG. Psychiatric aspects of traumatic brain injury. *Psychiatr Clin North Am.* 2002;25(1):43–69.

3. Dikmen SS, Temkin NR, Miller B, Machamer J, Winn HR. Neurobehavioral effects of phenytoin prophylaxis of posttraumatic seizures. *JAMA.* 1991;265(10):1271–1277.

4. Goldstein LB. Neuropharmacology of TBI-induced plasticity. *Brain Inj.* 2003;17(8):685–694.

5. Zhang L, Plotkin RC, Wang G, Sandel ME, Lee S. Cholinergic augmentation with donepezil enhances recovery in short-term memory and sustained attention after traumatic brain injury. *Arch Phys Med Rehabil.* 2004;85(7):1050–1055.

6. Whyte J, Hart T, Vaccaro M, et al. Effects of methylphenidate on attention deficits after traumatic brain injury: a multidimensional, randomized, controlled trial. *Am J Phys Med Rehabil.* 2004;83(6):401–420.

7. McDowell S, Whyte J, D'Esposito M. Differential effect of a dopaminergic agonist on prefrontal function in traumatic brain injury patients. *Brain.* 1998;121 (Pt 6):1155–1164.

8. Warden DL, Gordon B, McAllister TW, et al.; Neurobehavioral Guidelines Working Group. Guidelines for the pharmacologic treatment of neurobehavioral sequelae of traumatic brain injury. *J Neurotrauma.* 2006;23(10):1468–1501.

9. Feeney DM, Gonzalez A, Law WA. Amphetamine, haloperidol, and experience interact to affect rate of recovery after motor cortex injury. *Science.* 1982;217(4562):855–857.

10. Pope HG Jr, McElroy SL, Satlin A, Hudson JI, Keck PE Jr, Kalish R. Head injury, bipolar disorder, and response to valproate. *Compr Psychiatry.* 1988;29(1):34–38.

11. Hale MS, Donaldson JO. Lithium carbonate in the treatment of organic brain syndrome. *J Nerv Ment Dis.* 1982;170(6):362–365.

12. Young W. Review of lithium effects on brain and blood. *Cell Transplant.* 2009;18(9):951–975.

13. Butler PV. Diurnal variation in Cotard's syndrome (copresent with Capgras delusion) following traumatic brain injury. *Aust N Z J Psychiatry.* 2000;34(4):684–687.

14. Umansky R, Geller V. Olanzapine treatment in an organic hallucinosis patient. *Int J Neuropsychopharmacol.* 2000;3(1):81–82.

15. Lee HB, Lyketsos CG, Rao V. Pharmacological management of the psychiatric aspects of traumatic brain injury. *Int Rev Psychiatry.* 2003;15(4):359–370.

16. Brooke MM, Patterson DR, Questad KA, Cardenas D, Farrel-Roberts L. The treatment of agitation during initial hospitalization after traumatic brain injury. *Arch Phys Med Rehabil.* 1992;73(10):917–921.

17. Van Reekum R, Bayley M, Garner S, et al. N of 1 study: amantadine for the amotivational syndrome in a patient with traumatic brain injury. *Brain Inj.* 1995;9(1):49–53.

18. Price J, Cole V, Goodwin GM. Emotional side-effects of selective serotonin reuptake inhibitors: qualitative study. *Br J Psychiatry.* 2009;195(3):211–217.

40

Pain Management in Persons With Traumatic Brain Injury

Nathan D. Zasler

INTRODUCTION

There is limited, methodologically sound, evidence-based literature on the incidence, prevalence, epidemiology, etiology, assessment, and treatment of pain in persons with traumatic brain injury (TBI).

Pain, as defined by the International Association for the Study of Pain, is "an unpleasant sensory and emotional experience associated with actual or potential tissue damage, or described in terms of such damage" [1]. Pain should be considered as a multidimensional subjective experience mediated by cultural, emotional, and perceptual influences, among other factors that affect patient perception and coping ability.

PAIN GENERATORS IN PERSONS WITH TBI

There are often challenges with regard to accurately determining primary pain generators; frequently multiple pain generators can be identified in this population.

- In the acute care phase, the primary pain generators are more likely to involve such phenomena as fractures, intra-abdominal injuries, peripheral nerve injuries, soft tissue injuries, and pain associated with invasive procedures [2].
- In the chronic phase, spasticity/hypertonicity, myostatic contracture, myofascial pain, fibromyalgia, complex regional pain syndrome, central pain syndrome, central sensitization, skin breakdown, and tissue hypoxemia, among other phenomena, may be causes of pain [2].
- In persons with disorders of consciousness, pain must be adequately assessed; however, controversies remain regarding the methods for assessment and management, including differentiation between reflex and conscious pain responses [3].

PAIN ASSESSMENT

History

The primary points to address in the context of taking a pain history [4] include

- Time of onset of pain
- Progression of pain over time
- Treatment history relative to pharmacological and nonpharmacological approaches that have either helped pain and/or made it worse
- Frequency of pain
- Severity of pain, typically rated using some type of pain scale (i.e., pain faces)
- "COLDER" mnemonic—character, onset, location, duration, exacerbation, relief
- Functional consequences of pain (i.e., how this pain affects ability to perform work- and non–work-related activities)
- In the context of assessing pain, it is always important to determine if the patient had similar pain complaints predating the injury and, if so, whether they have been altered by the injury in any way (i.e., better or worse)
- Review relevant medical records to increase understanding of potential pain generators
- Interview corroboratory sources, as persons with TBI may not have adequate insight into, or memory regarding, their condition and/or its functional consequences.

There are also a number of well-validated and reliable pain assessment batteries that can be considered for use to supplement information derived during the interview, including measures of behavioral and cognitive coping, measures of general health functioning, specific pain domain inventories, and/or general psychological measures, in particular, the Minnesota Multiphasic Personality Inventory (MMPI; [5]). There are also additional pain assessment measures with built-in response bias indicators [5].

Clinicians should be familiar with nonorganic indicators on interview that may suggest the need for further assessment of functional contributors to the pain presentation.

Examination

- Conduct a holistic evaluation including inspection, palpation, and appropriate neuromusculoskeletal examination.

- Evaluate for response bias (e.g., MMPI-II validity scales, Word Memory Test), particularly when there are obvious secondary gain motivators such as personal injury litigation [6].

Diagnostic Assessment

The main clinical tests pertinent to assessment of pain include imaging, electrophysiological testing, affective status testing, response bias testing, pain psychology and coping testing, and general functional assessment testing. Tests should only be ordered when it is anticipated that the results will have an impact on clarifying a diagnosis and/or treatment plan or facilitating prognostication [4,5,7].

PAIN MANAGEMENT

Primary Goals in Pain Management

- Modulate and ideally negate associated physical and psychological signs and symptoms associated with the pain condition/disorder [7].
- Prevent chronicity and secondary complications thereof, such as central sensitization and/or chronic affective and maladjustment issues.
- Reduce functional disability and facilitate productive activity including, as possible, return-to-work.
- Establish realistic treatment end points for the specific pain disorder.
- Educate regarding treatment options including risks versus benefits.
- The simplest, least invasive, lowest risk, and most cost effective management approaches that allow for optimization of patient compliance and maximal functional restoration should be used whenever possible.
- When pharmacological agents are used, analgesia should be delivered with minimal adverse effects and inconvenience to the patient, with clearly defined treatment expectations, including education regarding medication side-effects [7].
- Proper communication should be maintained between the patient, the caregiver, and treater regarding response to individual pain treatment interventions.
- The treating clinician should maintain ongoing communication with any other clinicians involved with the patient's health management to adequately coordinate clinical care.
- Try to avoid use of opiates to modulate pain unless other options have failed.
- Remember that not all pain is opiate sensitive; musculoskeletal pain generators tend to respond better to opiates than neurogenic/neuropathic pain generators.

- Institute appropriate screening (i.e., Opiate Risk Tool) and monitoring procedures (including use of opiate agreements and random urine screens) [8].

Pharmacological Methods of Treatment

General Guidelines
Pharmacological approaches should be hierarchically divided based on the intensity and type of pain being treated.

Mild Mild pain medicines that should be considered typically include aspirin, acetaminophen, and nonsteroidal anti-inflammatory drugs (NSAIDs).

Moderate Moderate pain medications include high-dose aspirin or acetaminophen, high-dose standard NSAIDs, newer generation NSAIDs such as cyclooxygenase-II inhibitors, injectable nonsteroidal anti-inflammatories, mixed narcotic analgesics with aspirin or acetaminophen (with or without caffeine), compounded topical medications, whether trademark or compounded, and Tramadol.

Severe Medications to consider would include parenteral narcotics, with Morphine Sulfate being considered the standard, mixed agonist antagonists such as pentazocine, partial opiate agonists such as buprenorphine, ketamine, antidepressants, anticonvulsants, continuous local anesthetic, peripheral nerve block, and/or atypical agents including cannabinoids. Other agents can be considered as adjutants including atypical antipsychotic agents and N-methyl D-aspartate antagonists such as memantine [7].

Medications that have been used for opioid insensitive pain include NSAIDs, tricyclic antidepressants, newer generation antidepressants such as venlafaxine or duloxetine, anticonvulsants including carbamazepine derivatives, gabapentin, pregabalin, leviracetam, and lamotrogine, as well as less commonly used agents such as mexiletine. Other agents that have more recently been recognized as potential adjutants in the pharmacological management of pain include tizanidine and sodium amobarbital [7,8].

Evidence-based guidelines and meta-analyses should be referred to as guides to the specific use of pharmacological and nonpharmacological interventions for specific pain disorder conditions as available.

Attempts should be made to minimize polypharmacy as this will improve compliance, decrease drug-drug interactions, and improve quality of life at the same time as decreasing cost to patient. In addition, whenever possible, use of medications whose mechanism of action may impede neural plasticity (e.g., opiates, barbiturates, certain anticonvulsants) should be minimized or avoided [9].

Nonpharmacological Methods

Physical Approaches

- Physical agents such as superficial heat and cold can be used to modulate pain.
- There are a number of electrical stimulation techniques used in pain management [10]:
  - Transcutaneous electrical nerve stimulation and iontophoresis are commonly employed as adjutants for pain control.
  - Cranioelectrical stimulation is an FDA-approved treatment for pain reduction that can complement other interventions.
- Acupuncture may also serve as an adjunctive treatment for pain management [11].
- Physical modalities tend to play a more predominant role in the treatment of pain complaints of musculoskeletal origin, and may include traction, manual medicine techniques, as well as massage.
- Injection therapy, including intra-articular, periarticular, peritendinous, ligamentous/fibrous tissue, and trigger point injections, can all be used in various types of musculoskeletal pain disorders [12].
  - Older techniques such as prolotherapy and newer techniques such as injection of platelet-rich plasma seem promising for treatment of posttraumatic musculotendinous pain [7,13].
  - Anesthetic injections, either alone or in conjunction with steroids, may be helpful in certain posttraumatic, neuralgic, or neuritic pain conditions.
  - Axial injections (e.g., epidural, zygapophyseal, sympathetic) may be relevant considerations for particular posttraumatic pain disorders.
- Exercise is an underprescribed treatment intervention in pain management. Beneficial effects can include pain modulation on both a central and peripheral basis, weight control, positive affective modulation, benefits to brain function, improvement of general sense of well-being, and improved general state of health.
- Appropriate prescription of adaptive equipment, as well as an ergonomically modified work environment, may also add to overall management of posttraumatic pain conditions to facilitate greater pain modulation and tolerance.
- Novel techniques, such as vestibular stimulation and deep brain stimulation, are also being used for treatment of certain types of pain conditions [14,15].

Psychological Approaches

- A variety of psychological methods may be appropriate to consider in the context of pain management, either in conjunction with other interventions or as the sole intervention. Psychological interventions are underutilized treatment options for patients with chronic post-traumatic pain disorders [10].

- Behavioral treatment interventions for pain in persons with TBI should focus on coping with pain, modulation of affective responses to chronic pain and associated disability, as well as primary pain modulation. Behavioral interventional techniques including biofeedback, relaxation training, operant treatments, cognitive behavioral interventions, as well as social and assertiveness skills and training, imagery and hypnosis, and habit reversal should also be considered [5,10].

CONCLUSIONS

Appropriate pain management in persons with TBI requires not only an understanding of the impact TBI may have on the pain neuromatrix but also an understanding of the myriad pain generators that may occur after TBI, cranial trauma, cervical injury, and polytrauma in general. Clinicians must have an understanding of the literature relevant to this area of treatment, the numerous assessment challenges and tools (including the importance of taking an adequate history), and the various management options, including caveats for treatment in this population of patients.

ADDITIONAL READING

Electronic References

http://pain-topics.org/guidelines_reports/current_guidelines.php#acutepain
http://pain-topics.org/guidelines_reports/current_guidelines2.php
http://www.ninds.nih.gov/disorders/chronic_pain/chronic_pain.htm

Textbooks/Chapters

Martelli MF, Zasler ND. Post-traumatic pain disorders: psychological assessment and management. In: Zasler N, Katz D, Zafonte R, eds. *Brain Injury Medicine: Principles and Practice*. New York: Demos Medical Publishing; 2007.

Zasler ND, Horn L, Martelli MF, Nicholson K. Post-traumatic pain disorders: medical assessment and management. In: Zasler N, Katz D, Zafonte R, eds. *Brain Injury Medicine: Principles and Practice*. New York: Demos Medical Publishing; 2007:697–722.

Zasler ND, Martelli MF. Chronic pain. In: Silver JM, McAllister TW, Yudofsky SC, eds. *Textbook of Traumatic Brain Injury*. 2nd ed. Washington, DC: American Psychiatric Publishing, Inc. 2011:375–396.

Journal Articles

Dobscha SK, Clark ME, Morasco BJ, et al. Systematic review of the literature on pain in patients with polytrauma including traumatic brain injury. *Pain Med.* 2009;10(7):1200–1217.

Ivanhoe CB, Hartman ET. Clinical caveats on medical assessment and treatment of pain after TBI. *J Head Trauma Rehabil.* 2004;19(1):29–39.

Martelli MF, Zasler ND, Bender MC, Nicholson K. Psychological, neuropsychological and medical considerations in assessment and management of pain. *J Head Trauma Rehabil.* 2004;19(1):10–28.

Nampiaparampil DE. Prevalence of chronic pain after traumatic brain injury. *JAMA.* 2008;300(6):711–719.

REFERENCES

1. IASP Task Force on Taxonomy. In: Merskey H, Bogduk N, eds. *Classification of Chronic Pain.* 2nd ed. Seattle, WA: IASP Press, 1994:209–214.
2. Ivanhoe CB, Hartman ET. Clinical caveats on medical assessment and treatment of pain after TBI. *J Head Trauma Rehabil.* 2004;19(1):29–39.
3. Schnakers C, Zasler ND. Pain assessment and management in disorders of consciousness. *Curr Opin Neurol.* 2007;20(6):620–626.
4. Zasler ND, Martelli MF. Chronic pain. In: Silver JM, McAllister TW, Yudofsky SC, eds. *Textbook of Traumatic Brain Injury.* 2nd ed. Washington, DC: American Psychiatric Publishing, Inc. 2011:375–396.
5. Martelli MF, Zasler ND, Bender MC, Nicholson K. Psychological, neuropsychological, and medical considerations in assessment and management of pain. *J Head Trauma Rehabil.* 2004;19(1):10–28.
6. Martelli MF, Nicholson K, Zasler ND. Assessment of response bias. In: Zasler N, Katz D, Zafonte R, eds. *Brain Injury Medicine: Principles and Practice.* New York: Demos Medical Publishing; 2007:1183–1124.
7. Zasler ND, Horn L, Martelli MF, Nicholson K. Post-traumatic pain disorders: medical assessment and management. In: Zasler N, Katz D, Zafonte R, eds. *Brain Injury Medicine: Principles and Practice.* New York: Demos Medical Publishing; 2007:697–722.
8. Manchikanti L, Atluri S, Trescot AM, Giordano J. Monitoring opioid adherence in chronic pain patients: tools, techniques, and utility. *Pain Physician.* 2008;11(2 suppl):S155–S180.
9. Walker WC. Pain pathoetiology after TBI: neural and nonneural mechanisms. *J Head Trauma Rehabil.* 2004;19(1):72–81.
10. Martelli MF, Zasler ND. Post-traumatic pain disorders: psychological assessment and management. In: Zasler N, Katz D, Zafonte R, eds. *Brain Injury Medicine: Principles and Practice.* New York: Demos Medical Publishing; 2007:723–742.
11. Barlas P, Lundeberg T. Transcutaneous electrical nerve stimulation and acupuncture. In: McMahon SB, Koltzenburg M. *Wall and Melzack's Textbook of Pain.* Philadelphia, PA: Elsevier; 2006:583–590.
12. Lennard TA. *Physiatric Procedures in Clinical Practice.* Philadelphia, PA: Hanley & Belfus; 1995.
13. Rabago D, Best TM, Beamsley M, Patterson J. A systematic review of prolotherapy for chronic musculoskeletal pain. *Clin J Sport Med.* 2005;15(5):376–380.
14. Ramachandran VS, McGeoch PD, Williams L, Arcilla G. Rapid relief of thalamic pain syndrome induced by vestibular caloric stimulation. *Neurocase.* 2007;13(3):185–188.
15. Garonzik I, Samdani A, Ohara S, et al. Deep brain stimulation for the control of pain. *Epilepsy and Behavior.* 2001;2(3);S55–S60.

41

Practical Guidelines for Prognostication After Traumatic Brain Injury

Sunil Kothari

INTRODUCTION

- Families report that they rarely receive the prognostic information they desire after traumatic brain injury (TBI) [1–3].
- Subjective estimates of prognosis based solely on a clinician's personal experience are far less accurate than evidence-based prognoses derived from well-designed studies [4–6].
- Recently published evidence-based guidelines on prognosis after severe TBI have been updated for this chapter and are summarized in the following sections. Additional details about the methodology used are available elsewhere [7].
- These guidelines are designed to facilitate prognostication in individual patients by using readily available information (*predictor variables*) to predict the likelihood of long-term outcomes.

EVIDENCE-BASED GUIDELINES: BACKGROUND

- The guidelines are meant for *adults with severe TBI*. Information on both mild TBI as well as pediatric TBI is found elsewhere in this volume.
- The primary *outcomes* include classification according to the Glasgow Outcome Scale (GOS), independent living, and vocational reentry, all assessed at 6 months or later.
- The *Glasgow Outcome Scale* is the most widely used measure of outcome after TBI; the guidelines assume a basic familiarity with its main categories (Table 41.1).
- The primary *predictor variables* include age, initial Glasgow Coma Scale (GCS) score, duration of coma (as measured by the time to follow commands), early neuroimaging (both computed tomography [CT] and magnetic resonance imaging), and duration of posttraumatic amnesia (PTA).

TABLE 41.1 Glasgow Outcome Scale

- Dead
- Vegetative state ("alive but unconscious")
- Severe disability ("conscious but dependent")—unable to live alone for more than 24 hours: the daily assistance of another person at home is essential as a result of physical and/or cognitive impairments
- Moderate disability ("independent but disabled")—independent at home; able to utilize public transportation; able to work in a supported environment
- Good recovery ("mild to no residual deficits")—capacity to resume normal occupational and social activities, although there may be minor residual physical or mental deficits

- Several of the predictor variables were found to have *threshold values,* which are values above or below which a particular outcome was especially unlikely. For example:
  - If PTA lasts *more* than 3 months, a person is very unlikely to achieve a "good recovery" on the GOS.
  - If PTA lasts *less* than 2 months, a person is very unlikely to be severely disabled as defined by the GOS.
- Clinicians can use these *threshold values as milestones* in a patient's recovery. For instance, as the length of a patient's PTA extends beyond 3 months, rehabilitation clinicians can counsel family members about realistic expectations for the future. On the other hand, if 2 months have not yet elapsed since the injury, clinicians can give hope to families, even if the patient is still in PTA.
- Although they are well supported by research, these *threshold values are not absolute*; there is a degree of statistical uncertainty in their use. In particular, the upper limit of the confidence interval averaged approximately 10%. This means that approximately 10% of individuals will prove to be exceptions to the guidelines.

EVIDENCE-BASED GUIDELINES: RESULTS

- The results of the studies reviewed are summarized in Table 41.2. The final guidelines are presented in Table 41.3.
- The duration of PTA is a more powerful predictor of outcome than the length of coma. If both are available, one should rely on the duration of PTA when prognosticating [7].
- A large, recently published study (n=1332) based on the Traumatic Brain Injury Model System database reports threshold values for the

Table 41.2 Summary of Studies of Nonpenetrating Traumatic Brain Injury

Glasgow Coma Scale

- Lower scores associated with worse outcomes
- No threshold values

Length of coma

- Longer duration associated with worse outcomes
- Threshold values:
    - Severe disability unlikely when less than 2 weeks
    - Good recovery unlikely when more than 4 weeks

Posttraumatic amnesia

- Longer duration associated with worse outcomes
- Threshold values:
    - Severe disability unlikely when less than 2 months
    - Good recovery unlikely when more than 3 months

Age

- Older age associated with worse outcomes
- Threshold values:
    - Good recovery unlikely when more than 65 years

Neuroimaging

- Certain features (e.g., depth of lesions) associated with worse outcomes
- Threshold values:
    - Good recovery unlikely when bilateral brainstem lesions present on early magnetic resonance imaging

From Ref. [7].

Table 41.3 Summary of Evidence-Based Guidelines for Prognostication After Severe Nonpenetrating TBI[*]

Severe disability (according to GOS) is unlikely when
- Time to follow commands is less than 2 weeks
- Duration of PTA is less than 2 months

Good recovery (according to the GOS) is unlikely when
- Time to follow commands is longer than 1 month
- Duration of PTA is more than 3 months
- Age is more than 65 years

Up to 10% of patients may be exceptions to these guidelines.
GOS, Glasgow Outcome Scale; PTA, posttraumatic amnesia; TBI, traumatic brain injury.

From Ref. [7].

duration of PTA similar to those summarized here. In particular, it found that (1) good recovery is unlikely when PTA lasts more than 2 months and (2) severe disability is unlikely when PTA lasts less than 40 days [8].

PENETRATING INJURIES

- Although the mortality rate from penetrating injuries is much higher than with closed head injuries, survivors are less likely to be vegetative or severely disabled.
- In general, after penetrating missile injury, lower GCS scores and CT findings of bilaterality or transventricular injury are associated with worse outcomes. Moreover, patients with a postresuscitation GCS score of 8 or less are unlikely to achieve a good recovery [7].

MODERATE TBI

- More than 90% of individuals with moderate TBI (GCS 9–12) will achieve either a moderate disability or good recovery [9,10].
- Risk factors associated with poorer outcomes: GCS score of 9 or 10, older age, and abnormalities on CT scan. When these are present, patients are more likely to have a moderate disability (or, infrequently, severe disability) rather than good recovery [9,10].

RECENT DEVELOPMENTS

- Our ability to prognosticate after TBI may improve as a result of recent advances in technology such as magnetic resonance spectroscopy, serum markers (e.g., s100b), and neural networks. Although promising, there is not yet enough evidence to support the use of these modalities in routine clinical practice [11].

Table 41.4 General Guidelines for Communicating Prognostic Information

---

- Begin with the family's *desire for information* as well as their *current beliefs*
- Ensure that the meaning and content of the *outcomes* are understood
- Present *quantitative information* in a manner that can be understood (see Table 41.5)
- Foster *hope*
- Pay attention to the *process* of communication (see Table 41.6)

From Ref. [7].

Table 41.5 Guidelines for the Communication of Quantitative Information

- Try to use "natural frequencies" when communicating probabilistic information *(e.g., "Eight out of 10 people with this type of injury will make a good recovery")*
- Present information both qualitatively as well as quantitatively *(e.g., "There is a very good chance of a good recovery")*
- Attempt to "frame" information in both a positive and negative manner *(e.g., "That is the same as saying that 2 out of 10 people with this type of injury will not make a good recovery")*
- When possible, consider presenting the information visually
- Ask person to restate, in their own words, their understanding of the information provided

From Ref. [7].

Table 41.6 Guidelines for the Communication Process

- Find a quiet, comfortable room without interruptions
- Sit close and speak face to face
- Have the family member's support network present, if they desire
- Present the information at a pace the family can follow
- Periodically summarize the discussion to that point
- Periodically ask family member to repeat or summarize what was said
- Keep the language simple but direct, without euphemism or jargon
- Allow time for questions

From Ref. [7].

COMMUNICATING PROGNOSES

- Formulating a prediction is only the first step in prognostication; this information must then be conveyed to the family. Tables 41.4–41.6 provide some suggestions for communicating prognostic information.

ADDITIONAL READING

Electronic Reference
https://www.braintrauma.org/pdf/protected/prognosis_guidelines.pdf

Textbook/Chapter

Kothari S. Prognosis after severe TBI: a practical, evidence-based approach. In: Zasler N, Katz D, Zafonte R, eds. *Brain Injury Medicine: Principles and Practice;* New York: Demos Medical Publishing. 2007:169–199.

Journal Articles

Technologies of Prognostication. Theme Issue of the *J Head Trauma Rehabil.* 2006 (July/August);21(4):293–374.

Walker W, Ketchum J, Marwitz J, et al. A multicentre study on the clinical utility of post-traumatic amnesia duration in predicting global outcome after moderate-severe traumatic brain injury. *J Neurol Neurosurg Psychiatry.* 2010;81:87–89.

REFERENCES

1. Consensus conference. Rehabilitation of persons with traumatic brain injury. NIH consensus development panel on rehabilitation of persons with traumatic brain injury. *JAMA.* 1999;282:974–983.

2. Holland D, Shigaki CL. Educating families and caretakers of traumatically brain injured patients in the new health care environment: a three phase model and bibliography. *Brain Inj.* 1998;12(12):993–1009.

3. Junqué C, Bruna O, Mataró M. Information needs of the traumatic brain injury patient's family members regarding the consequences of the injury and associated perception of physical, cognitive, emotional and quality of life changes. *Brain Inj.* 1997;11(4):251–258.

4. Perkins HS, Jonsen AR, Epstein WV. Providers as predictors: using outcome predictions in intensive care. *Crit Care Med.* 1986;14(2):105–110.

5. Poses RM, Bekes C, Copare FJ, Scott WE. The answer to "What are my chances, doctor?" depends on whom is asked: prognostic disagreement and inaccuracy for critically ill patients. *Crit Care Med.* 1989;17(8):827–833.

6. Chang RW, Lee B, Jacobs S, Lee B. Accuracy of decisions to withdraw therapy in critically ill patients: clinical judgment versus a computer model. *Crit Care Med.* 1989;17(11):1091–1097.

7. Kothari S. Prognosis after severe TBI: a practical, evidence-based approach. In: Zasler N, Katz D, Zafonte R, eds. *Brain Injury Medicine: Principles and Practice.* New York: Demos Medical Publishing. 2007;169–199.

8. Walker WC, Ketchum JM, Marwitz JH, et al. A multicentre study on the clinical utility of post-traumatic amnesia duration in predicting global outcome after moderate-severe traumatic brain injury. *J Neurol Neurosurg Psychiatr.* 2010;81(1):87–89.

9. van der Naalt J. Prediction of outcome in mild to moderate head injury: a review. *J Clin Exp Neuropsychol.* 2001;23(6):837–851.

10. Stein SC. Outcome from moderate head injury. In: Narayan RK, Wilberger JE, Povlishock JT, eds. *Neurotrauma.* New York: McGraw-Hill; 1996:755–765.

11. Technologies of Prognostication. *J Head Trauma Rehabil.* 2006 (July/August);21(4):315–333.

42

Sexuality After Traumatic Brain Injury

Angelle M. Sander

GENERAL BACKGROUND

- Sexual dysfunction is a frequent occurrence in persons with traumatic brain injury (TBI), with many studies documenting sexual problems in more than half of their participants [1–3].
- Decreased frequency of, and/or satisfaction with, sexual activity has been noted among males and females [1–9].
- Failure to address sexuality can lead to emotional difficulties, low self-esteem, and relationship problems.

COMMON TYPES OF SEXUAL PROBLEMS AFTER TBI

- Decreased desire or drive [4,6,7]
- Decreased arousal: characterized by difficulty obtaining or maintaining an erection in males [2,4–7] and by decreased vaginal lubrication in females [6]
- Decreased ability to achieve orgasm [5–7]
- Ejaculatory dysfunction in males [8,9]
- Hypersexuality—drastic increase in sexual drive, accompanied by disinhibition and inappropriate sexual behaviors, or sexual behavior in inappropriate settings; occurs rarely, but results in significant distress for rehabilitation staff and family members [8,10]

CAUSES OF SEXUAL DYSFUNCTION AFTER TBI

Primary causes—direct result of changes to brain structure or function

- Frontal lobe damage or damage to related subcortical structures [10,11]
  - Dorsolateral frontal damage: apathy and decreased initiation and/or interest in sex
  - Orbitofrontal damage: disinhibited and impulsive sexual behavior

- Damage to temporal lobe or related limbic structures, including amygdala [11,12]
  - Temporo-limbic dysfunction in epileptics is associated with hyposexuality [13].
  - Bilateral anteromedial temporal lobe damage: Kluver-Bucy type syndrome, with disinhibited sexual behavior [14,15].
- Damage to subcortical structures (thalamus, hypothalamus, or hippocampus) [12,16,17]
- Damage to afferent (sensory) and efferent (motor) pathways in the brainstem [12]
- Disruption of neurochemical system (dopamine, serotonin) [12]
- Neuroendocrine dysfunction (hypothalamic-pituitary-gonadal system) [12,18]
  - Damage to hypothalamus and pituitary common with TBI
  - Disruption of hormone levels (testosterone, progesterone, and estrogen)
  - Can lead to disruptions in menstrual cycle and decreased fertility in women
  - Can lead to decreased sperm production and infertility in men

Secondary causes—due to indirect effects of other changes resulting from TBI

- Medication side effects [11,19]
  - Anticonvulsants—can result in decreased sex drive and impotence
  - Antidepressants—can result in decreased sex drive, erectile and ejaculatory dysfunction for men, and delayed orgasm for women
  - Anticholinergics—can reduce sex drive and result in erectile and ejaculatory dysfunction
  - Serotonergic agonists—can result in decreased sex drive
- Physical impairments [11]
  - Motor impairments (e.g., spasticity, hemiparesis, or decreased balance)—can lead to difficulty with positioning and to pain during sexual activity
  - Sensory impairments—can affect arousal and ability to achieve orgasm
- Cognitive impairments
  - Impaired attention and concentration can affect sexual arousal and ability to sustain attention during a sexual encounter [20].
  - Impaired memory can affect ability to recall sexual encounters and/or dates that can lead to sexual opportunity [10,21].
  - Impaired initiation affects frequency of sexual activity and can be interpreted as disinterest by partner [11].

- Impaired social communication/pragmatics results in decreased awareness of the impact of actions on others, decreased ability to read non-verbal cues and gestures, decreased ability to interpret others' emotions, decreased empathy, and decreased ability to initiate conversation [22].
- Impaired planning and goal-directed behavior may result in difficulty accomplishing social planning leading to opportunities for sexual relationships (e.g., can't make a date, plan date activities, set up a romantic environment) [11].
- Impaired cognitive flexibility and abstract thinking limit the ability to fantasize, which is important for drive and arousal [11].

- Emotional changes—including depression, low self-esteem, poor body image, child-like and dependent behaviors, self-centeredness, apathy, aggression, and impulsivity [20]
- Relationship issues—marital dysfunction, loss of friendships and social networks/social isolation [23]

TREATMENT

- The most important thing that you can do for your patients is to create an atmosphere of openness and comfort regarding the discussion of sexuality. Let them know that sexual problems are not infrequent after TBI. Emphasize that problems are treatable.
- Integrate 1 or 2 questions on sexuality into your intake or follow-up interview.
  - "Are you sexually active and/or are you satisfied with your sexual functioning?"
  - "Do you have any questions or concerns about the impact of TBI on sex?"
- Conduct a comprehensive medical examination, referring out and/or treating as appropriate:
  - Screen for other medical illnesses that could contribute to sexual dysfunction (e.g., diabetes, heart disease, kidney disease, and thyroid dysfunction).
  - Obtain hormone levels and investigate possibility of pituitary dysfunction.
  - Conduct or refer for urological examination and/or obstetrics/gynecology examination.
  - Review medications for side effects affecting sexual function.
  - Rule out pain as a cause of sexual problems.
  - Rule out motor problems as a contributor to sexual dysfunction.
- Provide specific suggestions to improve sexual functioning:
  - A change in positioning during sexual activity can reduce impact of motor problems, balance problems, and pain.

- Assist men with investigating drugs to enhance sexual performance and/or prosthetic devices to compensate for erectile dysfunction.
- Assist women with investigating lubricants and/or dilators to compensate for lack of vaginal lubrication.
- Altering the environment during sexual encounters can reduce the impact of distractibility and other cognitive deficits (e.g., arranging a quiet environment, with minimal background noise).
- Use of erotic movies or books to assist with arousal.
- Investigation of ways to increase social networks can increase the opportunity to form intimate relationships (e.g., local Y.M.C.A., church groups, and other social organizations). Have a list of these available in your clinic.
- Provide information on safe sex practices, including birth control and prevention of HIV and other sexually transmitted diseases.

- Refer for other services as appropriate:
  - Postacute cognitive rehabilitation to address cognitive deficits that can affect sexual functioning, particularly social communication
  - Individual counseling/psychotherapy to address emotional issues
  - Marital or couples therapy to address relationship issues
  - Licensed sex therapy to directly address sexual problems
  - Bibliotherapy—reading about sexuality and alternative ways for sexual fulfillment—books, or Internet; includes information on sexual prostheses

ADDITIONAL READING

Electronic References
General information about sexuality and
sexual health after TBI

Alberta Health Services. http://www.calgaryhealthregion.ca/programs/sexual-health/facts/disability/headinjury.htm

Better Health Channel. http://www.betterhealth.vic.gov.au/bhcv2/bhcarticles.nsf/pages/Traumatic_brain_injury_and_sexual_issues

Adaptable sexual aides

Comeasyouare.com

Mypleasure.com/education/disability/index.asp

Podcast: *Sexuality after Traumatic Brain Injury* hosted by Gerry Brooks, Northeast Center for Special Care, March 2009. http://www.northeastcenter.com/podcast-traumatic-brain-injury-029.htm

Textbooks/Chapters
Aloni R, Katz S. *Sexual Difficulties After Traumatic Brain Injury and Ways to Deal With It.* Springfield, IL: Charles C. Thomas Publisher; 2003.

Blackerby WF. *Head Injury Rehabilitation: Sexuality After TBI.* HDI Publishers; 1994.

Sandel ME, Delmonico R, Kotch MJ. Sexuality, reproduction, and neuroendocrine disorders following TBI. In: Zasler ND, Katz DI, Zafonte RD, eds. *Brain Injury Medicine*. New York: Demos Medical Publishing; 2007:673–695.

Journal Articles

Aloni R, Katz S. A review of the effect of traumatic brain injury on the human sexual response. *Brain Inj.* 1999;13(4):269–280.

Ducharme S, Gill KM. Sexual values, training, and professional roles. *J Head Trauma Rehabil.* 1990;5(2):38–45.

Horn LJ, Zasler N. Neuroanatomy and neurophysiology of sexual function. *J Head Trauma Rehabil.* 1990;5(2):1–13.

Ponsford J. Sexual changes associated with traumatic brain injury. *Neuropsychol Rehabil.* 2003;13(1/2):275–289.

REFERENCES

1. Kosteljanetz M, Jensen TS, Nørgård B, Lunde I, Jensen PB, Johnsen SG. Sexual and hypothalamic dysfunction in the postconcussional syndrome. *Acta Neurol Scand.* 1981;63(3):169–180.

2. Kreutzer JS, Zasler ND. Psychosexual consequences of traumatic brain injury: methodology and preliminary findings. *Brain Inj.* 1989;3(2):177–186.

3. Ponsford J. Sexual changes associated with traumatic brain injury. *Neuropsychol Rehabil.* 2003;13(1/2):275–289.

4. Aloni A, Keren O, Cohen M, Rosentul N, Romm M, Groswasser Z. Incidence of sexual dysfunction in TBI patients during the early post-traumatic inpatient rehabilitation phase. *Brain Inj.* 1999;13(2):89–97.

5. Garden FH, Bontke CF, Hoffman M. Sexual functioning and marital adjustment after traumatic brain injury. *J Head Trauma Rehabil.* 1990;5(2):52–59.

6. Hibbard MR, Gordon WA, Flanagan S, Haddad L, Labinsky E. Sexual dysfunction after traumatic brain injury. *NeuroRehabilitation.* 2000;15(2):107–120.

7. Kreuter M, Dahllöf AG, Gudjonsson G, Sullivan M, Siösteen A. Sexual adjustment and its predictors after traumatic brain injury. *Brain Inj.* 1998;12(5):349–368.

8. Sabhesan S, Natarajan M. Sexual behavior after head injury in Indian men and women. *Arch Sex Behav.* 1989;18(4):349–356.

9. Sandel ME, Williams KS, Dellapietra L, Derogatis LR. Sexual functioning following traumatic brain injury. *Brain Inj.* 1996;10(10):719–728.

10. Zencius A, Wesolowski MD, Burke WH, Hough S. Managing hypersexual disorders in brain-injured clients. *Brain Inj.* 1990;4(2):175–181.

11. Gervasio AH, Griffith ER. Sexuality and sexual dysfunction. In: Rosenthal M, Griffith ER, Kreutzer JS, Pentland B, eds. *Rehabilitation of the Adult and Child with Traumatic Brain Injury.* 3rd ed. Philadelphia, PA: F.A. Davis Company; 1999:479–502.

12. Horn LJ, Zasler N. Neuroanatomy and neurophysiology of sexual function. *J Head Trauma Rehabil.* 1990;5(2):1–13.

13. Herzog AG, Russell V, Vaitukaitis JL, Geschwind N. Neuroendocrine dysfunction in temporal lobe epilepsy. *Arch Neurol.* 1982;39(3):133–135.

14. Herzog AG, Seibel MM, Schomer DL, Vaitukaitis JL, Geschwind N. Reproductive endocrine disorders in men with partial seizures of temporal lobe origin. *Arch Neurol.* 1986;43(4):347–350.

15. Herzog AG, Seibel MM, Schomer DL, Vaitukaitis JL, Geschwind N. Reproductive endocrine disorders in women with partial seizures of temporal lobe origin. *Arch Neurol.* 1986;43(4):341–346.

16. Miller BL, Cummings JL, McIntyre H, Ebers G, Grode M. Hypersexuality or altered sexual preference following brain injury. *J Neurol Neurosurg Psychiatr.* 1986;49(8):867–873.

17. MacLean P. Brain mechanisms of primal sexual functions and related behavior. In: Sandler M, Gessa G, eds. *Sexual Behavior: Pharmacology and Biochemistry.* New York: Raven Press, 1975.

18. Sandel ME, Delmonico R, Kotch MJ. Sexuality, reproduction, and neuroendocrine disorders following TBI. In: Zasler ND, Katz DI, Zafonte RD, eds. *Brain Injury Medicine.* New York: Demos Medical Publishing; 2007:673–695.

19. Zasler ND. Traumatic brain injury and sexuality. In: Monga TN, ed. *Sexuality and Disability.* Philadelphia, PA: Hanley and Belfus; 1995:361.

20. Aloni R, Katz S. *Sexual Difficulties After Traumatic Brain Injury and Ways to Deal With It.* Springfield, IL: Charles C. Thomas Publisher Ltd; 2003.

21. Blackerby WF. A treatment model for sexuality disturbance following brain injury. *J Head Trauma Rehabil.* 1990;5(2):73–82.

22. Marsh NV. Social skills deficits following traumatic brain injury. In: McDonald S, Togher L, Codse C, eds. *Communication Disorders Following Traumatic Brain Injury.* Hove, UK: Psychology Press; 1990:175–210.

23. Lezak M. Psychological implications of traumatic brain injury for the patient's family. *Rehabil Psychol.* 1986;31:241–250.

43

Assessment of Decisional Capacity

Rebecca Brashler

GENERAL PRINCIPLES

Definitions

- Medical competence is generally referred to as "decisional capacity," "decision-making capacity" or just "capacity."
- "Competency" is a legal concept. It can only be formally determined by the courts, although in practice, the terms capacity and competency are often used interchangeably [1].
- There is no universally accepted definition of competence and no universally accepted method of assessing a patient's decisional capacity [1].

Decisional Capacity Implications and Assumptions

- There is a presumption that every adult patient is competent unless proven otherwise.
- Competent patients are believed to have the authority to provide informed consent and act autonomously when making medical decisions [1].
- Competent patients have the right to refuse unwanted (even life-saving) medical care and make what we might think are bad or risky decisions [3].
- Patients judged to be incompetent by the courts will have a legal decision maker appointed (a guardian) and they may lose certain rights such as the right to vote, the right to marry, and the right to enter into contractual agreements.

ASSESSING CAPACITY

Background

- Patients with brain injuries (along with the elderly, patients with mental illness, mental retardation, and aphasia) should receive formal assessments of their capacity. They should not be deemed to be incompetent based solely on their medical diagnosis or condition.
- Patients who disagree with their healthcare providers often have their capacity questioned more frequently than those who are compliant and agree to the recommended treatment plan.
- Decisional capacity is situation specific. A patient may have the capacity to make some simple decisions but remain unable to make more complex decisions. When assessing capacity the clinician should explicitly state which decision is being tested (i.e., "this patient is being assessed for her ability to make decisions about having a shunt revision this week to relieve intracranial pressure").
- Decisional capacity is not static. A patient's capacity fluctuates and is influenced by mood, time of day, metabolic status, fatigue, pain, medications, and other factors.
- Sliding scale: Most ethicists agree that the more probable or serious the risk inherent in the decision, the more stringent the standard of capacity should be [3]
  - Routine decisions
  - Invasive procedures/clinical trials
  - Life and death decisions

Decisional Capacity Assessment Instruments

- *MacArthur Competence Assessment Tool for Treatment (MacCAT-T).* A guide developed by Applebaum and Grisso to assist clinicians in rating responses during a structured assessment interview [4].
- *Aid to Capacity Evaluation.* An assessment tool, available online, developed by the University of Toronto Joint Center for Bioethics [5].
- *Hopkins Competency Assessment Test.* A brief method for evaluating patients' capacity to provide informed consent based on a short essay and a questionnaire [6].
- *Capacity to Consent to Treatment Instrument.* An instrument that asks patients to respond to hypothetical oral and written vignettes in order to determine general capacity to consent to medical treatment [7].

The Decisional Capacity Structured Interview

The Decisional Capacity Structured Interview. Whether or not a specific tool is used to rate the patient's responses, assessing capacity involves a structured conversation or interview between a clinician and the patient. The following elements should be considered:

- Alertness: Patients must have a level of alertness that allows for the assessment to take place. Comatose and vegetative patients are easily adjudicated and are universally viewed as incompetent.
- Orientation: May include a Mini Mental Status Examination as well as orientation to situation and appreciation of the need to participate in decision making.
- Ability to communicate a choice: Patients must be able to express a preference via verbal or nonverbal means. They cannot have a level of ambivalence so extreme that choices cannot be determined. Stability of choice is relevant and can be tested by asking the same questions at different times/days.
- Understanding of relevant information: Includes the ability to receive, store, and remember information. Deficits in intelligence, memory, and attention span can interfere with this element. Clinicians can test understanding by asking the patient to paraphrase what they have been told about the treatment or life decision.
- Appreciation of the situation and its consequences: Can the patient grasp the probable outcomes of the treatment and the consequences of its refusal? Pathological denial, delusional perceptions, and affective/cognitive deficits may interfere with this ability.
- Rational manipulation of information: Can the patient engage in a risk/benefit analysis? This involves the ability to reach conclusions that are logically consistent with the starting premise. The chain of reasoning and not the conclusion should be the focus.

DECISION MAKING AFTER TBI: CHALLENGES AND ETHICAL CONCERNS

Neuropsychological Testing and Decisional Capacity

- Institutions and courts traditionally rely on neuropsychological testing alone when making determinations about capacity, although as noted by Kothari & Kirschner, "there is no clear way to determine what pattern of test findings preclude adequate decision making" [8].
- During the early stages of recovery and emergence from coma, a patient's capacity may change rapidly. It is impractical to repeat full neuropsychological batteries while a patient's status is in flux.

Decisional Capacity Versus Performative Capacity

- Many patients with traumatic brain injury (TBI) demonstrate a discrepancy between decisional capacity and performative capacity [9]. They may be able to describe what they want to do in a particular situation but they may not be able to act accordingly when that situation arises.

- Most capacity tools focus on a patient's ability to provide consent for medical treatment while on brain injury units. We often need to assess a patient's capacity to make decisions about practical life situations—such as a decision to choose to live independently or a decision to drive a car. This usually necessitates moving beyond a structured interview to some type of simulated testing environment where observable behaviors can be incorporated into the assessment.

Personhood

Families often tell us that patients with TBI seem like "different people" and demonstrate uncharacteristic behaviors/beliefs after their injuries. They may be impulsive, lack initiative, or be interpersonally provocative. Ethically it may be difficult to know how to respond when a patient who appears to have some limited capacity makes decisions that their loved ones know to be profoundly different from those they made prior to their injury.

- If previous wishes were documented, particularly if they were written in a formal advance directive, the premorbid preferences will hold greater legitimacy.

- A tendency to minimize the severity of cognitive deficits, while not necessarily denying the fact that they sustained an injury—a hallmark of many patients with TBI—may be a reason to place greater weight on previously demonstrated preferences, particularly around practical life choices.

- If current behaviors/choices place the patient at high risk for further injury or if they potentially place others at risk, a more stringent capacity standard should be met.

ADDITIONAL READING

Electronic Reference
University of Toronto Joint Centre for Bioethics (ACE). http://www.jointcentre-forbioethics.ca/tools/ace.shtml

Textbooks/Chapters
Grisso T. *Evaluating Competencies: Forensic Assessments and Instruments*. 2nd ed. New York: Springer; 2002.

Grisso T, Appelbaum PS. *Assessing Competence to Consent to Treatment: A Guide to Physicians and Other Health Professionals.* New York: Oxford University Press; 1998.

Kothari S, Kirschner K. Decision-making capacity after TBI: clinical assessment and ethical implications. In Zasler N, Zafonte R, Katz D, eds. *Neurorehabilitation of Traumatic Brain Injury.* 2nd ed. New York: Demos Medical Publishing; 2007:1205–1222.

Journal Articles

Applebaum PS, Grisso T. Assessing patients' capacities to consent to treatment. *N Engl J Med.* 1988;319(25):1635–1638.

Cooney LM, Kennedy GJ, Hawkins KA, Hurme SB. Who can stay at home? *Arch Intern Med.* 2004;164(2):357–360.

Etchells E. Assessment of patient capacity to consent to treatment. *J Gen Intern Med.* 1999;14(1):27–34.

Ganzini L, Volicer L, Nelson WA, Fox E, Derse AR. Ten myths about decision-making capacity. *J Am Med Dir Assoc.* 2004;7/8:263–267.

Kothari S, Kirschner K. Beyond consent: assent and empowerment in brain injury rehabilitation. *J Head Trauma Rehabil.* 2003;18(4):379–382.

Naik AD, Dyer CB, Kunik ME, McCullough LB. Patient autonomy for the management of chronic conditions: a two-component re-conceptualization. *Am J Bioeth.* 2009;9(2):23–30.

Vesney BA. A clinician's guide to decision making capacity and ethically sound medical decisions. *Am J Phys Med Rehabil.* 1994;73(3):219–226.

REFERENCES

1. Applebaum PS. Assessment of patients' competence to consent to treatment. *N Engl J Med.* 2007;357:1834–1840.

2. Beauchamp TL, Childress JF. *Principles of Biomedical Ethics.* 6th ed. New York: Oxford University Press; 2009.

3. Jonsen AR, Siegler M, Winslade WJ. *Clinical Ethics: A Practical Approach to Ethical Decision in Clinical Medicine.* 5th ed. New York: McGraw-Hill; 2002.

4. Grisso T, Applebaum PS. *MacArthur Competence Assessment Tool for Treatment (MacCAT-T).* Sarasota, FL: Professional Resource Press; 1998.

5. Etchells E. http://www.utoronto.ca/jcb/_ace.htm

6. Janofsky JS, McCarthy RJ, Folstein MF. The Hopkins Competency Assessment Test: A brief method for evaluating patient's capacity to give informed consent. *Hosp Community Psychiatry.* 1991;43:132–136.

7. Marson DC, Ingram KK, Cody HA, Harrell LE. Assessing the competency of patients with Alzheimer's disease under different legal standards. A prototype instrument. *Arch Neurol.* 1995;52(10):949–954.

8. Kothari S, Kirschner K. Beyond consent: assent and empowerment in brain injury rehabilitation. *J Head Trauma Rehabil.* 2003;18(4):379–382.

9. Cooney LM, Kennedy GJ, Hawkins KA, Hurme SB. Who can stay at home? *Arch Intern Med.* 2004:164(2):357–360.

44

Community Integration

James F. Malec and Anne M. Moessner

GENERAL PRINCIPLES

The concept of *community integration* is best understood via the four categories [1] listed below:

- *Assimilation*—The individual with brain injury (BI) fully participates in community life but special needs resulting from BI *are not* identified and supported by the community;
- *Integration*—The individual fully participates; needs *are* identified or supported;
- *Segregation*—The individual does not fully participate; needs *are* identified or supported;
- *Marginalization*—The individual does not fully participate; needs *are not* identified or supported.

The degree of acculturation may differ across needs. For instance, integration is more common after BI for medical needs than for vocational needs.

Early Intervention

Early rehabilitation intervention, ideally within days of injury onset, is typically more efficient, promotes recovery, leads to less supervision and hours of care needed later, and is less expensive over a lifetime when compared to rehabilitation that is delayed [2]. However, rehabilitation provided later, even years post injury, can still be effective in reducing disability, care, and supervision needs [3]. Most survivors of BI will return to the community [4,5]; often overlooked during early recovery is the need to provide a long-term perspective to families that includes eventual return to community.

Coordinated Care by Specialized Providers

For patients with complex injuries, coordinated care provided by specialists encourages return to community [2,6]. Care coordinators can serve as continuous, knowledgeable, and accessible points of contact and assure the patient receives services from well-qualified practitioners in specialized facilities.

Long-Term Follow-Up and Care

Recovery following severe BI is often measured in months to years. In light of the trend toward reduced rehabilitation lengths of stay (LOS; TBI Model Systems rehabilitation LOS: 1990=48 days; 2000=29 days; 2010=19 days) [4], much of this recovery will occur in the community or other posthospital settings. This trend has increased the importance of rehabilitation programs either directly offering long-term outpatient treatment and follow-up, or referring to affiliated reputable programs that do so. Adapting to change after BI is oftentimes challenging. Even as progress is made and successful community living with or without supports has been realized, a change in family status, health, work, external supports, or environment can result in renewed need for rehabilitation services. A system of care that allows for long-term follow-up is critical.

Family Education

Families may be the sole providers of community-based care for individuals with BI. Behavioral, cognitive, and emotional residuals following BI significantly interfere with successful community living. Teaching families about these and other common issues, and imparting problem-solving and advocacy skills, fosters successful coping and integration.

Education for families in formal settings, such as structured classes, or more informally, via BI support groups, can be helpful, as can use of multimedia and web-based education approaches.

Community Partnerships

Connecting patients and families with community services, peers, and advocacy organizations is essential for successful community integration. Examples of traditional services include: social services, state department of vocational rehabilitation, public education, public health, health care funding (Medicaid, Medicare), subsidized accessible housing, and independent living centers. These services are not available in all locales, particularly small town and rural communities. An individualized network of community supports may need to be constructed involving, for instance, family and friends, social and church groups. Such social support networks promote positive outcomes after BI [7]. Lack of transportation is a common obstacle to employment; family and friends are often the most reliable providers of transportation.

Resource Facilitation

Resource facilitation (RF) is a process by which a coordinator provides assistance and advocacy to "break down barriers, increase access, and facilitate timely, coordinated management of resources" [8] to support the individual with BI's return to full participation in family and community life. The RF coordinator assists the individual with BI to develop a self-directed plan for community re-entry, identify and gain access to needed services and supports, and develop a sustainable network of these services and supports. The Brain Injury Association in many states of the United States provides RF.

Social Versus Medical Model Interventions

RF represents a *social model* intervention [9]. In the social model of disability, the target of interventions is the physical and social environment in which the person with disability lives and works. The goal of social model interventions is to reduce physical and social environmental obstacles to participation in community life following disability. These types of interventions are in contrast to *medical model* interventions in which the target is the disease or impairment that creates illness or disability. These models are not mutually exclusive. To the contrary, our best recommendation for assisting individuals with BI in community re-entry is an individualized approach that combines elements of both models.

NEEDS ASSESSMENT

Community re-entry should be considered throughout the person's hospitalization, inpatient and outpatient rehabilitation, and follow-up. *Begin with the end in mind* [10]. The type and intensity of services to support community re-entry will be highly individualized. Needs will change over the continuum of care and therefore need to be continuously assessed. Correct "dosing" of services optimizes outcome and responsible stewardship of the health care dollar. The indicators described in the following sections should be considered in recommending the intensity and extent of services along the continuum of care.

Severity of Injury Versus Severity of Disability

Initial injury severity has traditionally been important for determining acute medical and surgical intervention and rehabilitation. Assessment of disability at the time of hospital discharge, however, (assessed, for example, by Discharge FIM [11] or Mayo-Portland Adaptability Inventory [MPAI-4]) [12] will give a better indication of the extent and intensity of future services required [13].

Time Since Injury

Chronic injuries typically require greater intensity of service provision, but extended chronicity does not preclude capacity to benefit from those services [3].

Self-Awareness

Impaired self-awareness has a negative impact on outcome and is associated with poorer compliance and participation in treatment, need for more intense rehabilitation services, and longer LOS [14]. However, treatment studies suggest that this can be mitigated by comprehensive holistic rehabilitation and specific interventions [15].

Depression

Depression is prevalent following BI (40%–70% are diagnosed within 2 years of injury) and negatively affects outcome [16].

Substance Abuse

Those with a preinjury history of substance abuse are at higher risk for return to abuse post injury; substance abuse negatively affects outcome [17].

Preinjury Issues

Preinjury unemployment, limited education, preinjury chemical dependency, and/or psychiatric history negatively affect outcome [18].

Family Issues

Preinjury family dysfunction is present in more than 25% of families at the time of injury and is likely exacerbated by stresses related to injury [19].

The negative impact of emotional, substance-related, family, and some preinjury issues can be mitigated with early detection and specific treatment.

INTERVENTION

Successful community re-entry requires the integration of community-based services with rehabilitation services. Malec and Basford [20] identified four major categories of programs following inpatient rehabilitation:

(1) *neurobehavioral*—pharmacologic and behavioral treatment for patients with severe behavioral disturbances in a highly restricted environment; (2) *residential*—rehabilitation and community services in an environment with professional supervision throughout the day; (3) *comprehensive-holistic day treatment*—intensive, integrated, interdisciplinary BI rehabilitation for those with severe and pervasive disabilities typically including impaired self-awareness; and (4) *outpatient community integration*—focused rehabilitation for individuals with circumscribed and self-identified goals. Most patients, even after severe BI, are appropriate for one of the latter two types of outpatient programs. A number of reviews describe such programs and endorse their effectiveness [21–23].

Rehabilitation Intensity

Those with more severe and pervasive disabilities generally require more intensive rehabilitation. Pre- or postinjury factors that contribute to severity of disability include: severely impaired self-awareness, depression, other pre- or postinjury psychiatric or personality disorder, current or past substance abuse, or other disabling conditions. Family, social, or environmental disadvantages may also enhance overall disability. Rehabilitation can be effectively delivered either in outpatient clinic settings or in the community [24]. Intensive holistic day programs, although not available in many areas, can achieve superior outcomes (for instance, 60%–70% of participants ultimately transition into community-based employment) [15].

Facilitative Services

RF and specialized vocational services (SVS) are also typically required for successful community re-entry. RF and SVS may be sufficient in some cases without outpatient rehabilitation.

Vocational Re-entry

Successful vocational reintegration often requires RF, SVS, and supported employment [6,9,25]. Please see Chapter 67 for a detailed discussion of this topic.

ADDITIONAL READING

Electronic Reference
Ashley, M, O'Shanick, G, Kreber, L. *Early vs. Late Treatment of Traumatic Brain Injury*. Vienna, VA: Brain Injury Association of America, 2009.

http://www.biausa.org/LiteratureRetrieve.aspx?ID=49033&A=SearchResult
&SearchID=1895185&ObjectID=49033&ObjectType=6

Textbook/Chapter

High WM, Sander AM, Struchen MA, Hart KA, eds. *Rehabilitation for Traumatic Brain Injury.* New York, NY: Oxford University Press; 2005.

Journal Article

Malec JF, Buffington ALH, Moessner AM, Degiorgio L. A medical/vocational case coordination system for persons with brain injury: an evaluation of employment outcomes. *Arch Phys Med Rehabil.* 2000;81:1007–1015.

REFERENCES

1. Minnes P, Buell K, Nolte ML, McColl MA, Carlson P, Johnston J. Defining community integration of persons with brain injuries as acculturation: a Canadian perspective. *NeuroRehabilitation.* 2001;16(1):3–10.

2. Worthington AD, Matthews S, Melia Y, Oddy M. Cost-benefits associated with social outcome from neurobehavioural rehabilitation. *Brain Inj.* 2006;20(9):947–957.

3. Malec JF, Degiorgio L. Characteristics of successful and unsuccessful completers of 3 postacute brain injury rehabilitation pathways. *Arch Phys Med Rehabil.* 2002;83(12):1759–1764.

4. NIDRR Traumatic Brain Injury Model Systems National Data and Statistical Center. Traumatic brain injury model systems national database update, 2010. http://www.tbindsc.org/Documents/2010%20TBIMS%20National%20 Database%20Update.pdf. Accessed August 1, 2010.

5. Mellick D, Gerhart KA, Whiteneck GG. Understanding outcomes based on the post-acute hospitalization pathways followed by persons with traumatic brain injury. *Brain Inj.* 2003;17(1):55–71.

6. Malec JF, Buffington AL, Moessner AM, Degiorgio L. A medical/vocational case coordination system for persons with brain injury: an evaluation of employment outcomes. *Arch Phys Med Rehabil.* 2000;81(8):1007–1015.

7. Rauch RJ, Ferry SM. Social networks as support interventions following traumatic brain injury. *NeuroRehabilitation.* 2001;16(1):11–16.

8. Trexler LE, Trexler LC, Malec JF, Klyce D, Parrott D. Prospective randomized controlled trial of resource facilitation on community participation and vocational outcome following brain injury. *J Head Trauma Rehabil.* 2010;25(6):440–446.

9. Malec JF, Moessner AM. Replicated positive results for the VCC model of vocational intervention after ABI within the social model of disability. *Brain Inj.* 2006;20(3):227–236.

10. Covey SR. *The Seven Habits of Highly Effective People.* Carlsbad, CA: Hay House; 2003.

11. Ottenbacher KJ, Hsu Y, Granger CV, Fiedler RC. The reliability of the functional independence measure: a quantitative review. *Arch Phys Med Rehabil.* 1996;77(12):1226–1232.

12. Manual for the Mayo-Portland Adaptability Inventory, 2008. www.tbimis. org/combi/mpai. Accessed August 1, 2010.

13. Bush BA, Novack TA, Malec JF, Stringer AY, Millis SR, Madan A. Validation of a model for evaluating outcome after traumatic brain injury. *Arch Phys Med Rehabil.* 2003;84(12):1803–1807.

14. Sherer M. Rehabilitation of impaired awareness. In: High WM Jr, Sander AM, Struchen MA, Hart KA, eds. *Rehabilitation for Traumatic Brain Injury.* New York, NY: Oxford University Press; 2005:31–46.

15. Malec JF. Impact of comprehensive day treatment on societal participation for persons with acquired brain injury. *Arch Phys Med Rehabil.* 2001;82(7):885–895.

16. Malec JF, Brown AW, Moessner AM, Stump TE, Monahan P. A preliminary model for posttraumatic brain injury depression. *Arch Phys Med Rehabil.* 2010;91(7):1087–1097.

17. Corrigan JD. Substance abuse. In: High WM Jr, Sander AM, Struchen MA, Hart KA, eds. *Rehabilitation for Traumatic Brain Injury.* New York, NY: Oxford University Press; 2005:133–155.

18. Gordon WA, Zafonte R, Cicerone K, et al. Traumatic brain injury rehabilitation: state of the science. *Am J Phys Med Rehabil.* 2006;85(4):343–382.

19. Sander AM, Sherer M, Malec JF, et al. Preinjury emotional and family functioning in caregivers of persons with traumatic brain injury. *Arch Phys Med Rehabil.* 2003;84(2):197–203.

20. Malec JF, Basford JS. Postacute brain injury rehabilitation. *Arch Phys Med Rehabil.* 1996;77(2):198–207.

21. Cicerone KD, Dahlberg C, Kalmar K, et al. Evidence-based cognitive rehabilitation: recommendations for clinical practice. *Arch Phys Med Rehabil.* 2000;81(12):1596–1615.

22. Cicerone KD, Dahlberg C, Malec JF, et al. Evidence-based cognitive rehabilitation: updated review of the literature from 1998 through 2002. *Arch Phys Med Rehabil.* 2005;86(8):1681–1692.

23. Geurtsen GJ, van Heugten CM, Martina JD, Geurts AC. Comprehensive rehabilitation programmes in the chronic phase after severe brain injury: a systematic review. *J Rehabil Med.* 2010;42(2):97–110.

24. Glenn MB, Selleck EA, Goldstein R, Rotman M. Characteristics of home-based community integration programmes for adults with brain injury. *Brain Inj.* 2005;19(14):1243–1247.

25. Malec JF. Vocational rehabilitation. In: High WM Jr, Sander AM, Struchen MA, Hart KA, eds. *Rehabilitation for Traumatic Brain Injury.* New York: Oxford University Press; 2005:176–202.

PART 5

Traumatic Brain Injury–Related Medical Complications

45

Cranial Nerve Palsies

Flora Hammond

GENERAL PRINCIPLES

Epidemiology

True incidence of cranial nerve (CN) injuries is not certain.

- Most frequently injured—CN I, followed next by CN VII and CN VIII
- Less commonly injured—optic (CN II) and oculomotor (CN III) nerves
- Rarely injured—trigeminal (CN V) and lower cranial nerves

Etiology

Etiology includes acceleration-deceleration, shearing, skull fracture, intracranial hemorrhage, intracranial mass lesion, uncal herniation, infarct, and vascular occlusion.

Mechanism of Injury

- Mechanisms include compression, traction, transection, and ischemia.
- Central (nuclear) CN injury occurs from brainstem damage; peripheral CN injury results from fracture or local injury.
- CNs are at particular risk for injury, because they traverse over bony protuberances and canals, or by direct injury from skull fracture.

Prognosis

- *Olfactory* (I)—Reported prognosis is: 33% recovery, 27% worsened, and 40% no change [1]. Recovery is usually noticed within the first 6 months and complete by 12 months post injury [2], with later recoveries (up to 5 years) reported [3]. Parosmia (sensation of smell in absence of stimulus) may be the first sign of return.
- *Optic* (II)—The optic nerve is a direct extension of the brain and docs not regenerate.

- *Oculomotor* (III)—Recovery usually takes 6 to 12 months. Return of function is usually incomplete, with complete recovery in 40% [3].
- *Facial* (VII)—With delayed-onset palsy, CN VII is usually structurally intact and recovers in 8 weeks [2].

EVALUATION

Risk Factors

Risk factors include skull fractures due to close proximity to CN (especially CN: I, II, III, IV, V [first two branches], VII, and VIII); and increased intracranial pressure, causing compression (CN III).

Clinical Presentation

- *Olfactory* (I)—altered sense of smell
- *Optic* (II)—altered visual acuity and/or visual fields
- *Oculomotor* (III)—ptosis, lack of accommodation, dilated and fixed pupil, divergent strabismus, diplopia, and the eye only moving laterally. When looking straight ahead, the affected eye turns outward and slightly down. When looking inward, the affected eye can move only to the middle and cannot look up or down
- *Trochlear* (IV)—diplopia (especially when descending stairs); affected eye rotated out with inability to turn eye in and down, compensatory head tilt away from affected side
- *Trigeminal* (V)—scleral injection due to corneal abrasions and drying, decreased facial sensation and/or neurogenic pain, weakness with chewing
- *Abducens* (VI)—impaired ability to turn affected eye outward, affected eye turns inward when looking straight ahead, diplopia with looking toward the affected side, esotropia (strabismus in which one or both eyes turn inward) worsened by lateral gaze, and head turned laterally toward paretic side
- *Facial* (VII)—weakness of face and lid closure, and loss of taste sensation on anterior two-thirds of the tongue. Facial muscle weakness may affect mastication with impaired oropharyngeal swallowing phase
- *Vestibulocochlear* (VIII)—hearing loss, vertigo, nystagmus, and/or impaired balance; commonly associated with temporal bone fracture, mastoid fracture, Battle's sign, otorrhea, bleeding from the ear, and hemotympanum
- *Glossopharyngeal* (IX)—loss of taste over posterior third of the tongue, deviation of the uvula contralaterally, decreased salivation, and slight dysphagia

- *Vagus* (X)—palate paralysis with loss of the gag reflex, dysphagia, and aphonia or hypophonia due to unilateral paralysis of the vocal fold. Bilateral vagal disruption is fatal
- *Spinal* (XI)—inability to turn the head to the opposite side, and ipsilateral shoulder drooping, which may result in shoulder dysfunction and pain
- *Hypoglossal* (XII)—inability to protrude tongue on the affected side; may lead to dysphagia

Physical Examination

Diagnosis is generally based on physical examination of CN functions. Examination may need to be repeated or completed as consciousness recovers.

- *Olfactory* (I)—Test detection of familiar, non-noxious smells with eyes closed. Giving the person choices may help overcome word-finding problems.
- *Optic* (II)—Assess visual acuity, visual fields, pupillary reactivity, and perform ophthalmoscopic examination. Complete monocular blindness with preservation of normal pupillary reflexes is usually a sign of malingering or other types of functional (nonorganic) disorders.
- *Oculomotor* (III)—Assess tracking in the six cardinal positions, convergence on near targets, pursuit movements, saccades, pupillary reaction, and eyelid elevation. CN III palsy is indicated by difficulty moving the eye in, or up and down, with preserved outward movement, and may be associated with pupillary dilatation and ptosis. Doll's eye maneuver and pupillary light reflex are used for assessment if unconscious. A fixed and dilated pupil signals herniation as the nerve runs medial to the temporal lobe at the tentorium edge.
- *Trochlear* (IV)—Assess adduction in conjunction with downward gaze of the involved eye. Individuals with CN IV palsy cannot look downward when the eye is adducted.
- *Trigeminal* (V)—Test facial sensation, corneal reflex, and motor function of the jaw.
- *Abducens* (VI)—Look for deficiency in lateral gaze when testing movement of the eyes through the full extent of the horizontal plane.
- *Facial* (VII)—Test the five main functions: facial expression (smile, wrinkle forehead, puff cheeks, close eyes tightly), taste identification on anterior two-third of the tongue, external ear sensation, stapedius muscle function, and lacrimal and salivary gland function.
  - Upper motor neuron lesion—facial weakness contralateral to the lesion with sparing of forehead wrinkle because of the bilateral innervation of the frontalis muscle

- Lower motor neuron lesion—ipsilateral facial weakness inclusive of flattened forehead wrinkle; inability to close eye
- Pontine lesion (CN VII nucleus)—complete ipsilateral facial paralysis along with contralateral hemiparesis, and frequently accompanied by ipsilateral CN VI palsy

- *Vestibulocochlear* (VIII)—Examine tympanic membrane for tears, and test eye movement for nystagmus, postural responses, and hearing.
- *Glossopharyngeal* (IX)—Test sensation of posterior palate and gag reflex.
- *Vagus* (X)—Test palate elevation and gag reflex.
- *Spinal* (XI)—Test resisted head rotation to opposite side and ipsilateral shoulder shrug.
- *Hypoglossal* (XII)—Look for ipsilateral atrophy, tongue fasciculations, and deviation with tongue protrusion. The tongue deviates to the side of the lesion because of the unopposed, contralateral muscles.

Diagnostic Evaluation

- *Olfactory* (I)—Evaluation may include imaging the anterior cranial structures, ethmoid tomography to detect basal skull fracture, and electroencephalography (EEG) in cases of parosmia.
- *Optic* (II)—Consider EEG to evaluate for occipital seizures. Visual evoked response (VER) may be considered to evaluate the integrity of the visual system from the eye to the occipital cortex.
- *Oculomotor* (III)—CN III palsy may be a sign of impending neurologic compromise, and as such, diagnostic imaging studies (CT/MRI) are generally needed emergently to evaluate cause.
- *Trochlear* (IV) and *Abducens* (VI)—CT or MRI may help assess location of associated pathology.
- *Facial* (VII)—Electromyography and nerve conduction can provide prognostic data. Brain imaging may be warranted to aid in distinguishing between central and peripheral lesions.
- *Vestibulocochlear* (VIII)—CT of the temporal bones may be indicated to assess for skull fracture in the region of the auditory canal. Audiometry helps detect, characterize, and quantify hearing loss, and guide treatment decisions. Brainstem auditory evoked responses (BAER) may be useful in those who are unable to cooperate with audiometry.

MANAGEMENT

Measures are needed to prevent secondary injury, and a variety of treatments may be aimed at promoting recovery and improving function.

- *Olfactory* (I)—There are no established effective treatments. Safety measures and education are needed, including: awareness of potential risks (e.g., inability to detect smoke, spoiled foods, or toxins), use of smoke alarms on all floors, labeling food, and need for hygiene routines.

- *Optic* (II)—Evaluation by a neuro-opthalmologist or optometrist is warranted. Steroids and/or optic canal decompression may be beneficial in selected cases. Special optics may help visual field defects [4]. Visual training may help visual spatial disorders [5].

- *Oculomotor* (III)—Occlusive therapy resolves diplopia during patching, but does not produce long-term effects. Pleoptics (eye exercises) do not appear to be effective [6]. Strabismus surgery may be performed to correct cosmetic deformity, although it should be delayed 6 to 9 months after injury to allow for spontaneous recovery.

- *Trochlear* (IV)—Treatment depends on the cause. Ocular exercises may help. Sometimes strabismus surgery is necessary.

- *Trigeminal* (V)—Decreased corneal sensation with resulting risk of corneal abrasions requires frequent eye irrigation, lubricating gel, and patching of the affected eye, especially at night. If irritation continues, lateral or complete tarsorrhaphy is needed to avoid development of corneal ulceration and opacities. If trigeminal neuralgia develops, consider anticonvulsants or other agents and modalities used for neuropathic pain.

- *Abducens* (VI)—CN VI palsy due to traumatic brain injury usually resolves over time.

- *Facial* (VII)—Treatment considerations for facial nerve swelling within the facial canal may include corticosteroid administration, otolaryngology consultation, and facial nerve decompression. Complete facial nerve disruption may be helped with surgical techniques. Inadequate lid closure requires frequent topical lubricant, and may require an eye pad/taping or tarsorrhaphy. In cases of oral-motor weakness, speech therapy may be needed to assess swallowing safety and administer exercises for oral-motor strengthening.

- *Vestibulocochlear* (VIII)—Vestibular treatment is aimed at the system's capacity to habituate to stimuli [2]. Refer to a physical therapist well versed in vestibular rehabilitation. Labyrinthine exercises are used to decrease vestibular sensitivity [7]. Medications for vestibular dysfunction are discouraged because of potential sedation, cognitive side effects, and prevention of central adaptation [2]. Unilateral hearing loss may be helped with contralateral routing of signal (CROS) type hearing aid [2]. Sensorineural hearing loss is not amenable to surgery or hearing aids. Surgical repair may help conductive hearing loss that fails to recover spontaneously [8]. Masking sound devices and biofeedback may help tinnitus [2].

- *Glossopharyngeal* (IX)—Treat symptomatically, and assess risk for aspiration. May need speech pathology to assist with oral-motor exercises.

- *Vagus* (X)—Identify alternative feeding techniques for those at risk for aspiration. Pharyngeal exercises may improve mild dysarthria [7]. Glottic incompetence may be improved with procedures that augment vocal cord bulk. For high vagal lesions, aggressive surgical procedures (e.g., thyroplasty and arytenoids adduction) may be beneficial [9].

- *Spinal* (XI)—Aggressive physical therapy should be initiated as soon as possible. Surgical nerve repair after sectioning may be possible in selected cases.
- *Hypoglossal* (XII)—Dysarthria exercises may improve coordination and strength. Assess for dysphagia, possible need for swallowing precautions or oral-motor exercises.

ADDITIONAL READING

Electronic Reference

http://library.med.utah.edu/neurologicexam/html/cranialnerve_normal.html

Textbook/Chapter

Hammond FM, Masel B. Cranial nerve disorders. In: Zasler N, Katz D, Zafonte R, eds. *Brain Injury Medicine: Principles and Practice.* 1st ed. New York, NY: Demos Medical Publishing; 2006:529–544.

Journal Article

Jin H, Wang S, Hou L, et al. Clinical treatment of traumatic brain injury complicated by cranial nerve injury. *Injury.* 2010;41(7):997–1002.

REFERENCES

1. Costanzo RM, Becker DFP. Sense of smell and taste disorders in head injury and neurosurgery patients. In: Meiselman HL, Rivlin RS, eds. *Clinical Management of Taste and Smell.* New York, NY: Macmillan Publishing; 1986:565–578.
2. Berrol S. Cranial nerve dysfunction. In: Horn LJ, Cope DN, eds. *Physical Medicine and Rehabilitation: State of the Art Reviews.* Philadelphia, PA: Hanley and Belfus; 1989:85–93.
3. Keane JR, Baloh RW. Posttraumatic cranial neuropathies. *Neurol Clin.* 1992;10(4):849–867.
4. Padula WV: Neuro-optometric rehabilitation for persons with a TBI or CVA. *Journal of Optometric Vision Development.* 1992;23:4–8.
5. Kerkhoff G. Rehabilitation of Visuospatial Cognition and Visual Exploration in Neglect: a Cross-over Study. *Restor Neurol Neurosci.* 1998;12(1):27–40.
6. Vaughn D, Asbury T. *General Ophthalmology.* Los Altos, CA: Lange Medical Publications; 1974:182.
7. Yorkston KM, Beukelman DR, Strand EA, Bell KR. *Management of Motor Speech Disorders.* 2nd ed. Austin, TX: Pro-ed; 1999.
8. Sismanis A. Post-concussive neuro-otological disorders. *Physical Medicine and Rehabilitation: State of the Art Reviews.* 1992;6(1):79–88.
9. Eibling DE, Boyd EM. Rehabilitation of lower cranial nerve deficits. *Otolaryngol Clin North Am.* 1997;30(5):865–875.

46

Hydrocephalus

David F. Long

GENERAL PRINCIPLES

Definition and Epidemiology

- Hydrocephalus is defined as "an active distension of the ventricular system of the brain related to inadequate passage of cerebrospinal fluid (CSF) from its point of production within the ventricular system to its point of absorption into the systemic circulation" [1].
- It is the most common treatable neurosurgical complication in traumatic brain injury (TBI) rehabilitation; occurs in up to 45% of severe TBI patients while in inpatient rehabilitation [2].
- Dynamic hydrocephalus can be difficult to distinguish from ex vacuo ventriculomegaly, a hallmark of severe diffuse brain injury [2,3].

Classification

- Communicating hydrocephalus—all ventricles are interconnected with free exit of CSF to subarachnoid space [1]; most posttraumatic hydrocephalus cases
- Noncommunicating hydrocephalus—obstruction between ventricles or preventing outflow from ventricles [1]; consider aqueductal stenosis decompensated by TBI when lateral and third ventricles are large but fourth ventricle is small or normal; lumbar puncture is contraindicated [2]

Pathophysiology of Hydrocephalus

- The processes causing the development of hydrocephalus are complex. Hydrocephalus is not necessarily associated with increased pressure, because when ventricles enlarge, the expanding force is distributed over a larger area, reducing the pressure. Also the size of the ventricles reflects the pressure within them relative to that of the surrounding tissues (just as the size of a balloon depends on the pressure inside compared with that outside) [2,3].

DIAGNOSIS

Clinical Presentation

- Risk factors—subarachnoid or intraventricular hemorrhage, meningitis, craniectomy [1,4].
- Acute hydrocephalus may present with headache, nausea, vomiting, lethargy, papilledema, bulging craniectomy flap, Cushing's triad (hypertension, bradycardia, and hypoventilation) [2].
- Normal-pressure hydrocephalus (NPH) may present with triad of gait "apraxia" (shuffling magnetic quality with reduced cadence, decreased step height, loss of counter-rotation), "subcortical" cognitive impairment, and urinary incontinence [5].
- Other presentations—akinetic mutism, bradykinesia, Parkinsonian syndrome, pretectal syndrome (loss of upgaze, lid retraction, impaired papillary reactivity, convergence retraction nystagmus), nonspecific deterioration in neurological status [2,5].

Computerized Tomography and Magnetic Resonance Imaging

- Typical appearance—progressive ventriculomegaly with convex frontal horns, enlarged temporal horns and third ventricle [2].
- Sulci are typically less prominent than ventricles, especially in high convexity, but the presence of enlarged sulci does not exclude hydrocephalus [2,5,6].
- Transependymal fluid may be present—smooth periventricular signal (MRI) or lucency (CT); predictive of a good response to shunting. Differential considerations—frontal contusions, cerebral infarctions or demyelination—are usually more irregular and asymmetric [2].

Supplemental and Invasive Assessment

- CSF tap—clinical improvement, especially in gait, after removal of 40 to 50 cc of CSF by lumbar puncture predicts good response to shunting, but low test sensitivity (26%–61%) means that a negative result cannot be used as an exclusionary test for hydrocephalus; many patients with a negative test can respond to shunting [7].
- Placement of a continuous external lumbar drain for 72 hours, if available in a specialized center, is both more sensitive and specific for diagnosing NPH than CSF tap [2,7].
- Cisternography—does not add to accuracy of diagnosis of hydrocephalus [8].

TREATMENT

Initial Management

Surgical Options

- Ventriculoperitoneal shunt—CSF drains from ventricular catheter, out of skull through a burr hole, through a one-way valve. Catheter passes under the skin terminating in the peritoneal space; the standard procedure for communicating managing hydrocephalus [2,9]
- Third ventriculostomy—for aqueductal stenosis, a hole can be created between the floor of the third ventricle and the adjacent cistern to allow passage of CSF without requiring a shunt [2]
- Other shunt types—include ventriculoatrial, ventriculopleural (with intra-abdominal process or to get lower pressure), lumboperitoneal (communicating hydrocephalus only) [2,9]

Basic Shunt Concepts

- Shunts typically have a one-way valve, either with fixed setting or programmable with an external magnet; very large ventricles may need a particularly low pressure valve setting [2].
- A palpable reservoir or pumping chamber will generate forward flow if there is a valve between it and the ventricle; if the valve is further downstream than the reservoir, pumping can generate retrograde flow into the ventricle, such as for intrathecal medication administration [2,9].
- Clinical improvement and reduction in ventricular size after shunting do not correlate well. Recent efforts with combined programmable and gravitational shunts seem to indicate that good clinical results can sometimes be obtained from shunting with little associated reduction in ventricular size [2].

Shunt Complications

Shunt Failure

- Incidence of shunt revision in adults is approximately 30% [2].
- Shunt failure symptoms include irritability, confusion, lethargy, headache, or acute neurologic change.
- Shunt palpation may show excessive resistance (distal occlusion) or inadequate refill (proximal obstruction). Unfortunately, one cannot determine with certainty whether a shunt is working by bedside palpation [10].
- Perform CT or MRI and look for increased ventricular size compared with prior scan.
- Distal shunt occlusion may also have fluid loculation or pseudocyst on abdominal CT [11].

- Shuntogram is most definitive—A needle is inserted into a safely perforable part of shunt, pressure measured, and contrast or isotope injected and followed down into peritoneal space [9]

Shunt Infection
- Insidious presentation—low grade fever, malaise, irritability; erythema over shunt; 70% occur in the first 2 months after insertion; *Staphylococcus epidermidis* is most common; diagnosis is by shunt tap, not lumbar puncture (unreliable) [2]
- Treatment—intravenous antibiotics, shunt removal or externalization [2]

Overdrainage
- Gravitational pressure of column of CSF between the valve and the distal end of the catheter frequently causes siphoning of CSF resulting in overdrainage [2,9].
- Acute overdrainage symptoms can include orthostatic headache, dizziness, vomiting, lethargy, and diplopia. Chronic overdrainage causes slit ventricle syndrome with nonpostural headache and intermittent proximal shunt malfunction [2].
- Overdrainage predisposes to development of subdural hematomas and hygromas—CSF drainage from ventricles creates increased potential subdural space. Subdural collections occur in 4.5% to 28% of shunted patients and are more likely with very large ventricles before shunting [2].

Additional Considerations

Programmable Shunts—Concepts and Use
- These allow bedside adjustment of the opening pressure of shunt valves by use of an external magnet to prevent underdrainage (poor clinical response) or overdrainage [2,9,12,13].
- Cost effective (often avoids reoperation) and adjustments can improve clinical course [12,13].
- Inadvertent valve resetting by MRI, magnets, valve filliping, or transcranial magnetic stimulation may occur [2,14,15]; MRI scans are not contraindicated, but valve settings need to be rechecked after MRI; some valves require confirmatory x-ray to verify setting [2,14,15].

Antisiphon Devices and Gravitational Shunts
- Antisiphon devices, gravitational valves, and gravitational units added to a shunt system attempt to prevent excessive CSF flow induced by siphoning [2,16].
- A gravitational unit in series with a programmable valve can decrease siphoning and allow adjustment with an external magnet [16].

Specific Programmable Shunts

- Codman Hakim Programmable Valve—first in United States, multiple clinical trials, 18 settings at 10 mm increments from 30 to 200 mm H_2O; MRI can reset valve, and determination of setting requires x-ray [2,12,14]
- Medtronic PS Medical Strata Valve—five settings from 0.5 to 2.5 for opening pressures 15 to 170 mm H_2O; MRI can reset, but valve can be read and adjusted at bedside [2,14]
- Sophysa Programmable Valves—new Polaris model has five positions and locking mechanism designed to prevent changes in valve by MRI [14,16]
- Aesculap-Miethke proGAV programmable shunt system—combines a gravitational unit in series with a programmable valve with a brake to prevent inadvertent MRI valve change; settings can be checked at bedside without x-ray [16]

ADDITIONAL READING

Electronic Reference

Website with information about how different programmable shunts respond to MRI. http://mrisafety.com/safety_article.asp?subject=175

Textbooks/Chapters

Long DF. Diagnosis and management of late intracranial complications of TBI. In: Zasler ND, Katz DI, Zafonte RD, eds. *Brain Injury Medicine: Principles and Practice.* New York, NY: Demos Medical Publishing; 2007:577–601.

Drake JM, Sainte-Rose C. *The Shunt Book.* Cambridge, MA: Blackwell Scientific; 1995.

Journal Articles

Lollis SS, Mamourian AC, Vaccaro TJ, Duhaime AC. Programmable CSF shunt valves: radiographic identification and interpretation. *AJNR Am J Neuroradiol.* 2010;31(7):1343–1346.

Marmarou A, Bergsneider M, Klinge P, Relkin N, Black PM. The value of supplemental prognostic tests for the preoperative assessment of idiopathic normal-pressure hydrocephalus. *Neurosurgery.* 2005;52(suppl 2):17–28.

Relkin N, Marmarou A, Klinge P, Bergsneider M, Black PM. Diagnosing idiopathic normal-pressure hydrocephalus. *Neurosurgery.* 2005:57(3 suppl):S4–S16.

Sprung C, Schlosser HG, Lemcke J, et al. The adjustable proGAV shunt: a prospective safety and reliability multicenter study. *Neurosurgery.* 2010;66:465–474.

REFERENCES

1. Rekate HL. A contemporary definition and classification of hydrocephalus. *Semin Pediatr Neurol.* 2009;16(1):9–15.

2. Long DF. Diagnosis and management of late intracranial complications of TBI. In: Zasler ND, Katz DI, Zafonte RD, eds. *Brain Injury Medicine: Principles and Practice.* New York, NY: Demos Medical Publishing; 2007:577–601.

3. Bigler ED. Neuroimaging correlates of functional outcome. In: Zasler ND, Katz DI, Zafonte RD, eds. *Brain Injury Medicine: Principles and Practice.* New York, NY: Demos Medical Publishing; 2007:201–224.

4. Waziri A, Fusco D, Mayer SA, McKhann GM II, Connolly ES Jr. Postoperative hydrocephalus in patients undergoing decompressive hemicraniectomy for ischemic or hemorrhagic stroke. *Neurosurgery.* 2007;61(3):489–493.

5. Relkin N, Marmarou A, Klinge P, Bergsneider M, Black PM. Diagnosing idiopathic normal-pressure hydrocephalus. *Neurosurgery.* 2005;57(3 suppl):S4–S16.

6. Ishikawa M, Oowaki H, Matsumoto A, Suzuki T, Furuse M, Nishida N. Clinical significance of cerebrospinal fluid tap test and magnetic resonance imaging/computed tomography findings of tight high convexity in patients with possible idiopathic normal pressure hydrocephalus. *Neurol Med Chir (Tokyo).* 2010;50(2):119–123.

7. Marmarou A, Bergsneider M, Klinge P, Relkin N, Black PM. The value of supplemental prognostic tests for the preoperative assessment of idiopathic normal-pressure hydrocephalus. *Neurosurgery.* 2005;52(suppl 2):17–28.

8. Vanneste J, Augustijn P, Davies GA, Dirven C, Tan WF. Normal-pressure hydrocephalus. Is cisternography still useful in selecting patients for a shunt? *Arch Neurol.* 1992;49(4):366–370.

9. Drake JM, Sainte-Rose C. *The Shunt Book.* Cambridge, MA; Blackwell Scientific; 1995:1–228.

10. Piatt JH Jr. Physical examination of patients with cerebrospinal fluid shunts: is there useful information in pumping the shunt? *Pediatrics.* 1992;89(3):470–473.

11. Chung JJ, Yu JS, Kim JH, Nam SJ, Kim MJ. Intraabdominal complications secondary to ventriculoperitoneal shunts: CT findings and review of the literature. *AJR Am J Roentgenol.* 2009;193(5):1311–1317.

12. Zemack G, Romner B. Do adjustable shunt valves pressure our budget? A retrospective analysis of 541 implanted Codman Hakim programmable valves. *Br J Neurosurg.* 2001;15(3):221–227.

13. Muramatsu H, Koike K, Teramoto A. Ventriculoperitoneal shunt dysfunction during rehabilitation: prevalence and countermeasures. *Am J Phys Med Rehabil.* 2002;81(8):571–578.

14. Lollis SS, Mamourian AC, Vaccaro TJ, Duhaime AC. Programmable CSF shunt valves: radiographic identification and interpretation. *AJNR Am J Neuroradiol.* 2010;31(7):1343–1346.

15. Lefranc M, Ko JY, Peltier J, et al. Effect of transcranial magnetic stimulation on four types of pressure-programmable valves. *Acta Neurochir (Wien).* 2010;152(4):689–697.

16. Sprung C, Schlosser HG, Lemcke J, et al. The adjustable proGAV shunt: a prospective safety and reliability multicenter study. *Neurosurgery.* 2010;66(3):465–474.

47

Posttraumatic Seizures

Puneet K. Gupta and Ramon Diaz-Arrastia

GENERAL PRINCIPLES

Definition

A seizure (sz) is a spontaneous, excessive synchronous discharge of cortical neurons that can result in clinical manifestations such as sensations, alteration in behavior or consciousness, and/or body movements

- Subclinical sz—"nonconvulsive sz"; no overt clinical features
- Simple partial sz (SPS)—no impairment of consciousness (i.e., intact memory)
- Complex partial sz (CPS)—impaired attention, awareness, and/or consciousness (i.e., impaired memory)
- Generalized tonic-clonic sz (GTCS)—loss of consciousness (LOC); can be primarily generalized or secondarily generalized (from SPS or CPS)

A posttraumatic sz (PTS) refers to a sz after traumatic brain injury (TBI)

- Immediate szs or "concussive convulsions" are acute symptomatic szs that occur within minutes of TBI; not predictive of posttraumatic epilepsy (PTE) [1]
- Early PTS are acute symptomatic szs occuring within 1 week after TBI
- Late PTS occur more than 1 week after TBI

PTE refers to a disorder of recurrent, unprovoked, late PTS

Epidemiology

- The prevalence of PTS in the United States is 2% to more than 50% depending on cohort and injury severity [2,17].
- About 80% of first PTS occur within 2 years, 50% to 60% within 1 year, and 40% within 6 months of TBI [4].
- Early PTS occur in 2% to 17% of all patients with head injuries, are more common in children, and correlate with TBI severity [2].

- The cumulative incidence of late PTS in the first 30 years after TBI is 2% for mild injuries, 4% for moderate injuries, 20% for severe closed head injuries, and more than 50% if the dura is penetrated [3,19].

Pathophysiology

- Physiological mechanisms causing szs after TBI are not completely understood [7,8,20].
- Both focal and diffuse brain insults often coexist in TBI patients. Focal insults (contusions or intracranial hematomas) result in neighboring neural inflammation, gliosis, sprouting, and neurogenesis, which are felt to result in epileptogenesis [9]. Diffuse insults can result in injury to susceptible brain regions, such as the hippocampus. Injury can lead to atrophy and sclerosis; up to one-third of PTE is of temporal lobe origin [9].

DIAGNOSIS

Risk Factors

- For early PTS—younger age (especially <5 years), acute ICH, acute subdural hematomas (SDH; in children), diffuse cerebral edema (in children), metal fragment retention, neurological deficits, depressed or linear skull fractures (in adults), and LOC or amnesia for >30 minutes [2]
- For late PTS—age > 65 years, early PTS (in adults), SDH, brain contusion, alcoholism, penetrating injury, retained metal fragments, depressed skull fracture, neurological deficits, brain tissue loss, and severe TBI [2,4,10] (see Annegers under Additional Reading)
- The risk of PTS decreases with time and reaches the baseline value for the population at 10 to 15 years after the head injury [4].
- A single late PTS has a 65% to 90% chance of progressing to PTE.
- The likelihood that PTE will go into remission is lower if PTS are frequent in the first year after TBI, if PTS onset is >4 years after TBI, or if there is intracranial hemorrhage (ICH) [10–12] (see Jennett under Additional Reading).

Clinical Presentation

- PTS may present as subclinical sz, partial sz (majority), symptomatic and secondarily generalized sz, or even as primary generalized szs (up to 5%) but not as generalized absence sz [10,11,18] (see Diaz-Arrastia under Additional Reading).
- Any partial onset sz (SPS or CPS) can secondarily generalize; more common with frontal than temporal lobe origin sz.

- Typical symptoms associated with SPS by location of sz origin:
  - Frontal lobe—rare auras; clonic or tonic posturing of body parts
  - Temporal lobe—autonomic (abdominal discomfort, nausea, abdominal rising feeling), psychic (fear or sense of impending doom, anxiety, feelings of déjà vu or jamais vu), or olfactory and gustatory hallucinations (usually of an obnoxious smell or taste)
  - Parietal lobe—vertiginous aura, elementary sensory symptoms (which can be painful)
  - Occipital lobe—elementary visual hallucinations (bright lights, zig-zagging colored lines, or kaleidoscopic shapes), formed visual hallucinations
- Typical symptoms associated with CPS by location of sz origin:
  - Frontal lobe CPS—hyperkinetic motor movements, bicycling, hip thrusting, thrashing, and asymmetric tonic posturing
  - Temporal lobe CPS—staring, unresponsiveness, automatisms (i.e., stereotyped behaviors such as chewing, lip smacking, self-polishing movements of fumbling with their clothes), or dystonic posturing of the extremitis.
- GTCS are characterized by tonic extensor posturing of the arms and legs, followed by rhythmic clonic movements of the arms, legs, and trunk. GTCS are often associated with transient apnea, vomiting, tongue biting, and sphincter incontinence.
- After a CPS or GTCS, there may be a post-ictal period (typically lasting <10 minutes), during which the patient is obtunded and difficult to arouse. Even after regaining consciousness, patients are often confused and amnestic for up to several more hours. Patients often report headaches, dizziness, and sleepiness after a sz, particularly GTCS.

Physical Examination

- Neurological findings, if present, may correlate with the epileptogenic zone.
- Immediately after a sz, transient focal neurological deficits (i.e., weakness that later resolves ["Todd's paralysis"] or aphasia) are often helpful in localizing sz onset.

Diagnostic Evaluation

- Differential diagnosis includes psychogenic nonepileptic szs (PNES) (i.e., "pseudoseizures"), syncope (e.g., concussive syncope), confusional states (i.e., delirium), acute memory disorders (e.g., fugue state), dizziness, and imbalance.
- In patients with moderate to severe TBI with refractory spells, about 30% were misdiagnosed as having PTE but actually had PNES [14]. Therefore, if atypical features are present and szs continue despite

treatment, the diagnosis of PTE should be verified by video electroen-cephalogram (VEEG).

Laboratory Studies

- Serum tests (i.e., chem panel, liver function tests, urine drug screen); EEG. Note that a single interictal (between sz) EEG has a low sensitivity (30%–50%, which approaches 80%–85% with serial EEGs) of capturing epileptiform activity. However, if captured, epileptiform discharges (spikes or sharp waves) are >97% specific for epilepsy.
- VEEG evaluation should be considered if seizures are disabling and do not respond to appropriate antiepileptic drugs (AEDs).

Radiographic Assessment

- Patients who present with an acute TBI and a sz should be imaged with a computed tomography (CT) scan immediately, and the study should be repeated if the condition of the patient does not improve or worsens.
- Head CT is more accessible and cheaper than magnetic resonance imaging (MRI) and, although less sensitive, is usually able to depict acute pathology (i.e., intracranial bleed) that needs urgent intervention.
- Brain MRI is the study of choice for nonacute evaluations of PTS or PTE. Transient diffusion weighted imaging (DWI) and/or Fluid-attenuated inversion-recovery imaging (FLAIR) changes may occur with sz and do not reflect structural injury.

TREATMENT

Guiding Principles

- Prophylaxis with AEDs is often initiated as soon as possible after moderate to severe TBI [16]. AEDs (i.e., phenytoin, levetiracetam) given within a day of injury prevent early PTS but not late PTS or PTE [17–19]. Chronic prophylactic use of AEDs is possibly associated with an increased risk for PTS. For these reasons, AEDs are widely recommended for a short time after head trauma (7 days) to prevent early but not late PTS (see Temkin under Additional Reading).
- Late PTS or PTE worsens functional outcome significantly, and therefore prevention of PTS is an important goal [20]. However, no treatment is established to prevent the development of epilepsy (e.g., antiepileptogenesis), but AEDs may repress sz if late PTS or PTE occur.
- In children, AEDs may be ineffective in preventing both early and late PTS.
- Treatment of PTE does not require hospitalization, but admission may be needed for the treatment of status epilepticus or for VEEG to assist in the diagnosis.

Initial Management

- PTS prophylaxis—See Guiding Principles.
- In those with a single unprovoked sz, the decision whether or not to begin AEDs depends on the risk of developing further szs (see Risk Factors).
- Early PTS—The recommendation is that early PTS should be treated promptly. Acutely, lorazepam, diazepam, fosphenytoin, sodium valproate, and levetiracetam are the drugs of choice and are usually effective in stopping an ongoing sz. There is little data on how long to continue therapy, but many continue AEDs for a few weeks to months, especially in those with moderate to severe TBI.
- Chronically, one first- or second-generation AED can be started. Typically, the second-generation medications are just as efficacious and better tolerated. No known randomized controlled studies have been performed to prove that one is better than the other. Phenytoin probably should be avoided, because it increases the risk of impairing cognitive function. Levetiracetam is better tolerated and just as effective as phenytoin in TBI.
- If sz control is not achieved with one drug, a second or even a third AED may be required to achieve sz control.
- Late PTS—The risk of sz recurrence after a first late PTS is high; chronic use of AEDs is recommended in these individuals. The choice of AEDs is the same as mentioned earlier.
- PTE—The choice of antiepileptic medications is the same as mentioned earlier.

Ongoing Care

Medical Care

- Regular follow-up (at least yearly) should be performed.
- Once a therapeutic medication regimen is achieved, the individual is typically maintained on the same dosage for a period of 2 years. After 2 years, the individual should be evaluated for the possibility of withdrawal from the antiepileptic therapy.
- Factors such as the presence of focal neurological deficits, CT evidence of structural brain disease, and persistent EEG abnormalities increase the risk of recurrence.
- If szs remain intractable, referral to an epilepsy specialist may be indicated, and consideration may need to be given to interventional approaches such as placement of a neurostimulator or epilepsy surgery.

Additional Considerations

- Patients must be warned to exercise caution during bathing, swimming, and climbing heights. They should never be alone during these activities.

- Patients must also be counseled about the limitations in driving, based on the laws in their state or country of residence.
- Psychological problems related to social isolation and the stigma of epilepsy must be addressed. Depression is a common comorbidity. Consultation with psychiatrists, counselors, and social workers should be considered when these issues are identified.

ADDITIONAL READING

Electronic Reference
AAN PTS Practice Guideline. http://www.neurology.org/cgi/reprint/60/1/10

Textbooks/Chapters
Jennett B. *Epilepsy After Non-Missile Head Injuries.* England: William Heinemann Medical Books; 1975:1–179.

Young B. Post-traumatic epilepsy. In: Barrow DL, ed. *Complications and Sequelae of Head Injury.* Park Ridge, IL: American Association of Neurological Surgeons; 1992:127–132.

Journal Articles
Annegers JF, Hauser A, Coan SP, et al. A population based study of seizures after traumatic brain injuries. *N Engl J Med.* 1998;338(1):20–24.

Caveness WF, Walker AE, Ascroft PB. Incidence of posttraumatic epilepsy in Korean veterans as compared with those from World War 1 and World War II. *J Neurosurgery.* 1962;19:122–129.

Diaz-Arrastia R, Agostini MA, Frol AB, et al. Neurophysiologic and neuroradiologic features of intractable epilepsy after traumatic brain injury in adults. *Arch Neurol.* 2000;57(11):1611–1616.

Temkin NR, Dikmen SS, Wilensky AJ. A randomized, double-blind study of phenytoin for the prevention of post-traumatic seizures. *N Engl J Med.* 1990;323(8):497–502.

REFERENCES

1. McCrory PR, Berkovic SF. Concussive convulsions. Incidence in sport and treatment recommendations. *Sports Med.* 1998;25(2):131–136.
2. Frey LC. Epidemiology of posttraumatic epilepsy: a critical review. *Epilepsia.* 2003;44 Suppl 10:11–17.
3. Caveness WF, Walker AE, Ascroft PB. Incidence of posttraumatic epilepsy in Korean veterans as compared with those from World War I and World War II. *J Neurosurg.* 1962;19:122–129.
4. Annegers JF, Hauser WA, Coan SP, Rocca WA. A population-based study of seizures after traumatic brain injuries. *N Engl J Med.* 1998;338(1):20–24.
5. Angeleri F, Majkowski J, Cacchiò G, et al. Posttraumatic epilepsy risk factors: one-year prospective study after head injury. *Epilepsia.* 1999;40(9):1222–1230.
6. Yablon SA. Posttraumatic seizures. *Arch Phys Med Rehabil.* 1993;74(9):983–1001.

7. D'Ambrosio R, Perucca E. Epilepsy after head injury. *Curr Opin Neurol.* 2004;17(6):731–735.

8. Panter SS, Sadrzadeh SM, Hallaway PE, Haines JL, Anderson VE, Eaton JW. Hypohaptoglobinemia associated with familial epilepsy. *J Exp Med.* 1985;161(4):748–754.

9. Diaz-Arrastia R, Agostini MA, Madden CJ, Van Ness PC. Posttraumatic epilepsy: the endophenotypes of a human model of epileptogenesis. *Epilepsia.* 2009;50 Suppl 2:14–20.

10. Salazar AM, Jabbari B, Vance SC, Grafman J, Amin D, Dillon JD. Epilepsy after penetrating head injury. I. Clinical correlates: a report of the Vietnam Head Injury Study. *Neurology.* 1985;35(10):1406–1414.

11. Jennett B. *Epilepsy After Non-Missile Head Injuries.* England: William Heinemann Medical Books; 1975:1–179.

12. Annegers JF, Hauser WA, Elveback LR. Remission of seizures and relapse in patients with epilepsy. *Epilepsia.* 1979;20(6):729–737.

13. Diaz-Arrastia R, Agostini MA, Frol AB, et al. Neurophysiologic and neuroradiologic features of intractable epilepsy after traumatic brain injury in adults. *Arch Neurol.* 2000;57(11):1611–1616.

14. Hudak AM, Trivedi K, Harper CR, et al. Evaluation of seizure-like episodes in survivors of moderate and severe traumatic brain injury. *J Head Trauma Rehabil.* 2004;19(4):290–295.

15. Vespa PM, Nuwer MR, Nenov V, et al. Increased incidence and impact of nonconvulsive and convulsive seizures after traumatic brain injury as detected by continuous electroencephalographic monitoring. *J Neurosurg.* 1999;91(5):750–760.

16. Chang BS, Lowenstein DH; Quality Standards Subcommittee of the American Academy of Neurology. Practice parameter: antiepileptic drug prophylaxis in severe traumatic brain injury: report of the Quality Standards Subcommittee of the American Academy of Neurology. *Neurology.* 2003;60(1):10–16.

17. Temkin NR, Dikmen SS, Wilensky AJ, Keihm J, Chabal S, Winn HR. A randomized, double-blind study of phenytoin for the prevention of posttraumatic seizures. *N Engl J Med.* 1990;323(8):497–502.

18. Temkin NR, Dikmen SS, Anderson GD, et al. Valproate therapy for prevention of posttraumatic seizures: a randomized trial. *J Neurosurg.* 1999;91(4):593–600.

19. Szaflarski JP, Meckler JM, Szaflarski M, Shutter LA, Privitera MD, Yates SL. Levetiracetam use in critically ill patients. *Neurocrit Care.* 2007;7(2):140–147.

20. Asikainen I, Kaste M, Sarna S. Early and late posttraumatic seizures in traumatic brain injury rehabilitation patients: brain injury factors causing late seizures and influence of seizures on long-term outcome. *Epilepsia.* 1999;40(5):584–589.

48

Heterotopic Ossification

Nora Cullen and Christina Taggart

BACKGROUND

Heterotopic ossification (HO) is a common sequela of traumatic brain injury (TBI) that often leads to pain and restricted joint range of motion (ROM), limiting a patient's ability to participate in rehabilitation and further adding to disability by reducing mobility and function.

Definition

The abnormal formation of mature lamellar bone within soft tissues such as tendons, ligaments, and muscles [1].

Epidemiology

The incidence of HO following TBI is 11% to 73.3%, reaching clinical significance in 10% to 20% of cases [2].

Classification

After Brooker et al. (1973) [3]:

- Class I—Islands of bone in the soft tissue
- Class II—Bone spurs leaving at least 1 cm between opposing surfaces
- Class III—Bone spurs leaving less than 1 cm between opposing surfaces
- Class IV—Ankylosis

Pathophysiology

Neurogenic Factors
Osteoblastic cells undergo inappropriate differentiation within soft tissues. They are likely stimulated by an osteogenic factor released by the injured brain [4–6], which affects prostaglandins (PG), leading to

abnormal regulation of bone metabolism. Other contributing factors include hypercalcemia, hypoxia, sympathetic imbalance, and disequilibrium of parathyroid hormone and calcitonin [7].

Enhanced Osteogenesis
Ectopic bone is highly metabolically active, with a rate of formation three times greater and an osteoclastic density twice that of normal age-matched bone [8].

Timeline
The ectopic organic osteoid matrix reaches full calcification within a matter of weeks. Osseous reorganization to mature trabecular bone occurs during subsequent months [4].

DIAGNOSIS

Early detection is imperative in preventing the progression of HO.

Risk Factors

There is an increased risk with skeletal trauma, spasticity, immobilization, and post-injury coma more than 2 weeks [5].

Clinical Presentation

Restricted joint ROM, swelling, and pain [9].

Timing
- Symptoms generally begin 2 months post-injury, but range from 2 weeks to 12 months [1].
- HO formation precedes symptom onset; decreased ROM is often the earliest clinical sign.

Location
HO can occur at any joint following TBI but most often develops at fracture sites or in bruised soft tissue. The most commonly affected joints are the hip, shoulder, elbow, and, rarely, the knee [9]. Ankylosis is most likely to occur at the elbow.

Physical Examination

Clinical exam often reveals a swollen, warm, and painful joint, with decreased ROM. Other findings may include erythema, para-articular mass, and fever. These clinical findings may be mistaken for deep venous thrombosis, infection, local trauma, or fracture [10], but should be considered in the differential diagnosis of HO.

Bloodwork

- Elevated serum alkaline phosphatase levels can occur from 7 weeks before [5] to 3 weeks after [11] appearance of clinical symptoms.
- Erythrocyte sedimentation rate and C-reactive protein may also become elevated early in the formation of HO [12].

Radiography

- Triple-phase bone scan with increased uptake during first and second phases is the diagnostic gold standard. HO can be detected as soon as clinical features appear [5].
- Plain radiographs may remain negative until 2 to 6 weeks after clinical symptoms begin [13].

MANAGEMENT

The aim is prevention of progression, pain management, and maximization of joint mobility.

Physical Modalities

- *Physiotherapy* involving assisted ROM exercises and gentle stretching is of benefit in relieving pain, maintaining mobility, and preventing ankylosis [5,14]. The joint should not be moved beyond its pain-free range of movement [15].
- Manipulation under anesthesia may help differentiate between spasticity and ankylosis and relax muscles enough to perform *forceful manipulation,* increasing ROM [16].
- *Continuous passive motion* can increase and maintain joint ROM at the knee both during HO development and after surgical excision [17].

Medical Management

Nonsteroidal Anti-Inflammatory Drugs [18]

Action   Minimize HO formation and patient discomfort in early and intermediate stages.

Mechanism   Most nonsteroidal anti-inflammatory drugs (NSAIDs) act as nonselective inhibitors of cyclooxygenase, thereby blocking the formation of PG.

Optimal drug Indomethacin

- Indomethacin is the gold standard in the prevention of HO following total hip arthroplasty (THA). Other NSAIDs, such as naproxen and diclofenac, have been shown to be equally effective and are considered alternative first-line treatments.
- Cyclooxygenase-2 inhibitors, such as rofecoxib and celecoxib, can also be used.

Potential side effects of NSAIDs Gastrointestinal complications, cardiovascular side effects, and delayed fracture healing.

Bisphosphonates [18]

Action Inhibitory effect on the formation of hydroxyapatite.

Mechanism Bisphosphonates block the aggregation, growth, and mineralization of hydroxyapatite, thereby retarding the ossification process.

Optimal drug Disodium etidronate

- When used in conjunction with NSAIDs, etidronate affects the osteoblasts that escape the inhibitory action of NSAIDs. It may also reduce the number of osteoclasts and alter their cellular morphology.
- Etidronate may have an anti-inflammatory effect.

Dosing Should be started as early as possible post-injury at a dose of 10 to 20 mg/kg/day, before significant ectopic bone begins to form, and administered for at least 6 months.

Potential side effects Gastrointestinal symptoms, hyperphosphatemia, and possibly osteomalacia.

Caution A *Cochrane Review* [19] suggests "there is insufficient evidence to recommend the use of disodium etidronate or other pharmacological agents for the treatment of acute HO." It has been suggested that disodium etidronate acts by delaying, rather than preventing, the mineralization of ectopic bone, which may then occur after treatment cessation.

Surgical Intervention

General Principles
Surgical excision of HO is an option if conservative treatment has failed. It has been shown to significantly improve joint mobility, ambulation, and patient comfort, as well as to reduce spasticity [12].

Timing
The optimal timing of surgical resection of HO following TBI is still controversial but it is usually not considered until 12 to 18 months after formation to reduce the likelihood of recurrence [20]. However, there is

increasing evidence that timing of surgical intervention does not affect recurrence rates [21–23]. Further, late surgical intervention may result in poorer functional outcomes by leading to an increased risk of ankylosis, disuse osteopenia, and associated iatrogenic intraoperative fracture [22].

Potential Complications
HO has a 36% recurrence rate, usually within 3 months of surgical excision [24]. Intraoperative fracture can also occur [22]. NSAIDs and etidronate may be useful in preventing HO recurrence following surgical excision [15].

Radiotherapy

Local radiotherapy has been used successfully to prevent HO after THA [5]. Its utility in TBI patients is less clear due to the difficulty in predicting the site of HO formation after a head injury. Radiotherapy has not been shown to be of benefit in reducing the volume of established ectopic bone in TBI patients.

ADDITIONAL READING

Electronic Reference
Teasell R, Hilditch M, Marshall S, Cullen N, Bayona N. Heterotopic ossification and venous thromboembolism. *Evidence-Based Review of Moderate to Severe Acquired Brain Injury.* 5th ed. Module 11. http://www.abiebr.com/modules/modules/9_12_files/category-module002311.html

Textbook/Chapter
Garland DE, Varpetian A. Heterotopic ossification in traumatic brain injury. In: Ashley MJ, ed. *Traumatic Brain Injury: Rehabilitative Treatment and Case Management.* 2nd ed. Boca Raton, FL: CRC Press; 2003:119–132.

Journal Articles
Cipriano CA, Pill SG, Keenan MA. Heterotopic ossification following traumatic brain injury and spinal cord injury. *J Am Acad Orthop Surg.* 2009;17:689–697.
Cullen N, Bayley M, Bayona N, Hilditch M, Aubut J. Management of heterotopic ossification and venous thromboembolism following acquired brain injury. *Brain Inj.* 2007;21:215–230.

REFERENCES

1. Cipriano CA, Pill SG, Keenan MA. Heterotopic ossification following traumatic brain injury and spinal cord injury. *J Am Acad Orthop Surg.* 2009;17(11):689–697.

2. Simonsen LL, Sonne-Holm S, Krasheninnikoff M, Engberg AW. Symptomatic heterotopic ossification after very severe traumatic brain injury in 114 patients: incidence and risk factors. *Injury.* 2007;38(10):1146–1150.

3. Brooker AF, Bowerman JW, Robinson RA, Riley LH Jr. Ectopic ossification following total hip replacement. Incidence and a method of classification. *J Bone Joint Surg Am.* 1973;55(8):1629–1632.

4. Pape HC, Lehmann U, van Griensven M, Gänsslen A, von Glinski S, Krettek C. Heterotopic ossifications in patients after severe blunt trauma with and without head trauma: incidence and patterns of distribution. *J Orthop Trauma.* 2001;15(4):229–237.

5. Pape HC, Marsh S, Morley JR, Krettek C, Giannoudis PV. Current concepts in the development of heterotopic ossification. *J Bone Joint Surg Br.* 2004;86(6):783–787.

6. Toffoli AM, Gautschi OP, Frey SP, Filgueira L, Zellweger R. From brain to bone: evidence for the release of osteogenic humoral factors after traumatic brain injury. *Brain Inj.* 2008;22(7–8):511–518.

7. Stover SL, Hataway CJ, Zeiger HE. Heterotopic ossification in spinal cord-injured patients. *Arch Phys Med Rehabil.* 1975;56(5):199–204.

8. Puzas JE, Brand JS, Evarts CM. The stimulus for bone formation. In: Brand RA, ed. *The Hip.* St Louis, MO: CV Mosby; 25–38.

9. Garland DE, Blum CE, Waters RL. Periarticular heterotopic ossification in head-injured adults. Incidence and location. *J Bone Joint Surg Am.* 1980;62(7):1143–1146.

10. Buschbacher R. Heterotopic ossification: a review. *Clin Rev Phys Med Rehabil.* 1992;4:199–213.

11. Kim SW, Charter RA, Chai CJ, Kim SK, Kim ES. Serum alkaline phosphatase and inorganic phosphorus values in spinal cord injury patients with heterotopic ossification. *Paraplegia.* 1990;28(7):441–447.

12. Teasell R, Hilditch M, Marshall S, Cullen N, Bayona N. Heterotopic ossification and venous thromboembolism. *Evidence-Based Review of Moderate to Severe Acquired Brain Injury.* 5th ed. Module 11. http://www.abiebr.com/modules/modules/9_12_files/category-module002311.html. Accessed April 12, 2010.

13. Orzel JA, Rudd TG. Heterotopic bone formation: clinical, laboratory, and imaging correlation. *J Nucl Med.* 1985;26(2):125–132.

14. Ellerin BE, Helfet D, Parikh S, et al. Current therapy in the management of heterotopic ossification of the elbow: a review with case studies. *Am J Phys Med Rehabil.* 1999;78(3):259–271.

15. Evans EB. Heterotopic bone formation in thermal burns. *Clin Orthop Relat Res.* 1991;(263):94–101.

16. Garland DE, Razza BE, Waters RL. Forceful joint manipulation in head-injured adults with heterotopic ossification. *Clin Orthop Relat Res.* 1982;(169):133–138.

17. Linan E, O'Dell MW, Pierce JM. Continuous passive motion in the management of heterotopic ossification in a brain injured patient. *Am J Phys Med Rehabil.* 2001;80(8):614–617.

18. Cullen N, Perera J. Heterotopic ossification: pharmacologic options. *J Head Trauma Rehabil.* 2009;24(1):69–71.

19. Haran M, Bhuta T, Lee B. Pharmacological interventions for treating acute heterotopic ossification. *Cochrane Database Syst Rev.* 2008;4:CD003321.

20. Garland DE. Surgical approaches for resection of heterotopic ossification in traumatic brain-injured adults. *Clin Orthop Relat Res.* 1991;(263):59–70.

21. Vanden Bossche L, Vanderstraeten G. Heterotopic ossification: a review. *J Rehabil Med*. 2005;37(3):129–136.
22. Genet F, Marmorat JL, Lautridou C, Schnitzler A, Mailhan L, Denormandie P. Impact of late surgical intervention on heterotopic ossification of the hip after traumatic neurological injury. *J Bone Joint Surg Br*. 2009;91(11):1493–1498.
23. Chalidis B, Stengel D, Giannoudis PV. Early excision and late excision of heterotopic ossification after traumatic brain injury are equivalent: a systematic review of the literature. *J Neurotrauma*. 2007;24(11):1675–1686.
24. Garland DE, Hanscom DA, Keenan MA, Smith C, Moore T. Resection of heterotopic ossification in the adult with head trauma. *J Bone Joint Surg Am*. 1985;67(8):1261–1269.

49

The Management of Endocrine Dysfunction in Traumatic Brain Injury

Lucy-Ann Behan and Amar Agha

INTRODUCTION

Posttraumatic hypopituitarism (PTHP) refers to any abnormality of the endocrine hypothalamic-pituitary axis following traumatic brain injury (TBI), including anterior pituitary hormone deficiency and posterior pituitary hormone deficiency.

EPIDEMIOLOGY

Based on published prospective studies the estimated frequency of long-term PTHP is 22.7% to 68.5% [1].

PITUITARY GLAND ANATOMY AND PHYSIOLOGY

The pituitary gland is located at the base of the skull within the sella turcica, and is joined to the hypothalamus by the infundibulum. The pituitary gland, measuring 8 mm by 10 mm, receives its blood supply from the internal carotid arteries, primarily via the superior hypophyseal artery and the long hypophyseal portal vessels, which arise above the diaphragma sella, while the inferior hypophyseal artery and short hypophyseal vessels enter below the diaphragma sella. The hormones produced by the pituitary and their peripheral targets are described in Table 49.1.

PATHOPHYSIOLOGY

The pathophysiology of PTHP is not completely understood. Current evidence suggests that multiple factors are involved in the development of PTHP including [2]

Table 49.1 Pituitary Physiology

Pituitary Hormone	Target Gland	Result
Anterior		
Growth hormone	Various end organs, liver	Mainly acts via insulin-like growth factor-1
Adrenocorticotropin hormone	Adrenal gland	Cortisol, androgens
Gonadotropins (FSH/LH)	Ovaries/testes	Estrogen/testosterone
Thyroid stimulating Hormone	Thyroid gland	Thyroid hormone
Prolactin	Mammary glands	Lactation and gonadal suppression
Posterior		
Antidiuretic hormone (vasopressin)	Distal nephron	Fluid and electrolyte balance
Oxytocin	Uterus and breast in females	No known role in males. Contracts pregnant uterus and contributes to lactation. No known adverse effects with deficiency of this hormone

FSH, follicle-stimulating hormone; LH, luteinizing hormone.

- Primary brain injury
  - Mechanical trauma may injure the gland, the infundibulum and/or the hypothalamus.
  - Skull base fractures, rotational and shearing injuries may compromise the blood supply to the pituitary. The long hypophyseal vessels along the infundibulum are particularly vulnerable.
  - Hemorrhage into the sella turcica or into the pituitary gland may also result in direct structural injury.
- Secondary insults
  - Hypoxia, hypotension, cerebral edema, or anemia may all contribute to pituitary ischemia.
  - Medications used following TBI may also contribute to PTHP by both direct effects on the hypothalamic/pituitary axis or by direct effect on the adrenal glands or cortisol metabolism. Those at risk of PTHP may not be able to compensate for any adrenal insult or altered cortisol metabolism. Medication effects are usually transient and reversible. Agents to be aware of include opiate derivatives,

phenytoin, etomidate, and high-dose pentobarbital and propofol, all of which can induce acute adrenal insufficiency.

- Note that severe brain injury is not required for the development of PTHP; several studies have demonstrated hypopituitarism following moderate TBI, mild TBI, and repetitive mild sports related injury [3].

ASSESSMENT AND MANAGEMENT OF ENDOCRINE STATUS FOLLOWING TBI

Anterior Pituitary Dysfunction in the Acute Phase (i.e., Hours to Days Post TBI)

- Adrenocorticotropic hormone (ACTH) deficiency
  - Glucocorticoid deficiency is potentially life threatening.
  - Suspicion should be high if any of the following are present: hypotension despite pressor support, hypoglycemia, or hyponatremia.
  - Morning serum cortisol <200 nmol/L in a subject in intensive care is inappropriately low and glucocorticoid replacement is necessary.
  - Morning serum cortisol between 200 and 500 nmol/L in a subject following TBI must be interpreted in the clinical context. Replacement should be considered if any of the above features are present.
  - Confirm the subject has received no exogenous steroids that may alter the interpretation of serum cortisol results, for example, dexamethasone.
  - The synthetic ACTH (Synacthen) test should NOT be used to diagnose adrenal insufficiency in the acute phase of TBI as adrenal atrophy has not yet developed; the diagnosis must be based on the aforementioned features.
- Assessment of the growth hormone (GH), gonadal, and thyroid axes are not necessary in the acute phase as there is currently no evidence to suggest replacement is beneficial.

Posterior Pituitary Dysfunction in the Acute Phase

- Diabetes insipidus (DI)
  - Due to antidiuretic hormone (ADH) deficiency
  - Defined by >3 L of dilute urine (urine osmolality <300 mOsm/kg) in 24 hours and plasma sodium >145 mmol/L
  - May be transient in this phase of TBI
  - Urine output >200 mL/hour for 2 consecutive hours may be suggestive.
  - Electrolyte abnormalities in this setting may be life threatening.
  - Adequate fluid replacement and ADH replacement (desmopressin) may be required and should be adjusted according to hourly urine output response and plasma sodium.

- SIADH
  - Characterized by euvolemic hyponatraemia in the absence of glucocorticoid deficiency or hypothyroidism.
  - Plasma osmolality <270 mOsm/kg, urine osmolality >100 mOsm/kg, and spot urinary sodium >40 mmol/L.
  - Treat with fluid restriction to 500 mL—1.5 L in 24 hours.
  - Rarely hypertonic saline infusion may be required. Note that rapid changes in plasma sodium increase the risk of cerebral pontine myelinolysis. Aim to correct sodium at a rate less than 0.5 mmol/L/hour.
- Cerebral salt wasting
  - A very rare differential diagnosis for hyponatraemia in the setting of TBI
  - Characterized by hypovolemic hyponatraemia
  - Plasma osmolality <270 mOsm/kg, urine osmolality >100 mOsm/kg, and spot urinary sodium >40 mmol/L, low central venous pressure/hypotension
  - Treat with isotonic saline administration to restore euvolemia. Aim to correct sodium at a rate less than 0.5 mmol/hour.

Pituitary Hormone Dysfunction in the Chronic Phase (i.e., >3 Months) After TBI

Screen all patients with moderate (Glasgow Coma Scale; GCS 9–12) and severe (GCS ≤8) TBI; screen subjects with mild TBI (GCS 13–15) if indicated based on clinical symptoms and signs.

- Glucocorticoid deficiency
  - Characterized by life threatening adrenal crisis, hypotension, fatigue, and recurrent infections
- GH deficiency
  - Impaired linear growth and abnormal body composition in children; in adults reduced lean body mass, decreased exercise capacity, reduced quality of life, impaired cardiac function, and reduced bone mineral density
- Gonadotropin deficiency
  - In males, testosterone deficiency is associated with reduced lean body mass, bone mineral density, erectile dysfunction, and muscle weakness. Estrogen deficiency in females leads to amenorrhea and reduced bone mineral density. Although 1.5% to 41% subjects following TBI will have chronic gonadotropin deficiency, there is no

available data regarding fertility outcomes. These patients should be referred to an endocrinologist for fertility assessment.

- Thyroid stimulating hormone (TSH) deficiency
  - Lethargy, fatigue, and neuropsychiatric manifestations
- Diabetes Insipidus (DI)
  - Polyuria, polydipsia, and excess thirst (in those with cognitive impairment clinicians must rely on urine output and biochemical markers to suggest this diagnosis)

All of these endocrine abnormalities may have serious adverse impact on patients with TBI and may impair recovery and rehabilitation. Untreated hypopituitarism in any population is associated with premature mortality and increased morbidity.

Subjects with moderate or severe TBI should undergo routine endocrine evaluation as described below between 3 and 6 months following TBI; hormone deficiencies should be replaced as appropriate (Figure 49.1).

- Synacthen (ACTH stimulation) test—adrenal reserve
- Basal free T4 and TSH
- Basal estrogen/testosterone and gonadotropins
- Serum sodium and clinical assessment of thirst, polyuria (>3 L/24 hours), polydipsia, and nocturia. If abnormal, formal water deprivation testing should be carried out under the guidance of a pituitary endocrinologist
- The GH–insulin-like growth factor-1 axis should not be assessed until at least 1 year post TBI, as changes before this time may be transient [4]. This requires dynamic stimulation tests and should be performed in specialist pituitary units. There is some evidence to suggest that GH replacement may improve quality of life and some metabolic parameters in this patient group; however, long-term prospective studies are lacking. GH replacement may be considered on an individual basis in conjunction with endocrine specialist advice

CONCLUSION

PTHP is a common, but underdiagnosed, complication of TBI and can contribute to the morbidity associated with this condition. An increased level of awareness among all disciplines caring for this patient group is vital in order to provide appropriate and timely hormone replacement. Subjects with moderate or severe TBI or those with clinical suggestion of hypopituitarism should be referred to a pituitary endocrinologist for evaluation.

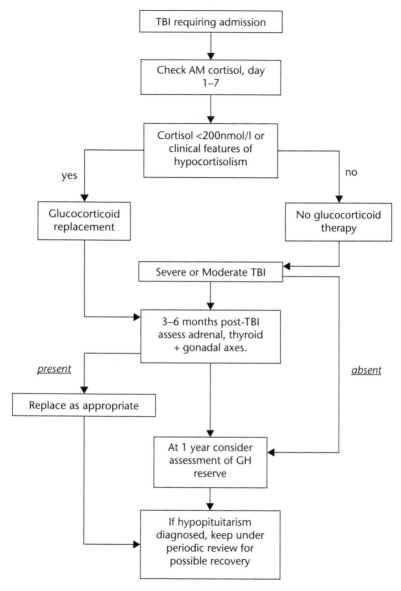

Figure 49.1 Algorithm for the endocrine assessment of patients following traumatic brain injury. GH, growth hormone; TBI, traumatic brain injury.

ADDITIONAL READING

Electronic Reference

Schneider HJ, Kreitschmann-Andermahr I, Ghigo E, et al. Hypothalamopituitary dysfunction following traumatic brain injury and aneurysmal subarachnoid hemorrhage: a systematic review. *http://jama.ama-assn.org/content/298/12/1429.full.pdf+html*

Textbook/Chapter

Sandel ME, Delmonico R, Kotch MJ. Sexuality, reprduction, and neuroendocrine disorders following TBI. In: Zasler ND, Katz D, Zafonte R, eds. *Brain Injury Medicine: Principles and Practice*. New York: Demos Medical Publishing; 2006:657–672.

Journal Articles

Ghigo E, Masel B, Aimaretti G, Leon-Carrion J, casanueva F, et al. Consensus guidelines on screening for hypopituitarism following traumatic brain injury. *Brain Injury*. 2005;19:711–724.

Kokshoorn NE, Wassenaar MJ, Biermasz NR, et al. Hypopituitarism following traumatic brain injury: prevalence is affected by the use of different dynamic tests and different normal values. *Eur J Endocrinol*. 2010;162:11–18.

REFERENCES

1. Behan LA, Phillips J, Thompson CJ, Agha A. Neuroendocrine disorders after traumatic brain injury. *J Neurol Neurosurg Psychiatr*. 2008;79(7):753–759.
2. Dusick JR, Wang C, Cohan P, Swerdloff R, Kelly DF. Chapter 1: pathophysiology of hypopituitarism in the setting of brain injury. *Pituitary*. 2008.
3. Tanriverdi F, Unluhizarci K, Kelestimur F. Pituitary function in subjects with mild traumatic brain injury: a review of literature and proposal of a screening strategy. *Pituitary*. 2010;13(2):146–153.
4. Agha A, Phillips J, O'Kelly P, Tormey W, Thompson CJ. The natural history of post-traumatic hypopituitarism: implications for assessment and treatment. *Am J Med*. 2005;118(12):1416.

Dysautonomia and Paroxysmal Autonomic Instability With Dystonia

Cherina Cyborski

BACKGROUND

- Dysautonomia and paroxysmal autonomic instability with dystonia (PAID) are terms used interchangeably for traumatic brain injury (TBI) patients with episodes of autonomic instability. PAID obligates dystonia as a part of the clinical picture, whereas dysautonomia can be applied more broadly. See Table 50.1 for proposed diagnostic criteria [1–3].
- Also known as sympathetic/autonomic storming, autonomic dysfunction syndrome, acute midbrain syndrome, hypothalamic-midbrain dysregulation syndrome, central fever, hyperpyrexia associated with muscle contraction, or acute hypothalamic instability

CLASSIFICATION

This varies among authors. Two proposed guidelines (Table 50.1):

- Baguley's diagnostic criteria for dysautonomia are simultaneous, paroxysmal episodes during which five of the seven listed parameters are met 2 or more weeks post injury [4].
- Blackman's diagnostic criteria for PAID apply only to patients Rancho Los Amigos level <IV who have one paroxysm per day for at least 3 days.
  - Blackman acknowledges that the syndrome is likely a continuum and these are restrictive criteria (only 1/3 of the patients in his database met full criteria) [3].
- Limitations of both: exclude patients who do not meet all of the criteria.
- Often episodes are triggered by a stimulus such as pain, endotracheal suction, constipation, urinary retention, and range of motion exercises.
- Cessation of episodes usually correlates with improving neurological status [5].

Table 50.1 Proposed Diagnostic Criteria

	Dysautonomia	**PAID**
Temperature (°C)	>39	>38.5
Blood pressure (systolic)	>160	>140
Heart rate (beats/minute)	>120	>130
Respiratory rate (breaths/minute)	>30	>20
Diaphoresis	+	+
Dystonia	+	+
Posturing	+	
Agitation		+

- Bottom line: no universal nomenclature or constellation of diagnostic features are recognized; however, the diagnosis should be considered in patients who demonstrate the aforementioned features

EPIDEMIOLOGY

Dysautonomia is more commonly seen in TBI patients who have diffuse axonal injury, cerebral hypoxemia, brainstem lesions, or bilateral diencephalic lesions, and those who are young [1].

INCIDENCE (IN MODERATE TO SEVERE TBI PATIENTS)

- Within the first 7 days post injury, elevated autonomic parameters in 92% (majority with hypertension and tachycardia) [6]
- 24% to 33% have dysautonomic features that are self-limiting and of short duration [6,7].
- 8% to 11.8% have prolonged and severe dysautonomia [6,8].
- Dysautonomia is seen in 5.3% of rehabilitation admissions [6].

PATHOPHYSIOLOGY

Pathophysiology is unknown. However, there are two theories:

- Paroxysms develop secondary to abnormal afferent stimulus processing [9].
- Disconnection between the cortex and hypothalamus/brainstem allows for paroxysms to be actively driven by diencephalic/brainstem impulses released from cortical control [3,10].

DIAGNOSIS

Clinical features—described in 3 phases:

- Phase 1—elevated autonomic parameters are indistinguishable between dysautonomic and non-dysautonomic patients. Retrospectively identified
- Phase 2—associated with cessation of sedation:
  - Initially—frequent, prolonged, and intense episodes of autonomic instability
  - Over time—Episodes become less pronounced and sweating pattern changes (whole body → upper trunk, head, neck) [11]
- Phase 3—marked by the cessation of sweating
  - Happens on average of 74 days post injury [1]
  - Continued dystonia/spasticity, but diaphoresis is resolved

Dysautonomia is a diagnosis of exclusion. Need to consider/rule out the following as appropriate: infection (most common cause of hyperthermia in TBI patients); seizures; acute hydrocephalus; increased intracranial pressure; neuroleptic malignant syndrome; serotonin syndrome; malignant hyperthermia; thyroid storm; venous thromboembolism; medication reaction; withdrawal from medications, illicit drugs, or alcohol; concomitant spinal cord injury → autonomic dysreflexia; and acute coronary syndrome.

TREATMENT

General Principles

Initiate treatment as early as possible because
- Core temperatures above 38°C to 39°C have produced neuronal death in animal models.
- An increased catabolic state may lead to loss of body weight.
- Dysautonomia is associated with an increased risk of developing critical illness polyneuropathy.
- Spasticity/dystonia can lead to contractures, pressure areas, and/or pain [12].

Environmental Management

- Decrease noxious stimuli: remove cervical collars as soon as possible, remove indwelling bladder catheters, prevent pressure areas, prevent constipation, use rubber tubes for suctioning.
- Minimize noise and activity around the patient.

Medication Management [10]

First-Line Agents [13]

Caution: all can be sedating, potentially impair cognition, and/or affect recovery/neuroplasticity.

1. β blockers

   - Propranolol: nonselective, β antagonist
   - Labetolol: nonselective, β and α1 antagonist
     - Both are lipophilic → cross blood brain barrier
     - Decrease circulating catecholamines, reduce cardiac work and catabolic drive
     - Decrease hypertension and hemodynamic abnormalities
     - Do not alter diaphoresis (mediated by sympathetic cholinergic neurons)

2. Gabapentin: exerts effect via voltage-dependent calcium channels [12]

   - Controls the autonomic symptoms and the dystonic posturing and may also be beneficial in treating neuropathic pain

3. Morphine: μ opioid receptor agonist

   - Decreases pain, which is a potential trigger for dysautonomic episodes [14]
   - Treats pulmonary edema and tachypnea, induces bradycardia [2]

Second-Line Agents

4. α2 agonist

   - Clonidine: acts centrally and peripherally
     - Modulates blood pressure and heart rate (through decreased plasma catecholamines) but not other aspects of dysautonomia
     - Considerations: causes sedation; studies in poststroke patients show that it impairs neuroplasticity [15]
   - Dexmedetomidine

5. Dopamine agonist

   - Bromocriptine: D2 agonist
     - One study demonstrated that bromocriptine improved hyperthermia and diaphoresis [5]; these results have not been replicated
   - Carbi/levodopa [13,14]

6. Direct-acting skeletal muscle relaxant

   - Dantrolene: inhibits calcium release in sarcoplasmic reticulum
     - Treats extensor posturing/spasticity with minimal effect on other symptoms

7. GABA-B agonist
   - Oral baclofen: no literature specifically studying use in dysautonomia
   - Intrathecal baclofen pump: in two case series, this approach appeared promising [16,17]—both spastic tone and dysautonomia improved
8. GABA-A agonists
   - Benzodiazepines: Anecdotal reports favor midazolam and diazepam [13]
     - Caution: negative impact on neuroplasticity; causes sedation and impairs cognitive processing [15]
9. A number of other agents have been tried (e.g., phenytoin, propofol, and prazosin), but there is insufficient evidence to recommend their use [13,14]

DURATION OF SYMPTOM PERSISTENCE (DESPITE MEDICATION USE)

- Study done in intensive care unit (ICU) setting showed 5.01 ± 1.57 dysautonomic episodes per day lasting 27.9 ± 11.3 minutes [18]
- Dysautonomia resolves over time: mean duration 2.5 to 5.9 months post injury [1,19]
- Preliminary evidence suggests that sympathetic overresponsiveness can be seen years after the injury in response to noxious stimuli [20]

PROGNOSIS

- TBI patients with dysautonomia have [6,13]:
  - Worse outcomes as measured by Glasgow Outcome Scale and Functional Independence Measure, characterized by (1) prolonged swallowing abnormalities; (2) prolonged posttraumatic amnesia; (3) longer hospital admissions, ICU stays, and mechanical ventilation [18]; and (4) greater overall healthcare costs.
- Show similar degrees of functional gain with active rehabilitation as non-dysautonomic patients [1]
- Patients with dysautonomia are at greater risk for developing heterotopic ossification [8].
- In patients in a vegetative state, those with dysautonomia have a greater likelihood (5×) of remaining in a vegetative state [19].

ADDITIONAL READING

Electronic Reference
http://emedicine.medscape.com/article/325994-overview

Textbook/Chapter

Mysiw WJ, Fugate LP, Clinchot DM. Assessment, early rehabilitation, intervention, and tertiary prevention. In: Zasler ND, Katz DI, Zafonte RD, eds. *Brain Injury Medicine: Principles and Practice.* New York: Demos Medical Publishing; 2007:290–291.

Journal Articles

Baguley IJ. Autonomic complications following central nervous system injury. *Semin Neurol.* 2008;28(5):716–725.

Baguley IJ, Cameron ID, Green AM, Slewa-Younan S, Marosszeky JE, Gurka JA. Pharmacological management of Dysautonomia following traumatic brain injury. *Brain Inj.* 2004;18(5):409–417.

Blackman JA. Paroxysmal autonomic instability with dystonia after brain injury—Erratum. *Arch Neurol.* 2004;61(6):980.

Blackman JA, Patrick PD, Buck ML, Rust RS Jr. Paroxysmal autonomic instability with dystonia after brain injury. *Arch Neurol.* 2004;61(3):321–328.

Crooks J, Gurka JA, Wade LD. Dysautonomia after traumatic brain injury: a forgotten syndrome? *J Neurol Neurosurg Psychiatry.* 1999;67(1):39–43.

REFERENCES

1. Baguley IJ, Nicholls JL, Felmingham KL, Crooks J, Gurka JA, Wade LD. Dysautonomia after traumatic brain injury: a forgotten syndrome? *J Neurol Neurosurg Psychiatr.* 1999;67(1):39–43.
2. Blackman JA, Patrick PD, Buck ML, Rust RS Jr. Paroxysmal autonomic instability with dystonia after brain injury. *Arch Neurol.* 2004;61(3):321–328.
3. Blackman JA. Paroxysmal autonomic instability with dystonia after brain injury—Erratum. *Arch Neurol.* 2004;61(6):980.
4. Baguley IJ, Nott MT, Slewa-Younan S, Heriseanu RE, Perkes IE. Diagnosing dysautonomia after acute traumatic brain injury: evidence for overresponsiveness to afferent stimuli. *Arch Phys Med Rehabil.* 2009;90(4):580–586.
5. Rossitch E Jr, Bullard DE. The autonomic dysfunction syndrome: aetiology and treatment. *Br J Neurosurg.* 1988;2(4):471–478.
6. Baguley IJ, Slewa-Younan S, Heriseanu RE, Nott MT, Mudaliar Y, Nayyar V. The incidence of dysautonomia and its relationship with autonomic arousal following traumatic brain injury. *Brain Inj.* 2007;21(11):1175–1181.
7. Rabinstein AA. Paroxysmal sympathetic hyperactivity in the neurological intensive care unit. *Neurol Res.* 2007;29(7):680–682.
8. Hendricks HT, Geurts AC, van Ginneken BC, Heeren AJ, Vos PE. Brain injury severity and autonomic dysregulation accurately predict heterotopic ossification in patients with traumatic brain injury. *Clin Rehabil.* 2007;21(6):545–553.
9. Baguley IJ. The excitatory:inhibitory ratio model (EIR model): An integrative explanation of acute autonomic overactivity syndromes. *Med Hypotheses.* 2008;70(1):26–35.
10. Baguley IJ, Heriseanu RE, Cameron ID, Nott MT, Slewa-Younan S. A critical review of the pathophysiology of dysautonomia following traumatic brain injury. *Neurocrit Care.* 2008;8(2):293–300.
11. Bullard DE. Diencephalic seizures: responsiveness to bromocriptine and morphine. *Ann Neurol.* 1987;21(6):609–611.

12. Baguley IJ, Heriseanu RE, Gurka JA, Nordenbo A, Cameron ID. Gabapentin in the management of dysautonomia following severe traumatic brain injury: a case series. *J Neurol Neurosurg Psychiatr.* 2007;78(5):539–541.

13. Baguley IJ. Autonomic complications following central nervous system injury. *Semin Neurol.* 2008;28(5):716–725.

14. Baguley IJ, Cameron ID, Green AM, Slewa-Younan S, Marosszeky JE, Gurka JA. Pharmacological management of Dysautonomia following traumatic brain injury. *Brain Inj.* 2004;18(5):409–417.

15. Goldstein LB. Neuropharmacology of TBI-induced plasticity. *Brain Inj.* 2003;17(8):685–694.

16. Cuny E, Richer E, Castel JP. Dysautonomia syndrome in the acute recovery phase after traumatic brain injury: relief with intrathecal Baclofen therapy. *Brain Inj.* 2001;15(10):917–925.

17. Becker R, Benes L, Sure U, Hellwig D, Bertalanffy H. Intrathecal baclofen alleviates autonomic dysfunction in severe brain injury. *J Clin Neurosci.* 2000;7(4):316–319.

18. Fernández-Ortega JF, Prieto-Palomino MA, Muñoz-López A, Lebron-Gallardo M, Cabrera-Ortiz H, Quesada-García G. Prognostic influence and computed tomography findings in dysautonomic crises after traumatic brain injury. *J Trauma.* 2006;61(5):1129–1133.

19. Dolce G, Quinteri M, Leto E, et al. Dysautonomia and clinical outcome in vegetative state. *J Neurotrauma.* 2008;25:1079–1082.

20. Baguley IJ, Heriseanu RE, Nott MT, Chapman J, Sandanam J. Dysautonomia after severe traumatic brain injury: evidence of persisting overresponsiveness to afferent stimuli. *Am J Phys Med Rehabil.* 2009;88(8):615–622.

51

Movement Disorders

Cherina Cyborski and Cindy Zadikoff

BACKGROUND

- Definition: A movement disorder is a condition that affects the ability to generate or control movement.
- Epidemiology: The few published studies on posttraumatic movement disorders (most of which are in the pediatric population) demonstrate a wide range of incidence—13% to 66% of severe traumatic brain injury (TBI) patients.
- Pathophysiology:
  - Generally characterized by delayed onset, up to years post injury, which may be due to sprouting, remyelination, ephaptic transmission, inflammatory changes, oxidative reactions, central synaptic reorganization, or neurotransmitter sensitivity [1]
- Risk factors:
  - Genetic predisposition may contribute to development of posttraumatic movement disorders [2].
- General principles of treatment:
  - Movement disorders cannot be treated in isolation because other sequelae of TBI (e.g., balance, cognitive deficits) may be exacerbated by usual movement disorder treatments [3].
  - Importantly, some movement disorders, such as hemiballism, will typically resolve spontaneously, so it is important to withdraw medications after several months to determine whether medications are still necessary.

HYPERKINETIC MOVEMENT DISORDERS

Tremor

Rhythmic, oscillatory movement due to co-contraction of agonist/antagonist muscles [4]

- Epidemiology: 10% to 20% of posttraumatic movement disorders [5]
- Subtypes

- Resting—present when body part is inactive
- Postural—present when maintaining body part in an antigravity position
- Kinetic—present when moving from one position to another
- Intention—only present when nearing goal of movement ("end-point tremor")

- Risk factor: prolonged coma
- Timing: often appears in first weeks after injury when voluntary movement begins to recover, but can develop years after injury [3]
- Exam findings: usually bilateral [6], affects the upper > lower extremities, and commonly associated with ataxia of the affected limb [2]. Evaluate the limb in different postures; characterize frequency and amplitude of tremor
- Differential diagnosis: seizure; rigors; tremor due to hyperthyroidism, hepatic failure, hypercapnia, or medication side effect (e.g., metoclopramide, amiodarone, lithium, typical and atypical neuroleptics or antipsychotics)
- Treatment:
  - Medications—No studies have been done to show efficacy; anecdotal literature suggests little benefit with medication use [3]. Primidone, β-blockers (e.g., propanolol), benzodiazepines (e.g., clonazepam), antiepileptics (e.g., leviteracetam, gabapentin), anticholinergics, L-dopa/carbidopa, isoniazid, and botulinum toxin injections have been used.
  - Physical modality—Light weights on affected limb to dampen tremor
  - Surgery—Consider 1 year after onset of tremor:
    - Deep brain stimulation: Posttraumatic tremors respond less predictably/less effectively than in essential tremor or Parkinson's tremor [7]; no consensus as to the best anatomical location for stimulation
    - Stereotactic surgery (e.g., radiofrequency lesioning or γ-knife thalamotomy): radio frequency lesioning in ventrolateral thalamus in one study showed improvement in 88% [6] with a decrease in both kinetic/postural and rest tremor; postoperative increase in dysarthria and/or gait disturbance in up to 90% immediately and 63% persistently
- Prognosis: In a small minority, tremor may lessen spontaneously within 1 year after onset [4]. For the majority, however, refractory tremor remains a persistent problem [2].

Dystonia

Involuntary, sustained patterned muscle contraction of opposing muscles resulting in repetitive twisting movements or abnormal postures; can be present with spasticity and rigidity and is usually *exacerbated or elicited by* voluntary activity.

- Epidemiology: 4.8% to 16% of posttraumatic movement disorders, probably underreported [5]
  - More common in men
- Subtypes: focal, segmental, generalized, hemidystonia [8]
- Risk factors: younger age at time of trauma (first 2 decades of life) [9] and severe TBI. Frequently preceded by, or associated with, ipsilateral hemiparesis [2]
- Timing: onset likely to be delayed (1 month to 9 years), mean latency = 20 months [8]. Initially slow progression with spread over months to years followed by eventual stabilization
- Exam findings: may be present at rest but usually exacerbated with voluntary movement. Characterized by maintaining the affected body part in an involuntary sustained contraction
- Differential diagnosis [3]: Evaluate for muscular, joint, or bone injuries causing abnormal posturing and evaluate for ocular or vestibular abnormalities that lead to head or trunk tilt. Rule out toxic or metabolic conditions (e.g., Wilson's disease) if uncertain etiologic link to TBI.
- Treatment:
  - Medications [3]: variably effective
    - Anticholinergics (e.g., trihexyphenidyl)—better tolerated in pediatric population
    - Tetrabenazine—major side effects include sedation, parkinsonism, and depression
    - Neuroleptics—often effective but may interfere with brain plasticity/recovery in TBI patients and carry long-term risk of tardive dyskinesias (should be avoided in TBI)
    - Antiepileptics (gabapentin, carbamazepine)—not usually effective but often tried
    - Benzodiazepine—may be useful as adjuvant, ineffective as sole agent; sedation often is rate limiting step; may interfere with neural plasticity/recovery in TBI
    - Botulinum toxin injections—for focal (not generalized) dystonia: has the advantage of fewer systemic side effects
    - Oral baclofen—sedation often a limiting factor
  - Physical modality: range of motion to prevent contractures
  - Surgery
    - Intrathecal baclofen pump—recommended for generalized dystonia associated with significant spasticity, not usually beneficial for isolated dystonia. Response to oral baclofen does not necessarily predict response to intrathecal baclofen
    - Functional stereotactic surgery—less effective for secondary dystonia (e.g., due to TBI) than for primary

- Deep brain stimulation—for generalized, focal segmental, and hemidystonia. Long-term follow-up is limited
- Thalamic radiofrequency lesioning (pallidotomy)—improvements may take up to months postoperatively
- Prognosis: spontaneous remission is unlikely

Myoclonus

Myoclonus is a sudden, brief, shock-like arrhythmic involuntary movement resulting from paroxysmal aberrant depolarization of individual or small groups of cortical motor neurons. Any disease process that causes cortical irritability can produce myoclonus; once the cortical irritability resolves, over weeks to months, myoclonus can also subside [3]

- Epidemiology: 0.5% of posttraumatic movement disorders [5]
- Subtypes [3]: focal, multifocal, subcortical, generalized
- Exam findings: Myoclonus is often stimulus induced (e.g., provoked by sudden loud noise). Look for segmental versus generalized presentation
- Differential diagnosis [3]: metabolic causes such as renal or hepatic failure or electrolyte shifts during hemodialysis; medications and toxins such as lithium, bismuth, propofol, antiepileptic mediations, serotonergic medications (including trazodone, buspirone, selective serotonin reuptake inhibitor [SSRIs]). Consider obtaining a brain magnetic resonance imaging and/or performing lumbar puncture to asses for new central nervous system (CNS) lesion/infection; consider obtaining an electroencephalogram to rule out myoclonic seizures.
- Treatment: medications (no evidence in literature): valproic acid, clonazepam, leviteracetam, tryptophan

Tics

Tics are semivoluntary repetitive simple or complex movements or vocalizations with associated premonitory urge to make movement or sound as well as relief associated with making movement/sound.

- Epidemiology: 0.9% of posttraumatic movement disorders [5]. Of six reported cases, all were male, mean age of 28 years, mild to moderate TBI in five, preceded by pain in the affected body part [10].
- Differential diagnosis: Rule out idiopathic tic disorder such as Tourette's syndrome.
- Treatment: Low-dose dopamine agonists, SSRIs, clonidine, neuroleptics (e.g., pimozide), CNS sedating agents, and dopa agonists should be avoided in TBI patients.

Other Hyperkinetic Movement Disorders

- Athetosis: slower phasic writhing of proximal extremities, "snake-like"
- Chorea: rapid unpredictable flowing, dance-like movements, predominantly in distal limbs, rarely can be associated with epidural or subdural hematomas
- Ballism: continuous, non-patterned purposeless movement; mostly involves proximal limbs. Can be forceful and of high amplitude and may be delayed in onset by weeks to months

Treatment

Treatment is as in dystonia except for the following:

- Chorea: consider amantadine. Deep brain stimulation and botulinum toxin injections are not recommended.
- Hemiballism: responsive to intrathecal baclofen in a single case report [11]

HYPOKINETIC MOVEMENT DISORDERS

Parkinsonism

This is characterized by bradykinesia, rigidity, resting tremor, and postural instability. It may occur in TBI due to injury to the substantia nigra. Lewy bodies, found in idiopathic Parkinson's disease, are not found in posttraumatic parkinsonism.

- Epidemiology: 0.9% of posttraumatic movement disorders [5]
- Risk factors: Studies have found that those with Parkinson's disease have a higher frequency of remote TBI; however, head trauma may result from, but not be a cause of, parkinsonism [1].
- Timing: Onset is typically within months after injury. TBI can also exacerbate parkinsonism transiently in those with Parkinson's disease without increasing/accelerating disability [2].
- Treatment:
  - Medications—similar to that for idiopathic Parkinson's disease, with dopaminergic medications including carbidopa-levodopa and dopamine agonists being the mainstay; however, less predictable response for posttraumatic parkinsonism than in idiopathic Parkinson's disease

Repeated Head Trauma

- That is, pugilistic parkinsonism or punch drunk syndrome: see Chapter 13

OTHER MOVEMENT DISORDERS

- Stereotypy: involuntary, patterned movement (e.g., self-caressing); 0.9% of posttraumatic movement disorders [5]
- Hyperekplexia: exaggerated startle response; 0.5% of posttraumatic movement disorders [5]
- Akathisia: inner sense of restlessness; 0.9% of posttraumatic movement disorder
    - Very difficult to treat. May respond to amantadine or propranolol

ADDITIONAL READING

Electronic Reference
http://www.northeastcenter.com/Podcast032.mp3

Textbook/Chapter
Krauss J, Jankovic J. Movement disorders after TBI. In: Zasler ND, Katz DI, Zafonte RD, eds. *Brain Injury Medicine: Principles and Practice*. New York: Demos Medical Publishing; 2007: 469–489.

Journal Articles
Krauss JK, Jankovic J. Head injury and posttraumatic movement disorders. *Neurosurgery*. 2002;50(5):927–939; discussion 939–940.

Krauss JK, Trankle R, Kopp KH. Posttraumatic movement disorders after moderate or mild head injury. *Mov Disord*. 1997;12(3):428–431.

Krauss JK, Trankle R, Kopp KH. Post-traumatic movement disorders in survivors of severe head injury. *Neurology*. 1996;47(6):1488–1492.

REFERENCES

1. Jankovic J. Post-traumatic movement disorders: central and peripheral mechanisms. *Neurology*. 1994;44(11):2006–2014.
2. Krauss JK, Jankovic J. Head injury and posttraumatic movement disorders. *Neurosurgery*. 2002;50(5):927–939; discussion 939.
3. O'Suilleabhain P, Dewey RB Jr. Movement disorders after head injury: diagnosis and management. *J Head Trauma Rehabil*. 2004;19(4):305–313.
4. Krauss J, Jankovic J. Movement disorders after TBI. In: Zasler ND, Katz DI, Zafonte RD, eds. *Brain Injury Medicine: Principles and Practice*. New York: Demos Medical Publishing; 2007: 469–489.
5. Krauss JK, Tränkle R, Kopp KH. Post-traumatic movement disorders in survivors of severe head injury. *Neurology*. 1996;47(6):1488–1492.
6. Krauss JK, Mohadjer M, Nobbe F, Mundinger F. The treatment of posttraumatic tremor by stereotactic surgery. Symptomatic and functional outcome in a series of 35 patients. *J Neurosurg*. 1994;80(5):810.
7. Deuschl G, Bain P. Deep brain stimulation for tremor [correction of trauma]: patient selection and evaluation. *Mov Disord*. 2002;17(suppl 3):S102–S111.

8. Krauss JK, Mohadjer M, Braus DF, Wakhloo AK, Nobbe F, Mundinger F. Dystonia following head trauma: a report of nine patients and review of the literature. *Mov Disord.* 1992;7(3):263–272.

9. Lee MS, Rinne JO, Ceballos-Baumann A, Thompson PD, Marsden CD. Dystonia after head trauma. *Neurology.* 1994;44(8):1374–1378.

10. Krauss JK, Jankovic J. Tics secondary to craniocerebral trauma. *Mov Disord.* 1997;12(5):776–782.

11. Francisco GE. Successful treatment of posttraumatic hemiballismus with intrathecal baclofen therapy. *Am J Phys Med Rehabil.* 2006;85(9):779–782.

52

Spasticity in Traumatic Brain Injury

Bamidele Adeyemo, John Lowry, and Ross Zafonte

BACKGROUND

Definition

Spasticity is a neuromuscular phenomenon manifested in patients with upper motor neuron syndrome, characterized by a velocity-dependent muscular resistance to passive joint range of motion (ROM) [1,2].

Pathophysiology

Spasticity refers to increased muscular tone that results from the disruption of exigent descending inhibitory modulation of α motor neurons. It results from aberrant neuronal pathway input from γ afferent motor neurons, reticulospinal and vestibulospinal input combined with exacerbations from irritant noxious stimuli [3]. Common precipitants of exacerbations in spastic tone include urinary tract infection, decubitus ulcers, fractures, ingrown toe nails, heterotopic ossification, catheter kinking and dislodgement, restrictive clothing, stool impaction, nephrolithiasis, or sources of physiologic or emotional stress [2,4].

ASSESSMENT

Clinical Manifestations

The sequelae of spasticity are grossly classified into beneficial and deleterious effects. The beneficial aspects of spasticity are the inadvertent functional and medical advantages conferred by the presence of increased tone: (1) facilitation of ambulation, standing, and transfers; (2) maintenance of muscle bulk; (3) promotion of venous return; (4) diminishment of deep venous thrombosis risk; (5) diminution of orthostatic hypotension; (6) prevention of osteoporosis; and (7) decrement of pressure ulcer formation. Conversely, the deleterious sequelae of spasticity include (1) pain, (2) immobility, (3) contractures, (4) increased energy expenditure, (5) muscle spasm, (6) fracture, (7) increased risk of heterotopic ossification, (8) joint subluxation or dislocation, (9) insomnia, and (10) interference in nursing care and hygiene [1–5].

Physical Examination

Spasticity is elicited by performing a passive motion maneuver across a joint on the affected limb: this motion induces an involuntary velocity-dependent activation of the stretch response. Occasionally, one may also see other corroborating signs such as the Westphal phenomenon, which is a passively activated stretched muscle response while in its shortened state. Passive stretch may also trigger "spasms" (or involuntary contractions) of agonist-antagonist groups, neighboring limb, girdle, and/or trunk muscles [5].

Assessment Scales

One of the first clinical scales employed to evaluate spasticity is the 1964 Ashworth Scale, modified by Bohannon and Smith in 1967 [5]. The Modified Ashworth Scale (MAS) is characterized as follows:

- 0: No increase in muscle tone with ROM
- 1: Slight increase in tone with or without a catch and release at the end of ROM
- 1+: Slight increase in muscle tone followed by slight resistance in the remainder of ROM
- 2: More marked increase in muscle tone through most of ROM
- 3: Considerable increase in tone, passive movement
- 4: Affected parts rigid in flexion or extension

The MAS is frequently criticized for its limited precision in detecting subtle effects of antispasmodic medications. A more practical validated assessment technique is to quantify the specific condition being treated, for example, pain, function, ambulation distance, gait analysis, or performance tests of the involved extremity [5].

Considerations

Indications for treatment of spasticity can be delineated via three categories [4]:

1. Patient-focused: The most discernable patient treatment marker is pain. Painful spasticity may impact adequate sleep, tranquility, and quality of life.

2. Medical and nursing management: Adequate spasticity control is essential in provision of nursing care, hygiene, pressure ulcer management, and seating positioning.
3. Function: Spasticity control can often improve gait, transfers, and self-care activities.

TREATMENT

Goal

Spasticity abolishment is often undesirable, as spasticity occasionally facilitates function. Therefore, the goal of treatment should be directed at the minimization of spasticity only as it relates to functional or symptomatic impairment. One should begin treatment by removing noxious stimuli, followed by minimally invasive interventions.

Nonpharmacologic Management

Positioning
The first step in managing spasticity is the maintenance of proper positioning. This may be implemented by piloting each limb through its full ROM multiple times a day. The maintenance of position may be further augmented with casting and splinting [5].

Physiotherapy and Modalities
Physiotherapy techniques (such as the Bobath and Brunnstrom programs) and modalities (such as cryotherapy) have been documented to be effective in spasticity management. In particular, a 15 to 20 minute application of cryotherapy to spastic muscles has been shown to enact a 35-degree improvement in ROM. Other modalities that may be employed for spasticity management include local heat, ultrasound, transcutaneous electrical nerve stimulation, electromyographic biofeedback, vibration, and feedback of tonic stretch reflex. Any modality should be used with caution, as traumatic brain injury (TBI) patients may have insensate dermatomes and/or impaired communication, which may limit the patient's ability to detect/communicate adverse effects of treatment [4,5].

Pharmacologic Management

Oral medications are frequently employed in the management of spasticity. Consideration of side effect profiles is the largest determinant of selection of an antispasmodic agent. Initiate any new medication slowly, followed by gentle dose escalation. Though often prescribed, the evidence for the efficacy of oral antispasmodics has not been well substantiated [3,5]. A description of commonly used antispasmodics follows:

Baclofen

This is the most frequently utilized oral antispasmodic agent [3]. It is an inhibitory GABA-B receptor agonist which presynaptically inhibits the release of excitatory neurotransmitters.

- Dosing: Start 5 mg two to three times a day and increase dose by 5 mg every 3 to 5 days. Max dose: 80 mg/day
- Side effects: hallucinations, convulsions, rigidity, lowered seizure threshold, and severe withdrawal syndrome (aka baclofen withdrawal syndrome) [3,5].
- Considerations: in widespread use despite paucity of evidence of efficacy [5].

Tizanidine

α2 adrenergic receptor agonist that targets supraspinal and spinal receptors [3,6].

- Dosing: Start 2 to 4 mg/day and increase to 8 mg three times a day; max dose: 36 mg/day
- Side effects: mirrors baclofen in most of its side effects, with sedation and asthenia being its most common dose-limiting adverse effect [3]. Note, however, that weakness is less frequently reported in comparison to baclofen and diazepam [6].
- Considerations: Studies have failed to demonstrate functional improvement [6].

Diazepam

This is the first antispasmodic agent described for the management of spasticity. It stimulates GABA-A neurotransmission resulting in presynaptic inhibition of stretch reflexes [6].

- Dosing: Start 2 mg twice a day; max dose: 60 mg/day; duration: long half-life at approximately 30 hours
- Side effects: cognitive diminution, sedation, drowsiness, memory and attention impairment, tolerance, dependence, weakness, and motor incoordination [6]
- Considerations: exacerbation of cognitive impairment and potential impediment of neurorecovery limit the recommendation of diazepam for the TBI population

Dantrolene

This is unique as an antispasmodic agent because it is peripherally acting. It inhibits calcium ion release from the muscular sarcoplasmic reticulum [3]. While this circumvents cognitive adverse effects of antispasmodics, dantrolene will nonspecifically weaken affected and nonaffected muscles alike.

- Dosing: Start 25 mg/day; max dose 400 mg/day; monitor liver function
- Side effects: gastrointestinal intolerance, sedation, and hepatotoxicity [3,6]
- Efficacy has been proven in placebo studies, but data supporting functional improvement is lacking [6].

Other less commonly used antispasmodic agents (e.g., clonazepam, ketazolam, tetrazepam, progabide, gabapentin, piracetam, clonidine, etc.) [2,3,6] are beyond the scope of this chapter. Please see the noted references for a more detailed discussion of these agents.

Interventional Approaches

Botulinum Toxin Injection

Botulinum toxin injection (BTI) is a common technique FDA-approved for the management of upper limb spasticity after stroke. Botulinum toxin is produced by *Clostridium botulinum* bacterium and acts at the neuromuscular junction to inhibit acetylcholine release [2,4,5,7]. Of the seven antigenically distinct serotypes of botulinum toxin, only serotypes A and B are available for commercial use [4]. Both serotypes have demonstrated efficacy for spasticity [7,8]. Serotype A is used more frequently, while serotype B is typically used for spasticity cases recalcitrant to serotype A [8]. An advantage of BTI in comparison with oral medications is its circumvention of systemic effects. Application requires identification of the muscle of interest followed by injection of the toxin solution. The onset of action is 1 to 3 days with a maximum effect in a few weeks and a duration of effect of 1 to 6 months [2,4]. The duration or magnitude of effect may decay with repeated applications due to antibody-mediated resistance [4,5].

The benefits of BTI effect may be enhanced by physiotherapy, splinting, or electrical stimulation [5]. Adverse effects include localized reaction, bleeding, infection, nerve trauma, and cervical dysphagia (rarely associated with cervical injection) [2,4]. Additional considerations include cost, transient nature of effect/necessity for repeated injections, and the paucity of evidence for functional efficacy [2–5]. Given its relative safety, and lack of systemic effects, botulinum offers "one of the most useful advances in the management of spasticity in recent years" [5].

Nerve Block

Nerve blocks ablate the culminant neurological input responsible for the spastic activity [4]. Temporary blocks may be effectuated using bupivocaine or lidocaine, while sustained blocks may be implemented using lytic agents such as phenol or ethanol [2,4,5]. Nerves are identified pre-procedurally using a variable intensity stimulator [4,5]. The duration of effect is between 3 and 9 months [4]. Adverse effects include weakness, sensitivity, injection site pain, phlebitis, central nervous system or cardiovascular compromise (rarely), phenol nerve fibrosis (which potentially adulterates anatomy for repeat injections), and (most distressing) dyesthesias [2,4]. Dyesthesias may also exacerbate spasticity; therefore, one should decrease this risk by limiting blockade to motor-only nerve branches [5].

Intrathecal Baclofen Pump
Intrathecal baclofen delivery can be an effective technique for managing spasticity recalcitrant to an oral regimen, or when adverse effects make use of oral agents untenable. A 50 µg test dose is typically administered via lumbar puncture or temporary catheter [4]. If efficacious, a subcutaneous medication pump is subsequently implanted [4]. Risks of use include infection, pump failure, nausea, sedation, hypotension, weakness, respiratory depression, and development of tolerance [2–5]. Catheter breakage or kinking can precipitate abrupt baclofen withdrawal syndrome, which can be life threatening. In select cases, intrathecal morphine and clonidine may be used as alternate agents [5].

Surgical Treatment

Permanent orthopedic and neurosurgical procedures are usually the last resort in tone management [4]. They include neurotomy, rhizotomy, dorsal root entry zone–otomy (DREZ-otomy), cordotomy, neurectomy, split tibialis transfer (SPLATT) procedure, tendon lengthening, and muscle tenotomies and transposition [2,4,5].

ADDITIONAL READING

Electronic Reference
http://www.biausa.org/LiteratureRetrieve.aspx?ID=48457&A=SearchResult&Se archID=1898471&ObjectID=48457&ObjectType=6

Textbook/Chapter
Barnes MP. Spasticity. In: Greenwood RJ, McMillan TM, Barnes MP, Ward CD, eds. *Handbook of Neurological Rehabilitation*. London: Psychology Press; 2003:157–169.

Journal Articles
Abbruzzese G. The medical management of spasticity. *Eur J Neurol*. 2002;9(suppl 1):30–34

Yablon SA. Botulinum neurotoxin intramuscular chemodenervation. Role in the management of spastic hypertonia and related motor disorders. *Phys Med Rehabil Clin N Am*. 2001;12(4):833–874.

REFERENCES

1. Barnes MP. An overview of the clinical management of spasticity. In: Barnes MP, Johnson GR, eds. *Upper Motor Neurone Syndrome and Spasticity— Clinical Management and Neurophysiology.* Cambridge: Cambridge University Press; 2001:1–11.

2. Elovic E, Baerga E, Cuccurullo S, et al. Associated topics in physical medicine and rehabilitation. In: Cuccurullo SJ, ed. *Physical Medicine and Rehabilitation Board Review.* New York: Demos Medical Publishing; 2004:641–700.

3. Abrams GM, Wakasa M. Chronic complications of spinal cord injury. In: Basow DS, ed. *UpToDate.* Waltham, MA: 2010.

4. Kaplan M. Upper motor neuron syndrome and spasticity. In: Nesathurai S, ed. *The Rehabilitation of People With Spinal Cord Injury.* Whitinsville, MA: AAP; 2003:75–80.

5. Bohannon RW, Smith MB. Inter-rater reliability of a modified Ashworth Scale of muscle spasticity. *Phys Ther.* 1987;67:206–207.

6. Abbruzzese G. The medical management of spasticity. *Eur J Neurol.* 2002;9(suppl 1):30–34; discussion 53.

7. Yablon SA. Botulinum neurotoxin intramuscular chemodenervation. Role in the management of spastic hypertonia and related motor disorders. *Phys Med Rehabil Clin N Am.* 2001;12(4):833–874, vii.

8. Francisco GE. Botulinum toxin for post-stroke spastic hypertonia: a review of its efficacy and application in clinical practice. *Ann Acad Med Singap.* 2007;36(1):22–30.

53

Mood Disorders

Ricardo E. Jorge

GENERAL PRINCIPLES

Background

Mood disorders occur in the context of profound changes in cognitive and emotional processing following traumatic brain injury (TBI). Recent studies have described the detrimental effect of traumatic prefrontal injury on patients' performance in social cognition as well as in the identification and modulation of emotions [1]. These changes may result in poorly integrated self-representations and dysfunctional interpersonal relationships, increasing patients' vulnerability to develop affective disorders.

Epidemiology

Neuropsychiatric illness is a highly prevalent complication of TBI, with a published incidence of 49% following moderate to severe TBI and 34% following mild TBI [2]. Approximately half of TBI patients will develop some sort of mood disorder during the first year after a TBI [3–5].

Classification

Following the Diagnostic and Statistical Manual of Mental Disorders (DSM-IV) diagnostic nomenclature, mood disorders associated with TBI are categorized as *mood disorder due to TBI* with subtypes of (1) *with major depressive-like episode* (if the full criteria for a major depressive episode are met), (2) *with depressive features* (prominent depressed mood but full criteria for a major depressive episode are not met); or (3) *with manic or with mixed features*.

Pathophysiology

The changes in neuronal circuitry seen in TBI may constitute the neurological substrate of cognitive and behavioral deficits that are frequently seen following injury. Mood disorders may result from deactivation of lateral and dorsal frontal cortex and increased activation in ventral limbic and paralimbic structures including the prelimbic cortex and the amygdala [6,7]. High levels of amygdala activation may be associated with an increased prevalence of anxiety symptoms and negative affect. Moreover, faulty prefrontal modulation of medial limbic structures could explain the impulsive and aggressive behavior frequently observed in these patients [8].

ASSESSMENT

Risk Factors

- Genetic polymorphisms modulating central dopaminergic pathways can affect prefrontal function following TBI. However, a recent study failed to demonstrate an association between 5-HTT polymorphisms and depression following TBI [9].
- Personal history of mood and anxiety disorders, and previous poor social functioning are associated with the occurrence of major depression in the aftermath of TBI [3,10].
- A history of alcohol misuse increases the risk of developing a mood disorder during the first year post TBI. It is plausible that alcohol toxicity and TBI interact to produce more severe structural brain damage and more profound changes in the ascending aminergic pathways that modulate reward, mood, and executive function [11].

Clinical Presentation and Symptoms

Mood disorders due to TBI are frequently associated with other behavioral disorders. For instance, anxiety disorders coexist with mood disturbance in up to two-thirds of the cases. In addition, clinically significant aggression and alcohol misuse coexist in approximately half of the patients who develop a mood disorder following TBI [11,12].

Differential Diagnosis

- The differential diagnosis of *post-TBI major depression* includes adjustment disorder with depressed and/or anxious mood, apathy, and emotional lability or pathological laughter and crying (PLC).
  - Patients with adjustment disorders develop short-lived and relatively mild emotional disturbances within 3 months of a stressful life event. Although they may present with depressive symptoms, they do not meet DSM-IV criteria for major depression.

- PLC is characterized by the presence of sudden and uncontrollable affective outbursts (e.g., crying or laughing), which may be congruent or incongruent with the patient's mood. These emotional displays are recognized by the patient as being excessive to the underlying mood and can occur spontaneously or may be triggered by minor stimuli. This condition lacks the pervasive alteration of mood, as well as the specific vegetative symptoms associated with a major depressive episode.

- Apathetic syndromes—A recent study of TBI patients referred to a neuropsychiatric clinic because of behavioral disturbance showed that 71% were apathetic. 85% of these apathetic patients were also depressed [13]. Apathy is frequently associated with psychomotor retardation and emotional blunting.

- A diagnosis of *mood disorder with manic or mixed features* should not be made if the mood disturbance occurs only during the course of agitation or delirium. The latter is characterized by sudden onset, fluctuating level of consciousness, disorientation, and prominent attention deficits. The differential diagnosis includes the following:

  - *Substance-induced mood disorder*—This may occur as a result of intoxication or withdrawal from drugs. It is usually identified by a careful clinical interview and/or toxicological screening.

  - *Psychosis associated with epilepsy*—This may be observed in patients with epileptic foci located in limbic or paralimbic cortices. Psychotic episodes may be temporally linked to seizures or may have a more prolonged interictal course. In the latter case, the clinical picture is characterized by the presence of partial and/or complex-partial seizures, and of a schizoaffective syndrome. EEG and functional neuroimaging studies (e.g., SPECT and PET) will usually define ictal and interictal disturbances.

  - *Personality change due to TBI*—This may include mood instability, disinhibited behavior, and hypersexuality. These patients lack, however, the pervasive alteration of mood that characterizes secondary manic syndromes.

TREATMENT

Guiding Principles

Patients with brain injury are more sensitive to the side effects of medications, especially psychotropic drugs. Doses of psychotropic drugs must be prudently increased, minimizing side effects (i.e., start low, go slow). However, the patient must receive an adequate therapeutic trial with regard to dosage and duration of treatment. Brain-injured patients must be frequently reassessed to determine changes in treatment schedules. Special care must be taken in monitoring drug interactions. Finally, if there is evidence of a partial response to a specific medication, augmentation therapy may be warranted, depending upon the augmenting drug's mechanism of action and potential side effects [15].

Treatment of mood disorders occurring after TBI involves different pharmacological and nonpharmacological strategies. Unfortunately, there is a lack of evidence-based scientific foundation to provide a solid basis for neuropsychiatric treatment. Selection among competing antidepressants is usually guided by their side effect profiles. Mild anticholinergic activity, minimal lowering of seizure threshold, and low sedative effects are the most important factors to be considered in the choice of an antidepressant drug in this population.

Specific Recommendations for Treating Depression

- Tricyclic antidepressants (TCAs) such as desipramine may be effective for treating depression in patients with severe TBI [16]. TCAs with significant anticholinergic effects (e.g., amitriptyline) should be avoided, however.
- Selective serotonin reuptake inhibitors:
  - Sertraline—A small study in patients with mild TBI showed statistically significant improvement in psychological distress, anger, and aggression as well as in the severity of postconcussive symptoms [17]. Sertraline may also lead to a beneficial effect on cognitive functioning [18].
  - Citalopram—A recent study suggested that citalopram may be effective in treating major depression occurring in the setting of TBI [19].

Specific Recommendations for Treating Manic Syndromes

There have been no systematic studies of the treatment of manic syndromes.

Lithium, carbamazepine, and valproate therapies have been reported to be efficacious in individual cases [15]. It has been proposed that both lithium and valproate have neuroprotective effects, which would certainly constitute an important therapeutic effect among brain-injured populations [20]. However, data from the only controlled trial of valproate in TBI fail to identify a beneficial effect on cognitive and functional outcomes [21]. The role of other anticonvulsants such as lamotrigine or topiramate as mood stabilizers has not been tested in TBI populations. A recent case report, however, reported adequate control of problematic behaviors with lamotrigine treatment [22]. In addition, there have been recent brief reports that suggest a beneficial effect of quetiapine on aggression and mania following TBI [23,24].

ADDITIONAL READING

Electronic References

http://www.biausa.org/LiteratureRetrieve.aspx?ID=43189&A=SearchRe
sult&SearchID=1898488&ObjectID=43189&ObjectType=6

Textbooks/Chapters

Sadock BJ, Sadock VA, Ruiz P, eds. *Kaplan and Sadock's Comprehensive Textbook of Psychiatry.* 9th ed. Philadelphia, PA: Wolters Kluwer Health/Lippincott Williams and Wilkins; 2009.

Silver JM, McAllister TW, Yudofsky SC. *Textbook of Traumatic Brain Injury.* 1st ed. Washington, DC: American Psychiatric Pub; 2005:xix, 771.

Journal Articles

Achte KA, Hillbom E, Aalberg V. Psychoses following war brain injuries. *Acta Psychiatr Scand.* 1969;45(1):1–18.

Lishman WA. Psychiatric disability after head injury: the significance of brain damage. *Proc R Soc Med.* 1966;59(3):261–266.

MacLean PD. The triune brain in conflict. *Psychother Psychosom.* 1977;28(1–4):207–220.

REFERENCES

1. Adolphs R. Cognitive neuroscience of human social behaviour. *Nat Rev Neurosci.* 2003;4(3):165–178.
2. Fann JR, Burington B, Leonetti A, Jaffe K, Katon WJ, Thompson RS. Psychiatric illness following traumatic brain injury in an adult health maintenance organization population. *Arch Gen Psychiatry.* 2004;61(1):53–61.
3. Bombardier CH, Fann JR, Temkin NR, Esselman PC, Barber J, Dikmen SS. Rates of major depressive disorder and clinical outcomes following traumatic brain injury. *JAMA.* 2010;303(19):1938–1945.
4. Hibbard MR, Uysal S, Kepler K, Bogdany J, Silver J. Axis I psychopathology in individuals with traumatic brain injury. *J Head Trauma Rehabil.* 1998;13(4):24–39.
5. Seel RT, Kreutzer JS, Rosenthal M, Hammond FM, Corrigan JD, Black K. Depression after traumatic brain injury: a National Institute on Disability and Rehabilitation Research Model Systems multicenter investigation. *Arch Phys Med Rehabil.* 2003;84(2):177–184.
6. Drevets WC. Neuroimaging studies of mood disorders. *Biol Psychiatry.* 2000;48(8):813–829.
7. Mayberg HS. Defining the neural circuitry of depression: toward a new nosology with therapeutic implications. *Biol Psychiatry.* 2007;61(6):729–730.
8. Jorge RE, Robinson RG, Moser D, Tateno A, Crespo-Facorro B, Arndt S. Major depression following traumatic brain injury. *Arch Gen Psychiatry.* 2004;61(1):42–50.

9. Chan F, Lanctôt KL, Feinstein A, et al. The serotonin transporter polymorphisms and major depression following traumatic brain injury. *Brain Inj.* 2008;22(6):471–479.

10. Jorge RE, Robinson RG, Arndt SV, Starkstein SE, Forrester AW, Geisler F. Depression following traumatic brain injury: a 1 year longitudinal study. *J Affect Disord.* 1993;27(4):233–243.

11. Jorge RE, Starkstein SE, Arndt S, Moser D, Crespo-Facorro B, Robinson RG. Alcohol misuse and mood disorders following traumatic brain injury. *Arch Gen Psychiatry.* 2005;62(7):742–749.

12. Tateno A, Jorge RE, Robinson RG. Clinical correlates of aggressive behavior after traumatic brain injury. *J Neuropsychiatry Clin Neurosci.* 2003;15(2):155–160.

13. Kant R, Duffy JD, Pivovarnik A. Prevalence of apathy following head injury. *Brain Inj.* 1998;12(1):87–92.

14. Bigler ED. Neurobiology and neuropathology underlie the neuropsychological deficits associated with traumatic brain injury. *Arch Clin Neuropsychol.* 2003;18(6):595–621; discussion 623.

15. Warden DL, Gordon B, McAllister TW, et al. Guidelines for the pharmacologic treatment of neurobehavioral sequelae of traumatic brain injury. *J Neurotrauma.* 2006;23(10):1468–1501.

16. Wroblewski BA, Joseph AB, Cornblatt RR. Antidepressant pharmacotherapy and the treatment of depression in patients with severe traumatic brain injury: a controlled, prospective study. *J Clin Psychiatry.* 1996;57(12):582–587.

17. Fann JR, Uomoto JM, Katon WJ. Sertraline in the treatment of major depression following mild traumatic brain injury. *J Neuropsychiatry Clin Neurosci.* 2000;12(2):226–232.

18. Fann JR, Uomoto JM, Katon WJ. Cognitive improvement with treatment of depression following mild traumatic brain injury. *Psychosomatics.* 2001;42(1):48–54.

19. Rapoport MJ, Chan F, Lanctot K, Herrmann N, McCullagh S, Feinstein A. An open-label study of citalopram for major depression following traumatic brain injury. *J Psychopharmacol (Oxford).* 2008;22(8):860–864.

20. Gould TD, Quiroz JA, Singh J, Zarate CA, Manji HK. Emerging experimental therapeutics for bipolar disorder: insights from the molecular and cellular actions of current mood stabilizers. *Mol Psychiatry.* 2004;9(8):734–755.

21. Dikmen SS, Machamer JE, Winn HR, Anderson GD, Temkin NR. Neuropsychological effects of valproate in traumatic brain injury: a randomized trial. *Neurology.* 2000;54(4):895–902.

22. Pachet A, Friesen S, Winkelaar D, Gray S. Beneficial behavioural effects of lamotrigine in traumatic brain injury. *Brain Inj.* 2003;17(8):715–722.

23. Kim E, Bijlani M. A pilot study of quetiapine treatment of aggression due to traumatic brain injury. *J Neuropsychiatry Clin Neurosci.* 2006;18(4):547–549.

24. Oster TJ, Anderson CA, Filley CM, Wortzel HS, Arciniegas DB. Quetiapine for mania due to traumatic brain injury. *CNS Spectr.* 2007;12(10):764–769.

54

Sleep Disturbances

Felise S. Zollman and Eric B. Larson

BACKGROUND

What Is a Sleep Disturbance?

- Dyssomnias—disorders that result in insomnia (e.g., sleep apnea)
- Parasomnias—disorders of arousal or sleep stage transition (e.g., nightmares, sleep-walking)
- Sleep disorders caused by medical or psychiatric illness (e.g., traumatic brain injury (TBI), stroke, depression, chronic pain)

The focus of this chapter will be on the most common type of post-TBI sleep disturbance—insomnia. Another common problem often associated with sleep disturbances, fatigue, is addressed in Chapter 14. Although some authors have proposed an association between TBI and other sleep disorders such as sleep apnea, periodic limb movements, and narcolepsy, it is not clear to what extent these conditions may have been present prior to (and perhaps even contributed to the occurrence of) TBI [1]. Detailed discussion of these conditions is beyond the scope of this chapter.

Sleep Architecture

- Five stages—stages I to IV and rapid eye movement (REM) sleep
- Non-REM sleep—stages I to IV. Stage I is lightest; Stage IV is deep sleep.
- REM sleep—approximately 20% to 25% of total sleep time. During REM sleep, the brain exhibits heightened activity. This is associated with dreaming and with actively maintaining an atonic state, which is mediated by signaling between the pons and the medulla.

Neurophysiology of Sleep and Wakefulness

- Sleep and wakefulness is regulated by interaction between the ventrolateral preoptic nucleus (VLPO) of the hypothalamus and arousal centers in the hypothalamus and brainstem.

357

- Melatonin-producing cells in the suprachiasmatic nucleus (SCN) of the hypothalamus induce sleep and regulate circadian rhythms.
- Serotonin and norepinephrine pathways promote wakefulness and are thought to play a role in regulating the stages of non-REM sleep.
- Acetylcholine helps maintain arousal and plays a role in REM sleep.

Neuropharmacology and Sleep

- Stimulants (e.g., catecholaminergic medications like methylphenidate) increase wakefulness and decrease REM sleep.
- Caffeine shortens REM latency and decreases non-REM sleep time.
- Antihistamines (e.g., diphenhydramine) increase non-REM sleep via blocking a descending activating histaminergic pathway from the hypothalamus to the tegmentum.
- GABA-ergic drugs (e.g., benzodiazepines) decrease time to sleep onset and increase total sleep time, but this is at the expense of deep (Stage III–IV) sleep and perhaps also REM sleep.
- Melatonin agonists (e.g., ramelteon) decrease sleep onset latency and regulate circadian rhythms.

INSOMNIA

Definition

Insomnia can be clinically defined as the occurrence of trouble sleeping characterized by difficulty falling asleep (i.e., requiring more than 30 minutes to get to sleep), and/or difficulty maintaining sleep (i.e., more than 30 minutes of nocturnal awakening), which occurs at least 3 nights per week, and results in impairment in daytime functioning [2].

Epidemiology

The widely accepted prevalence figure for insomnia in the general population is 30%.

Diagnosis [2]

- Subjective means include self-report and clinician rating scales such as the Insomnia Severity Index, the Epworth Sleepiness Scale, or the Pittsburgh Sleep Quality Index.
- Objective means of quantifying sleep or insomnia include sleep logs (for inpatients), actigraphy, and polysomnograpy (PSG).
  - Sleep log—typically completed by a nurse on an inpatient unit. Patient is briefly observed on an hourly basis and notation of sleep versus wake status is noted for each hour. Drawback—report is

typically based observations of 5 minutes or less per hour. Such a limited sample can result in inaccurate data.

- Actigraphy—uses a small motion-sensing device; activity level is sampled every tenth of a second and aggregated at a constant interval referred to as an epoch. A computerized algorithm translates this data into a representation of time awake versus asleep. Drawback—accurate measurement requires (1) that the device be worn continuously during the period of interest and (2) that the individual have little or no motor impairment, the presence of which can compromise accurate reading of movement as a surrogate for awake time.
- PSG—gold standard for measurement of sleep. PSG monitors many body functions through electroencephalogram (EEG), electro-oculogram (EOG), electromyogram (EMG), and electrocardiogram (ECG) during sleep. Drawback—because of the complexity of the equipment required, PSG is costly, labor intensive, and not convenient for routine use.

INSOMNIA AND TBI

- Insomnia may occur immediately following injury and may continue for several years thereafter.
- Incidence is reported to be 36% to 81% [3–7]. The wide variability is in part due to variability in operational definitions of insomnia and due to challenges in accurately applying assessment technology.

Mechanism

- Acutely, insomnia results from diffuse disruption of cerebral functioning because of both direct physical damage to deep brain structures (including the hypothalamus and/or brainstem) and because of secondary neuropathological events, which may cause damage because of cerebral pathways essential for the maintenance of normal sleep architecture.
- Melatonin deficiency also appears to play a role, having been demonstrated in TBI patients in the ICU setting [8]. This observation raises the prospect that use of a melatonin agonist may be of specific benefit in this population.
- Chronically, behavioral and affective factors also come into play.

Clinical Presentation

TBI patients present with a variety of symptoms which may be a direct result of their injury or may be secondary to insomnia, including [5]:

- Fatigue

- Irritability
- Cognitive deficits
- Pain

The significant overlap between symptoms that may be due to TBI and those which may be due to insomnia makes the accurate diagnosis of insomnia in the setting of TBI challenging.

MANAGEMENT OF INSOMNIA IN TBI

Behavioral and Environmental Interventions

Sleep hygiene practices and environmental modifications that encourage sleep should be implemented early in the course of treatment:

- Time of awakening—Waking up at the same time each morning regardless of the time one goes to sleep helps maintain consistent circadian rhythms.
- Caffeine, alcohol, or nicotine use—Each of these substances interferes with normal sleep architecture and should be avoided. For regular caffeine users, recommend cutting back on daily intake and not having any caffeine past noontime.
- Environmental factors—Advise turning off lights and minimizing noise or other distractors (e.g., late night activity in an inpatient unit, a TV left on overnight).
- Regular exercise—Exercise may benefit sleep via anxiolytic and antidepressant effects, circadian phase-shifting effects, and elevating levels of adenosine [9].

Stimulus control, reducing practices that condition a patient to associate the bed with wakefulness, should also be encouraged early in treatment:

- Limit time in bed for waking daytime activities—As much as possible, when patients are active and awake (e.g., watching TV), they should be out of bed.
- Limit time in bed at night when unable to sleep—If it is safe to do so, patients who can not sleep within 15 minutes of bedtime should be encouraged to get out of bed and find another place to engage in relaxing activities (e.g., reading) until they become drowsy.

Pharmacological Treatment Options [10]

- Melatonin agonists (e.g., ramelteon)—decrease sleep latency and modestly improve total sleep time. Ramelteon should be a first line consideration in TBI because of its excellent side-effect profile.

- Benzodiazepines—mainstay treatment for insomnia in the general population. Approved for short-term use—not as a chronic treatment intervention. Benzodiazepines bind nonselectively to the GABA(A) receptor subtype, potentiating the inhibitory effect of GABA in the central nervous system (CNS). In those with TBI, benzodiazepine use is associated with contemporaneous impairment in cognitive function as well as impaired CNS recovery due to inhibition of neural plasticity. In the general population, chronic use has resulted in impairment in memory and learning—likely at least in part due to interfering with long-term potentiation—even after months of abstinence. For these reasons, the use of benzodiazepines in those with TBI is discouraged.

- Atypical GABA agonists (e.g., zolpidem)—selective for the GABA(A) receptor 1 subtype. Generally have fewer cognitive side-effects and shorter half-life than benzodiazepines; however, studies in normals have shown that this class of agent impairs short-term memory and psychomotor speed immediately after administration and in some cases for as long as 24 hours afterward. There is limited data available to assess to effect of these agents in those with neurological impairment; however, given the demonstrated adverse effects in normals, and the likelihood that these effects would be magnified in those with TBI, these agents should be used with caution in the TBI population.

- Antidepressants:
  - Those with significant anticholinergic side-effects (e.g., amitriptyline) are generally to be avoided in patients with TBI because of the risk of exacerbating cognitive impairment, daytime "hangover" effect, orthostatic hypotension, and urinary retention.
  - Selective serotonin reuptake inhibitors may be effective if insomnia is felt to be primarily due to depression.
  - Trazodone is a triazolopyridine derivative that is approved by the Food and Drug Administration as an antidepressant but that is also used off-label for treatment of insomnia. Trazodone is frequently used to treat insomnia in those with TBI, although no studies have been conducted to assess the effect of this agent on cognition in patients with neurological impairment. Trazodone is typically used in a dosage range from 50 to 200 mg nightly. Some studies of general populations have suggested that doses of 100 mg or more may result in modest cognitive impairment.

- Antihistamines (e.g., diphenhydramine)—generally not used in those with TBI because anticholinergic effects can cause CNS impairment, urinary retention, and orthostatic dizziness [7].

- Herbal supplements, including melatonin and valerian root can be considered:
  - The usual over-the-counter melatonin formulation comes in a 3 mg tablet, although at least one study has shown that one-tenth that dose, or 0.3 mg, may be optimally effective [11]. Higher doses may be associated with some degree of hypothermia, although the clinical implication of this is uncertain.
  - Data supporting the efficacy of valerian root has been inconsistent [12]; however, it generally has a favorable side-effect profile and so may be an appropriate consideration in some cases.

COMPLEMENTARY AND ALTERNATIVE MEDICINE OPTIONS

A recently published study addressing the use of acupuncture to treat insomnia in patients with TBI suggests that this modality is well tolerated, may have equal efficacy to medication use without introducing untoward CNS side effects, and may result in improvement in mood and cognitive function. [13] This may be a promising area for continued future exploration.

ADDITIONAL READING

Electronic Reference
http://www.craighospital.org/tbi/TBI_Sleep_LP.pdf

Textbook/Chapter
Thaxton LL, Patel AR. Sleep disturbances: epidemiology, assessment and treatment. In: Zasler N, Katz D, Zafonte R, eds. *Brain Injury Medicine: Principles and Practice*. New York, NY: Demos Medical Publishing;2006:557–576.

Journal Articles
Larson EB, Zollman FS. The effect of sleep medications on cognitive recovery from traumatic brain injury. *J Head Trauma Rehabil*. 2010;25(1):61–67.

Thaxton LL, Myers MA. Sleep disturbances and their management in patients with brain injury. *J Head Trauma Rehabil*. 2002;17(4):335–348.

REFERENCES

1. Orff HJ, Ayalon L, Drummond SP. Traumatic brain injury and sleep disturbance: a review of current research. *J Head Trauma Rehabil*. 2010;24(3):155–165.
2. Zollman FS, Cyborski C, Duraski SA. Actigraphy for assessment of sleep in traumatic brain injury: case series, review of the literature and proposed criteria for use. *Brain Inj*. 2010;24(5):748–754.

3. Ouellet MC, Beaulieu-Bonneau S, Morin CM. Insomnia in patients with traumatic brain injury: frequency, characteristics, and risk factors. *J Head Trauma Rehabil.* 2006;21(3):199–212.

4. Rao V, Rollings P. Sleep Disturbances Following Traumatic Brain Injury. *Curr Treat Options Neurol.* 2002;4(1):77–87.

5. Ouellet MC, Morin CM. Subjective and objective measures of insomnia in the context of traumatic brain injury: a preliminary study. *Sleep Med.* 2006;7(6):486–497.

6. Mahmood O, Rapport LJ, Hanks RA, Fichtenberg NL. Neuropsychological performance and sleep disturbance following traumatic brain injury. *J Head Trauma Rehabil.* 2004;19(5):378–390.

7. Thaxton L, Myers MA. Sleep disturbances and their management in patients with brain injury. *J Head Trauma Rehabil.* 2002;17(4):335–348.

8. Paparrigopoulos T, Melissaki A, Tsekou H, et al. Melatonin secretion after head injury: a pilot study. *Brain Inj.* 2006;20(8):873–878.

9. Montgomery P, Dennis JA. Physical exercise for sleep problems in adults aged 60+. *Cochrane Database Syst Rev.* 2002;4:CD003404.

10. Larson EB, Zollman FS. The effect of sleep medications on cognitive recovery from traumatic brain injury. *J Head Trauma Rehabil.* 2010;25(1):61–67.

11. Zhdanova IV, Wurtman RJ, Regan MM, Taylor JA, Shi JP, Leclair OU. Melatonin treatment for age-related insomnia. *J Clin Endocrinol Metab.* 2001;86(10):4727–4730.

12. Stevinson C, Ernst E. Valerian for insomnia: a systematic review of randomized clinical trials. *Sleep Med.* 2000;1(2):91–99.

13. Zollman FS, Larson EB, Wasek-Throm LK, Cyborski CM, Bode RK. Acupuncture for Treatment of Insomnia in patients with Traumatic Brain Injury: a Pilot Intervention Study. J Head Trauma Rehabil. Epub ahead of Print. Jan 2011.

55

Posttraumatic Headache

Henry L. Lew, Sara Cohen, and Pei-Te Hsu

GENERAL PRINCIPLES

Definition

Headache (HA) that develops within 1 week after head trauma (or within 1 week of regaining consciousness) is referred to as posttraumatic headache (PTH). PTH that lasts longer than 3 months is referred to as chronic PTH [1].

Epidemiology

30% to 90% of traumatic brain injury (TBI) patients may develop some form of HA [2].

Classification

- Most common—majority are tension-type or migraine-type [2]
- Less common and benign—neuritic pain, musculoskeletal HA, dysautonomic HA, sinus HA, posttraumatic cluster HA, and medication overuse HA [3]
- Ominous—increased intracranial pressure (ICP), vascular injury, intracranial aneurysm, vasospasm, cerebrospinal fluid (CSF) fistula, dural sinus injury, posttraumatic hydrocephalus, abscess, and other structural neurological pathology [3,4]

Pathophysiology

Pathophysiology is poorly understood, but may be secondary to cerebral circulation abnormalities after TBI. There are similar biochemical alterations seen in both TBI and migraine, and a TBI may injure the trigeminovascular system that is implicated in migraines [5].

DIAGNOSIS

History [3]

- Quality of pain—COLDER (character, onset, location, duration, exacerbation, relief)
- Ask about severity, frequency, temporal associations, and postural relationships
- Associated symptoms—nausea, vomiting, dizziness, visual dysfunction, and auras
- Patients with family history of HA are more likely to develop PTH.

Clinical Presentation (Based on International Headache Society Classification of Headache)

Clinical presentation often comprises a hybrid rather than falling into only one of the following categories [3,5].

- *Migraine HA*—throbbing, unilateral, lasts 4 to 72 hours, may be associated with nausea or vomiting, may have aura. Basilar artery migraines can occur secondary to traction on the vertebral-basilar circulation from acceleration-deceleration injury.
- *Tension-type HA*—moderate diffuse nonpulsating pain in forehead or temples, often described as pressure, or band-like, which is not typically aggravated by activity
- *Neuritic pain*—sharp, shooting, electric pain. Most commonly originating from greater or lesser occipital nerves, with pain located periocular and radiating from back to front of head.
- *Musculoskeletal HA*—"cap-like" in quality, improves with nonsteroidal anti-inflammatory medications (NSAIDs). Patient may have history of skull fracture or bruxism.
- *Cervicogenic HA*—typically originates in the cervical or occipital region and radiates rostrally. Often active trigger points can be identified, palpation of which reproduces the pain pattern.
- *Dysautonomic HA*—unilateral episodic throbbing pain associated with autonomic changes
- *Sinus HA*—localized to the sinuses and associated with sinus tenderness
- *Temporomandibular joint syndrome*—typically located in the temporal region; may be exacerbated by chewing or yawning

Ominous Symptoms That May Indicate Intracranial Pathology [3]

- *Increased ICP*—Worsening and constant cephalgia, associated nausea and vomiting, declining cognition. May be secondary to a space-occupying lesion (e.g., bleed), tension pneumocephalus, hydrocephalus, or shunt failure

- *Low ICP*—HA exacerbation in upright position. Usually secondary to shunt dysfunction or CSF leak
- Acute or delayed vascular dysfunction:
  - *Carotid artery injury*—focal pain, involving orbital or periorbital regions
  - *Vertebral artery injury*—severe pain in cervical or ipsilateral occipital regions
  - *Carotid cavernous fistula*—frontal HA, chemosis, proptosis, and diplopia

Physical Examination [3]

- Comparison to baseline (whenever possible) is key.
- *Migraine or tension HA*—Likely normal examination, but may have transient neurological changes during initial phase of a migraine attack.
- *Neuritic HA*—Palpation of affected nerve may reproduce HA pain.
  - Greater occipital nerve—best palpated below base of skull, off midline
  - Lesser occipital nerve—best palpated behind sternocleidomastoid, one-third of muscle length from mastoid
- *Sinus HA*—Sinuses may be tender with palpation.
- *Musculoskeletal and cervicogenic HA*—Identify trigger points that may reproduce pain; palpate muscles of mastication in temporomandibular joint.

Ominous Examination Findings Which May Indicate Intracranial Pathology

- Increased ICP—deterioration in mental status, focal neurological deterioration, and papilledema
- CSF leak—clear rhinorrhea, otorrhea that may worsen with Valsalva
- Vascular injury—external evidence of neck trauma, cervical carotid bruit, ocular bruit, and Horner's syndrome
- Infection—fever, nuchal rigidity, purulent drainage from wound or postsurgical site

Laboratory Studies

Limited utility—If infection is suspected, CSF may be studied [3].

Radiographic Assessment [3]

- *Migraine-type or tension-type HA*—routine use of neuroimaging not warranted. MRA of the head or neck may be considered if basilar artery migraine is suspected. If focal neurological findings are noted, computed tomography (CT) or magnetic resonance imaging (MRI) of the brain should be considered.
- *Musculoskeletal HA*—may want to obtain C-spine plain films (lateral, open-mouth, flexion-extension), C-spine MRI if disk disease suspected.
- *Sinus HA*—CT can be used to evaluate for sinusitis, and anatomic or structural problems.

If red flags (ominous symptoms and/or signs) exist:

- *Increased ICP*—CT of brain is imaging of choice because of the ease of obtaining study, and will also identify cerebral swelling and pneumocephalus. If situation is not acute, MRI is more sensitive.
- *Vascular injury*—MRI or MRA of neck will assess blunt carotid trauma. Ultrasound can also detect vascular lesions and vasospasm but is limited by technique. Angiography may be considered in selected cases (e.g., as a preop assessment).
- *Infection*—CT or MRI with contrast can identify abscesses.

TREATMENT

General Principles

- The mainstay of treatment is prevention of chronicity by using prophylactic medications, minimization of polypharmacy, and diminishing the risk of medication-induced rebound phenomenon [2].
- Treat the HA symptomatically, independent of history of trauma.
- For headaches because of identified intracranial pathology, address the underlying pathology directly.
- Evaluate for depression or other underlying medical diagnoses that may exacerbate PTH. Psychological factors are frequent contributors to pain [5,6].
- Identify and counsel patient on PTH triggers—sleep, caffeine, stress, exercise, or diet [7].
- Medication overuse HA should be suspected if analgesics are being used more than two times per week [8].
- It is important to provide support and reassurance about the injury [5].

Nonpharmacological Treatment

- Relaxation and biofeedback have shown favorable results in uncontrolled studies [2].

- Physical therapy may be useful if the PTH is caused by musculoskeletal or biomechanical dysfunction [2]. Myofascial pain can be addressed with trigger point injections [7].
- Neuritic pain may respond to local anesthetic block of the affected nerve or surgical decompression if warranted [7].
- Acupuncture has been shown to be effective as both an abortive and a prophylactic management approach for migraine headaches and for tension headache [9,10].

Pharmacological Treatment [7]

Abortive Agents

- NSAIDs—effective for musculoskeletal HA, migraine HA, and tension HA. Ibuprofen and naproxen are most effective, but indomethacin can be used for paroxysmal hemicranialis
- Muscle relaxants—use not supported
- Acetaminophen—effective for musculoskeletal and tension HA
- Narcotics—avoid use if possible because of high abuse potential and risk of sedation/cognitive impairment.
- Vasoactive medications—serotonin receptor agonists (sumatriptan) and ergotamine derivatives should be taken at first appearance of migraine HA pain, provided that no cerebrovascular or cardiovascular contraindications are present

Prophylactic Agents

- β-Blockers (propranolol, metoprolol)—primary choice for migraine prophylaxis in patients who do not have cognitive impairment due to TBI. Exercise caution in the setting of cognitive impairment
- Calcium channel blockers (verapamil, nifedipine)—can be used in prophylaxis against migraine and cluster HA
- Antidepressants—tricyclic antidepressants (nortriptyline, amitriptyline) and selective serotonin reuptake inhibitors (fluoxetine) are frequently used for migraine prophylaxis
- Anticonvulsants (e.g., valproate, gabapentin, topiramate) also may be beneficial in migraine prophylaxis [8].

Other Agents

- Fiorinal (butalbital-ASA-caffeine)—may be effective as an abortive agent; however, exercise caution in using this medication in someone with fatigue, lethargy, or cognitive impairment
- Pulsed corticosteroids—may abort an attack of intractable migraine
- Inhalation of 100% oxygen for cluster HA
- Antiemetics—can be considered for patients with severe nausea who cannot ingest other medications

Treatment Controversies [5,6]

- There may be an inverse correlation between TBI severity and the presence of PTH.
- Many patients with PTH have pending litigation; possibility of secondary gain may interfere with response to treatment.

ADDITIONAL READING

Electronic Reference
International Headache Society website. http://www.ihs-headache.org

Textbook
Silberstein SD, Lipton RB, Dodlick D. *Wolff's Headache and Other Head Pain.* 8th ed. New York, NY: Oxford University Press; 2007.

Journal Articles
Bell KR, Kraus EE, Zasler ND. Medical management of posttraumatic headaches: pharmacological and physical treatment. *J Head Trauma Rehabil.* 1999;14(1):34–48.

Formisano R, Bivona U, Catani S, et al. Post-traumatic headache: facts and doubts. *J Headache Pain.* 2009;10(3):145–152.

Lew HL, Lin PH, Fuh JL, et al. Characteristics and treatment of headache after traumatic brain injury: a focused review. *Am J Phys Med Rehabil.* 2006;85(7):619–627.

Packard RC. Epidemiology and pathogenesis of posttraumatic headache. *J Head Trauma Rehabil.* 1999;14(1):9–21.

Silberstein SD. Practice parameter: evidence-based guidelines for migraine headache (an evidence-based review): report of the Quality Standards Subcommittee of the American Academy of Neurology. *Neurology.* 2000;55:754–762.

Zafonte RD, Horn LJ. Clinical assessment of posttraumatic headaches. *J Head Trauma Rehabil.* 1999;14(1):22–33.

REFERENCES

1. Headache Classification Committee of the International Headache Society. The International Classification of Headache Disorders: 2nd edition. *Cephalalgia.* 2004;24(suppl 1):9–160.
2. Lew HL, Lin PH, Fuh JL, Wang SJ, Clark DJ, Walker WC. Characteristics and treatment of headache after traumatic brain injury: a focused review. *Am J Phys Med Rehabil.* 2006;85(7):619–627.
3. Zafonte RD, Horn LJ. Clinical assessment of posttraumatic headaches. *J Head Trauma Rehabil.* 1999;14(1):22–33.
4. Ruff RL, Ruff SS, Wang XF. Headaches among Operation Iraqi Freedom/ Operation Enduring Freedom veterans with mild traumatic brain injury associated with exposures to explosions. *J Rehabil Res Dev.* 2008;45(7):941–952.
5. Packard RC. Epidemiology and pathogenesis of posttraumatic headache. *J Head Trauma Rehabil.* 1999;14(1):9–21.

6. Formisano R, Bivona U, Catani S, D'Ippolito M, Buzzi MG. Post-traumatic headache: facts and doubts. *J Headache Pain.* 2009;10(3):145–152.

7. Bell KR, Kraus EE, Zasler ND. Medical management of posttraumatic headaches: pharmacological and physical treatment. *J Head Trauma Rehabil.* 1999;14(1):34–48.

8. Silberstein SD. Practice parameter: evidence-based guidelines for migraine headache (an evidence-based review): report of the Quality Standards Subcommittee of the American Academy of Neurology. *Neurology.* 2000;55(6):754–762.

9. Linde K, Allais G, Brinkhaus B, et al. Acupuncture for migraine prophylaxis (Review). *Cochrane Database Syst Rev.* 2009;(1):CD001218.

10. Linde K, Allais G, Brinkhaus B, et al, Acupuncture for tension-type headache. *Cochrane Database Syst Rev.* 2009;(1):CD007587.

56

Neurovascular Complications After Nonpenetrating Brain Injury

Sunil Kothari, Michael M. Green, and
Ana Durand-Sanchez

INTRODUCTION

Although uncommon, neurovascular complications of traumatic brain injury (TBI) can have devastating consequences.

This chapter will focus on three of the most often seen of these complications—arterial dissection, carotid-cavernous fistulas (CCFs), and traumatic aneurysms.

- Recognizing neurovascular sequelae of TBI is complicated by several factors:
  - Patients may be asymptomatic or may have nonspecific symptoms
  - Symptoms may be delayed in their presentation, sometimes for weeks to months
  - Symptoms (e.g., headache) may mistakenly be attributed to the TBI itself, rather than to a neurovascular problem
  - There is often no correlation between the severity of TBI and the development of neurovascular sequelae
- Clinicians need to maintain a high index of suspicion in order to expediently identify these conditions.

ARTERIAL DISSECTION

- Can occur as a result of stretch injury or direct trauma, resulting in a tear in the wall of an artery, which allows intrusion of blood within the layers of the arterial wall.
- The site of dissection may be either within the connective tissue and vasa vasorum of the media or, more commonly, intimal [1]. Intimal

disruption can lead to thrombus formation, which can result in vascular obstruction in situ and/or result in distal embolization. Expansion of the subintimal blood causes luminal narrowing, sometimes resulting in obstruction. Involvement of the media or adventitia can result in aneurysms, pseudoaneurysms, or fistulae.

- Dissections can occur intracranially or extracranially, either in the internal carotid artery or the vertebral artery; they occur extracranially more commonly than intracranially.
- Usually, there is no external evidence of trauma over the affected vessel.

Clinical Presentation

- Symptoms may be a result of local effects or due to ischemia.
- Often, but not always, local symptoms precede the development of ischemia. Therefore, early recognition of local symptoms may reduce the risk of the development of ischemia.

Local Symptoms—Extracranial Carotid Artery Dissection

- Headache and neck pain are usually the most prominent symptoms [1]. The pain is typically ipsilateral, sharp or constant, and affects the jaw and face or frontoparietal area.
- Patients may report pulsatile tinnitus or a subjective bruit.
- A partial Horner's syndrome (miosis and ptosis) can be seen on the ipsilateral side as a result of involvement of the sympathetic fibers that travel along the internal carotid artery.
- Ipsilateral cranial nerve palsies can also be seen. The lower cranial nerves are more often involved, with taste disturbance and tongue weakness being the most common manifestations [1].

Ischemic Symptoms—Extracranial Carotid Artery Dissection

- Ischemic symptoms (cerebral or retinal) are common in carotid dissections, occurring in the majority of patients [2] and resulting in either transient ischemic attacks or infarctions.
- Ischemic symptoms usually follow local symptoms by hours or days.
- Specific symptoms are referable to the vascular territories of the involved vessel and can include visual loss (e.g., amaurosis fugax), aphasia, hemiparesis, and so on.

Local Symptoms—Extracranial Vertebral Artery Dissection

- Neck pain, often severe, is the most prominent local symptom. The pain is primarily located in the ipsilateral occipitocervical region.

Ischemic Symptoms—Extracranial Vertebral Artery Dissection

- Ischemic symptoms may not occur if there is adequate collateral circulation.
- When ischemic symptoms occur, symptoms usually reflect involvement of brainstem or cerebellar structures and can include ataxia, vertigo, dysarthria, and diplopia.

Intracranial Dissections

- Ischemic symptoms, not local symptoms, are usually the first manifestation. Ischemic symptoms tend to be more severe than in extracranial dissection.
- Intracranial dissections are much more likely to rupture, resulting in subarachnoid hemorrhage [1].

Imaging

- Although catheter angiography remains the gold standard, noninvasive options are frequently used, at least for the initial diagnosis. These include CT angiography (CTA), MR angiography (MRA), and Doppler ultrasound.
- Choice of modality should take into consideration issues such as degree of suspicion, accessibility of modality, contraindications to modality (e.g., to contrast or magnetic fields), and so on.

Treatment

- Treatment is broadly divided into medical and interventional treatments.
- Medical treatment consists either of antiplatelet therapy or anticoagulation. Although anticoagulation has generally been viewed as the primary therapeutic approach, a recent Cochrane Review found that there is currently not enough evidence to definitively recommend one modality over another [2,3].
- Interventional treatment includes surgery as well as procedures such as stenting, balloon occlusion, and so on.
- Choice of treatment depends on many factors including the patient's symptoms, time course of symptom progression, nature of lesion, etiology of ischemia (e.g., embolic vs. vessel occlusion), patient's overall neurological status, contraindications to certain treatments (e.g., anticoagulation), availability of newer interventional modalities, and so on.

- Most patients will require follow-up imaging to monitor status of the dissection, especially if being treated medically.

CAROTID-CAVERNOUS FISTULAS (CCF)

Description

- Although fistulas can occur in any artery after dissection or occlusion, the most common posttraumatic fistula occurs between the internal carotid artery and the cavernous sinus [2].
- The cavernous sinuses contain a number of venous channels. They are located on either side of the sella turcica and posterior to the orbits.
- A number of important structures pass through the cavernous sinus, including the internal carotid artery and cranial nerves III, IV, V, and VI.
- Although there are several different types of Carotid-Cavernous fistulas (CCFs), by far the most common after trauma is one in which a fistula develops directly between the internal carotid artery and the cavernous sinus. These traumatic CCFs are known as Barrow type A CCF or direct CCF [4]. Traumatic CCFs represent high-flow shunts because there is shunting of blood between a high-flow arterial system and a low-flow venous system. The high-flow shunt created by the CCF increases venous resistance, which impedes the venous drainage into the cavernous sinus.
- Although traumatic CCFs can develop at the time of or shortly after the initial injury, they can also develop much later, when an initially injured internal carotid artery finally erodes or ruptures into the cavernous sinus.
- Bilateral traumatic CCFs have been reported [4].

Clinical Presentation

- The symptoms of traumatic CCF are a result of vascular congestion in the regions that are normally drained by the cavernous sinus.
- Orbital and periorbital manifestations are the most common and include ipsilateral chemosis, scleral injection, proptosis (sometimes pulsatile), and pain.
- An orbital or facial bruit may be auscultated [5,6].
- Extraocular palsy (especially of CN VI) and diminished visual acuity can also occur.
- Increased intraocular pressure (because of impaired aqueous humor drainage through the canals of Schlemm) may result in glaucoma and loss of vision (ischemic optic neuropathy) [5].
- In addition to orbital and ophthalmic symptoms, patients may complain of headache, epistaxis, upper facial numbness, and tinnitus (often described as buzzing or "swishing") [4].

- The possibility of significant or even complete visual loss (from retinal hypoxia and/or ischemic optic neuropathy) warrants early detection and management of a traumatic CCF [4]. Other serious complications include cerebral ischemia (because of "vascular steal") and hemorrhage, both subarachnoid as well as parenchymal.

Imaging

- The gold standard modality is four-vessel digital subtraction angiography (DSA). However, the use of CT (with contrast) and MRI/MRA has also been reported [4].

Treatment

- Traumatic CCFs are most often treated with endovascular techniques [2, 4]. These include the use of balloons and coils to achieve occlusion or embolization.
- Direct surgical repair may be indicated in some cases [2].
- Although closure of the fistula usually results in resolution of most symptoms, visual function may not return because of permanent injury to the optic nerve [6].

TRAUMATIC INTRACRANIAL ANEURYSMS

Description

- Traumatic intracranial aneurysms (TICA), although uncommon, are associated with significant morbidity and mortality rates of 50% after rupture [7].
- Although more often associated with severe TBI, they can occur after even mild head trauma [7].
- Traumatic aneurysms can be classified both by histological type and location.
  Histologically, TICA fall into one of three main categories:
  - True aneurysms involve disruption of the intima and media with preservation of the adventitia, which forms the aneurysm wall.
  - In false aneurysms (or pseudoaneurysms), all three layers (intima, media, and adventitia) are disrupted and the extravasated blood is contained only by arachnoid, brain parenchyma, or the hematoma itself.
  - Mixed aneurysms represent false aneurysms that are formed after the contained rupture of a true aneurysm.
- TICA are also classified by their anatomic location. In particular, they can be distinguished by whether they arise proximal or distal to the circle of Willis.

- Aneurysms that arise proximal to the circle of Willis can involve the carotid artery (either the supraclinoid or intraclinoid segment) or the vertebrobasilar arteries.
- Aneurysms that arise distal to the circle of Willis involve cortical or subcortical arteries (or their branches).

Clinical Presentation

- The clinical presentation depends on whether the aneurysm has ruptured or not. Unfortunately, most aneurysms are asymptomatic until rupture, thereby minimizing the possibility of early detection.
- Patients with supraclinoid carotid artery aneurysms can present with headache, memory disturbance, and visual loss before rupture. Patients with unruptured infraclinoid carotid artery aneurysms can present with cranial nerve deficits, diabetes insipidus, recurrent epistaxis, or symptoms of a CCF [7].
- Most traumatic aneurysms present after rupturing, resulting in subdural, subarachnoid, or intraparenchymal hemorrhages. Symptoms of a ruptured aneurysm typically include decreased level of consciousness, focal neurological deficit, and/or seizure.
- The average time from initial trauma to aneurysmal hemorrhage is approximately 21 days, although rupture can be delayed for months or even years [7].

Imaging

- Unruptured aneurysms are difficult to detect with routine, noncontrast CT or MRI scans. CT or MR angiography may be considered, especially given the cost and risk of complications associated with DSA, the diagnostic gold standard [7].
- After rupture, CT or MRI will demonstrate intracranial hemorrhage. DSA should be performed as soon as possible in order to identify the underlying lesion.

Treatment

- The goal of treatment is to exclude the aneurysm from the circulation by surgical or endovascular methods.
- Endovascular procedures are more difficult with traumatic aneurysms because of the lack of an aneurismal neck, the extent of the arterial wall involved, the fragile nature of these aneurysms, and the lack of a defined wall in cases of pseudoaneurysm. Despite this, endovascular techniques utilizing balloons or embolization with detachable coils have been used with some success [7].

- Surgical clipping has advantages in that it allows for removal of the hematoma, provides definitive isolation of the aneurysm, and allows for the reconstruction of the parent artery, if needed [7].
- Ultimately, considerations such as aneurysm structure, location, clinical status of the patient, and availability of appropriately skilled personnel will dictate the optimal treatment method.

ADDITIONAL READING

Electronic References

Vascular complications of penetrating brain injury. http://journals. lww. com/jtrauma/Fulltext/2001/08001/Vascular_Complications_of_ Penetrating_Brain_Injury.7.aspx#

Treatment of carotid dissection. http://www2.cochrane.org/reviews/en/ ab000255.html

Textbook/Chapter

Chandler J, Batjer H, Kuznits S, et al. Intracranial and cervical vascular injuries. In: Cooper P, Golfinos J, eds. *Head Injury*. 4th ed. New York, NY: McGraw-Hill; 2000:361–396.

Journal Article

DeWitt D, Prough D. Traumatic cerebral vascular injury: the effects of concussive brain injury on the cerebral vasculature. *J Neurotrauma*. 2003;20(9):795–825.

REFERENCES

1. Thanvi B, Munshi SK, Dawson SL, Robinson TG. Carotid and vertebral artery dissection syndromes. *Postgrad Med J*. 2005;81(956):383–388.
2. Guyot LL, Kazmierczak CD, Diaz FG. Vascular injury in neurotrauma. *Neurol Res*. 2001;23(2–3):291–296.
3. Lyrer P, Engelter S. Antithrombotic drugs for carotid artery dissection. *Cochrane Database Syst Rev*. 2010;10:CD000255.
4. Fattahi TT, Brandt MT, Jenkins WS, Steinberg B. Traumatic carotid-cavernous fistula: pathophysiology and treatment. *J Craniofac Surg*. 2003;14(2):240–246.
5. Phatouros CC, Meyers PM, Dowd CF, Halbach VV, Malek AM, Higashida RT. Carotid artcry cavernous fistulas. *Neurosurg Clin N Am*. 2000;11(1):67–84, viii.
6. De Keiser R. Carotid-cavernous and orbital arteriovenous fistulas. *Orbit*. 2003;22:121–142.
7. Larson PS, Reisner A, Morassutti DJ, Abdulhadi B, Harpring JE. Traumatic intracranial aneurysms. *Neurosurg Focus*. 2000;8(1):e4.

PART 6

Special Considerations and Traumatic Brain Injury Resources

57

Pediatric Considerations in Traumatic Brain Injury Care

Christopher Giza and Daniel Shrey

PEDIATRIC TRAUMATIC BRAIN INJURY— GENERAL PRINCIPLES

Definition

Pediatric traumatic brain injury (TBI) is injury to the brain from a biomechanical etiology occurring in patients below 18 years of age including inflicted abusive head trauma as well as sports-related concussions and excluding obstetrical complications.

Epidemiology

TBI is a leading cause of morbidity and mortality among pediatric patients, and it is responsible for the majority of trauma-related hospitalizations and deaths in the pediatric population. Although outcomes after TBI are generally viewed as better in children than adults, TBI sustained in younger age groups (<4 years) actually results in worse long-term prognosis [1].

Classification

Uses modified pediatric Glasgow Coma Scale (GCS; see Table 57.1):

- Mild—GCS 13 to 15, includes concussion, constitutes 75% to 85% of all head injuries
- Complicated mild—GCS 13 to 15 with evidence of intracranial pathology (contusions, hemorrhage, axonal injury, etc.)
- Moderate—GCS 9 to 12
- Severe—GCS 3 to 8 after initial resuscitation
- Limitations in pediatrics—difficult to assess verbal score in preverbal infants and older children with language or developmental delays

Table 57.1 Modified Glasgow Coma Scale for Infants and Children (Merck Manual)

Area Assessed	Infants	Children	Score
Eye opening	Open spontaneously	Open spontaneously	4
	Open in response to verbal stimuli	Open in response to verbal stimuli	3
	Open in response to pain only	Open in response to pain only	2
	No response	No response	1
Verbal response	Coos and babbles	Oriented, appropriate	5
	Irritable cries	Confused	4
	Cries in response to pain	Inappropriate words	3
	Moans in response to pain	Incomprehensible words or nonspecific sounds	2
	No response	No response	1
Motor response	Moves spontaneously and purposefully	Obeys commands	6
	Withdraws to touch	Localizes painful stimulus	5
	Withdraws in response to pain	Withdraws in response to pain	4
	Responds to pain with decorticate posturing (abnormal flexion)	Responds to pain with decorticate posturing (abnormal flexion)	3
	Responds to pain with decerebrate posturing (abnormal extension)	Responds to pain with decerebrate posturing (abnormal extension)	2
	No response	No response	1

Pathophysiology

Specific pediatric implications include:

- Abusive head trauma—major cause in infants, due to shaking and/or impact; may be recurrent or have delayed presentation, often with concurrent hypoxic-ischemic injury
- Concussion—often recurrent in child and adolescent contact sports
- Contusion—less common in infants and toddlers than in adolescents or adults

- Diffuse cerebral edema—more common in infants and toddlers than in adolescents or adults
- Diffuse axonal or shearing injury—frontal white matter networks (controlling attention and executive function) are not fully mature until early 20s. In infants, unmyelinated white matter may be particularly vulnerable.
- Hypoxia-ischemia—particularly associated with abusive head trauma
- Penetrating injuries—rare in pediatrics
- Seizures—more common in infants and younger children than in adolescents or adults
- Skull fractures—slightly more common in younger children

Mechanism

The most common mechanisms of pediatric TBI vary by age group.
- Infants—inflicted abusive head trauma, falls
- Toddlers—Falls
- Children and adolescents—motor vehicle accidents and sports-related concussions

MODERATE TO SEVERE PEDIATRIC TBI—ASSESSMENT

[NOTE: Initial management MUST start concurrently with initial assessment]

History

- Risk factors for worse outcome—developmental delay or learning disabilities, comorbid medical conditions (coagulopathy, epilepsy), low socioeconomic status, prior TBI
- Symptoms of TBI in pediatrics are essentially the same as those seen in adults, with the exception that subjective symptoms (pain, dizziness, etc.) may be challenging to assess in preverbal or developmentally delayed children. Parental assessment of whether the child is different from baseline is helpful.

Physical Examination

The following examination considerations are unique to the pediatric population:

- General physical examination for other signs of trauma
  - External signs of head injury—assess for bulging fontanelle
  - Other physical examination findings—retinal hemorrhages, burns, multiple old scars or bruises; may be an indication of abuse-related injury

- Neurological examination findings—assess Moro reflex, tonic neck reflex, and/or other age-specific reflexes

Laboratory Studies

- Complete blood count, chemistry panel, toxicology screen (particularly for adolescents)

Radiographic Assessment

- A skeletal survey may be indicated to rule out inflicted trauma.
- Imaging is otherwise similar to that performed in the adult population (see Chapters 13 and 24).

MODERATE TO SEVERE PEDIATRIC TBI—MANAGEMENT

Guiding Principles

2003 Guidelines for Acute Management of Severe TBI in Infants, Children, and Adolescents [2]. These pediatric guidelines are currently being updated (2010–2011).

Initial Management

- ABCs (airway, breathing, circulation, etc.)
- Assess GCS score—if 3 to 8, obtain head CT, insert ICP monitor, maintain CPP
- Stepwise approach to treating elevated ICP (see Chapter 28)
- If diffuse swelling on CT—consider decompression via craniectomy with duraplasty
- If active ictal focus on EEG—consider high-dose barbiturates
- If evidence of ischemia—consider moderate hypothermia (32°C to 34°C)

Supportive Care

- Acute seizure prophylaxis may be warranted (for first 7 days post injury only).
- Nutrition—caloric supplementation > 130% to 160% of resting metabolic requirements
- General care—oral hygiene, skin care or decubitus ulcer prevention, bowel or bladder regimen

Treatment Controversies

- Many sedatives and anticonvulsants show developmental toxicity in animal models (exceptions—topiramate, levetiracetam [3]).
- Hypothermia (24 hours, rapid re-warming) is deleterious for pediatric TBI [4]; pediatric TBI hypothermia trial with longer duration and more gradual re-warming is ongoing.

PEDIATRIC CONCUSSION—GENERAL PRINCIPLES

Definition

Pediatric concussion is defined as a traumatically induced disturbance of neurological function and mental state, occurring with or without loss of consciousness; generally occurs without evidence of structural pathology on acute neuroimaging and the functional disturbance resolves over time [5,6].

Epidemiology

It is estimated that 1.6 to 3.8 million sports concussions occur in the United States per year in all ages [7]. Among high school athletes, 5% to 6% of all injuries involve the head [8]. Youth athletes represent the largest at-risk population for sports concussion, with more than 63,000 high school athletes alone sustaining a concussion or mild TBI annually [8]. After a single concussion, the risk of sustaining another concussion during the same season increases threefold [9].

Pathophysiology

Multiple potential physiological mechanisms may occur following concussion [10–13]. These include spreading neuronal depression or migraine, seizure activity, changes in cerebral blood flow, perturbations of brain metabolism, altered neuronal activation, and/or axonal dysfunction.

PEDIATRIC CONCUSSION—ASSESSMENT

Signs and Symptoms

Symptoms are usually self-limited with the vast majority (80%–90%) resolving within 1 to 2 weeks.

- Acute symptoms and signs—Essentially mirror those seen in adults (see Chapters 8 to 10). Subjective symptoms are more challenging to assess in young children, and the practitioner should take care to avoid suggestibility that can bias symptom reporting.

PEDIATRIC CONCUSSION—MANAGEMENT

Guiding Principles

Concussion in Sports Group, Consensus Statement, 2008 [6]. There are no pediatric-specific guidelines for concussion management, but there is growing recognition of the need for age-related modifications to adult guidelines. Earlier neurological guidelines [14] are currently being updated (2011–2012).

Management of Sports-Related Concussion

This is discussed in Chapter 9. Issues unique to pediatric concussion include:

- School—may require adjustments for cognitive, behavioral, and/or fine motor deficits [15,16]
    - Initial support—School personnel should be alerted to injury, reintegration into school occurs gradually; provide extra assistance or time to facilitate completion of makeup work.
    - General school-based support—Monitor student carefully for a period following recovery, be aware of any developing or subtle cognitive or behavioral problems.
    - Specific classroom-based support—Delay or provide additional time for tests, offering flexibility for assignment due dates, provide preferential seating to allow for closer monitoring and decreased distractions, provide examples of completed work.
- Return to play—Concerns guiding return to play recommendations include risk of second impact syndrome (SIS) and/or worsened symptoms after repeated concussions (see Chapters 9, 11, and 16 for a more thorough discussion of these issues).

ADDITIONAL READING

Electronic References

Brain Trauma Foundation. http://www.braintrauma.org/pdf/protected/guidelines_pediatric.pdf

CDC concussion website. http://www.cdc.gov/concussion/HeadsUp/youth.html

Textbooks/Chapters

Kliegman R, Behrman R, Jenson H, Stanton BMD. *Nelson Essentials of Pediatrics.* 18th ed. Philadelphia, PA: Saunders; 2007.

Giza CC. Traumatic brain injury in children. In: Swaiman KF, Ashwal S, Ferriero DM, eds. *Pediatric Neurology: Principles and Practice.* 4th ed. Philadelphia, PA: Mosby; 2006:1401–1444.

Journal Articles

Adelson PD, Bratton SL, Carney NA, et al. Guidelines for the acute medical management of severe traumatic brain injury in infants, children, and adolescents. *Pediatric Critical Care Med.* 2003;4:S1–S75.

Kirkwood MW, Yeates KO, Wilson PE. Pediatric sport-related concussion: a review of the clinical management of an oft-neglected population. *Pediatrics.* 2006;117(4):1359–1371.

Madikians A, Giza CC. Treatment of traumatic brain injury in pediatrics. *Curr Treat Options Neurol.* 2009;11(6):393–404.

McCrory P, Meeuwisse W, Johnston K, et al. Consensus Statement on Concussion in Sport: the 3rd International Conference on Concussion in Sport held in Zurich, November 2008. *Br J Sports Med.* 2009;43(suppl 1):76–90.

REFERENCES

1. Anderson V, Catroppa C, Morse S, Haritou F, Rosenfeld J. Functional plasticity or vulnerability after early brain injury? *Pediatrics.* 2005;116(6):1374–1382.

2. Madikians A, Giza CC. Treatment of traumatic brain injury in pediatrics. *Curr Treat Options Neurol.* 2009;11(6):393–404.

3. Kaindl AM, Asimiadou S, Manthey D, Hagen MV, Turski L, Ikonomidou C. Antiepileptic drugs and the developing brain. *Cell Mol Life Sci.* 2006;63(4):399–413.

4. Hutchison JS, Ward RE, Lacroix J, et al. Hypothermia therapy after traumatic brain injury in children. *N Engl J Med.* 2008;358(23):2447–2456.

5. *AAN Practice Parameter. The Management of Concussion in Sports.* Quality Standards Subcommittee of the American Academy of Neurology; 1997.

6. McCrory P, Meeuwisse W, Johnston K, et al. Consensus Statement on Concussion in Sport: the 3rd International Conference on Concussion in Sport held in Zurich, November 2008. *Br J Sports Med.* 2009;43(suppl 1):76–90.

7. Langlois JA, Rutland-Brown W, Wald MM. The epidemiology and impact of traumatic brain injury: a brief overview. *J Head Trauma Rehabil.* 2006;21(5):375–378.

8. Powell JW, Barber-Foss KD. Traumatic brain injury in high school athletes. *JAMA.* 1999;282(10):958–963.

9. Guskiewicz KM, Weaver NL, Padua DA, Garrett WE Jr. Epidemiology of concussion in collegiate and high school football players. *Am J Sports Med.* 2000;28(5):643–650.

10. Ryan CA, Edmonds J. Seizure activity mimicking brainstem herniation in children following head injuries. *Crit Care Med.* 1988;16(8):812–813.

11. Sanford RA. Minor head injury in children. *Semin Neurol.* 1988;8(1):108–114.

12. Bergsneider M, Hovda DA, Lee SM, et al. Dissociation of cerebral glucose metabolism and level of consciousness during the period of metabolic depression following human traumatic brain injury. *J Neurotrauma.* 2000;17(5):389–401.

13. Giza CC, Hovda DA. The Neurometabolic Cascade of Concussion. *J Athl Train.* 2001;36(3):228–235.

14. Kelly JP, Rosenberg JH. Diagnosis and management of concussion in sports. *Neurology.* 1997;48(3):575–580.

15. Kirkwood MW, Yeates KO, Wilson PE. Pediatric sport-related concussion: a review of the clinical management of an oft-neglected population. *Pediatrics.* 2006;117(4):1359–1371.

16. Hawley CA, Ward AB, Magnay AR, Mychalkiw W. Return to school after brain injury. *Arch Dis Child.* 2004;89(2):136–142.

58

Special Considerations in Caring for the Workers' Compensation Patient

Felise S. Zollman

BACKGROUND

The need for a no-fault workers' compensation (WC) system came into being in the context of the emergence of modern industrial society. In the United States, the first state-specific WC legislation was enacted in Maryland in 1902 [1], followed by Congress' 1906 Employers' Liability Act [2]. This legislation shifted the traditional view that employees accepted the risk associated with the work they did, and could only sue if they could prove gross negligence on the part of the employer, to the notion that employers bore responsibility for providing a safe work environment. The first federal WC system in the United States was enacted in 1908 in the form of the Federal Employer Liability Act, which covered railway workers. The first state WC system was established in Wisconsin in 1911. The last state to put such a system in place was Mississippi, in 1948 [1,2].

The core concept of WC is that it is a no-fault compensation system in which the employee is entitled to collect a percentage of lost wages and have medical and rehabilitation care paid for by the employer or the employers' agent or insurer. In return, the employee may not sue the employer because of the injury.

WORKERS' COMPENSATION AND TRAUMATIC BRAIN INJURY

Much of the available data on the incidence, prevalence, and costs associated with traumatic brain injury (TBI) in the context of the WC system comes from a few select states such as Washington, because these states have created a single large State Fund, which covers the vast majority of workers in the state, and therefore have access to a large centralized database containing injury and claim-related information. A handful of large employers may opt out and serve as their own insurers, and these workers are not reflected in published data. Federal employees covered under federal WC programs are also not included.

Epidemiology

Studies have reported that work-related TBIs account for between 5% and 14% of all TBIs [3]. The average annual incidence of work-related TBI is approximately 10 per 100,000 full-time equivalent employees [4]. The top three causes of work-related TBI are falls, motor vehicle accidents, and being struck by an object [4]. The gender differential for occupational injuries is greater than it is in the civilian sector in general: various studies have suggested a ratio of men to women affected by work-related TBI ranging from 2:1 to 10:1 [4–6]. One Canadian mild TBI (MTBI) study, however, did find a higher *prevalence* of MTBI claims among female employees versus males (although the incidence was 2:1 male:female). In this study, the highest risk professions were in education, specifically teachers and janitors, with falls accounting for the majority of MTBI claims. The authors postulated that the reversal in gender ratio for prevalence of MTBI might be due to an observed longer duration of claims remaining open for female workers with MTBI [6]. The incidence of fatal work-related TBI is approximately 6%.

Costs

A study from Washington State published in 2006 reported an annual claim cost per TBI of $25,400. Medical costs were $12,600, time lost was $3200, and disabled pension benefits were $4000. Median claim cost was $61,000. The highest risk/most costly industries included logging, construction, janitorial services, and roofing [5].

MANAGEMENT OF WORK-RELATED TBI

Personnel

- In addition to the usual clinical care personnel, injured workers are usually followed by a medical case manager (MCM), typically an RN by training. The role of this individual is to direct and move the case forward through the medical or rehabilitation care process and see the case to closure. MCMs are guided by the Code of Professional Conduct for Case Managers (see Additional Reading).
- WC carriers will typically identify a primary treating physician (PTP) for an injured worker. This physician is the individual who is primarily responsible for managing the treatment of the injured worker. Some states set forth detailed guidelines for PTPs, including case coordination and reporting duties (see, for example: http://www.scif.com/pdf/TreatingMDguide.pdf).

- WC carriers will also typically assign an adjustor to each case, whose responsibility it is to manage the financial aspect of a claim. The adjustor will typically work in conjunction with the MCM on behalf of the insurance company in monitoring claims-related costs.

Management Approach

Typical injury cases would be expected to progress through a sequence of stages, from acute care to medical rehabilitation to vocational rehabilitation (VR). A recent study by Wrona revealed, however, that only 48% of TBI survivors seen for acute medical management (identified based on hospital discharge records) progressed to medical rehabilitation; 46% were referred for VR. Sixty-five percent of those referred for VR did ultimately return to the work force. The author hypothesized that the reason a minority of cases were referred for medical rehabilitation was because "most cases do not occur in the area served by clinical model treatment programs and do not follow the clinical trajectory of short intensive initial inpatient care, followed closely by intensive rehabilitation and referral for return to work" [7].

CONCLUSION

Injured workers are typically cared for under the auspices of the WC system. Coverage specifics vary from state to state; however, the basic premise of WC is the same throughout the industrialized world—workers are provided coverage for lost wages, medical and rehabilitation care; and employers are protected from lawsuits resulting directly from the injury (no-fault coverage). Injured workers typically progress from acute medical care through medical and vocational rehabilitation (VR). MCMs help steer cases through the system; PTPs direct medical care, and adjustors monitor the claim and associated costs. Ultimately, the majority of injured workers with TBI who are referred for VR do return to the work force in some capacity.

ADDITIONAL READING

Electronic References
Case Manager code of conduct:
http://ccmcertification.org/pdfs/CCMCode.pdf
Treating Physician guide (California):
http://www.scif.com/pdf/TreatingMDguide.pdf

Textbook/Chapter
Andersson GB, Cocchiarella L. *Guidelines to the Evaluation of Permanent Impairment.* 5th ed. American Medical Association; 2000.

Journal Article

Wrona RM. Disability and return to work outcomes after traumatic brain injury: results from the Washington State Industrial Insurance Fund. *Disabil Rehabil*. 2010;32(8):650–655.

REFERENCES

1. Ky P, Hameed H, Christo PJ. Independent Medical Examinations: facts and fallacies. *Pain Physician*. 2009;12(5):811–818.

2. Guyton GP. A brief history of workers' compensation. *The Iowa Orthopaedic Journal*. 1999;19:106–110.

3. Annegers JF, Grabow JD, Kurland LT, Laws ER. The incidence, causes, and secular trands of head trauma in Olmsted County, Minnesota, 1935–1974. *Neurology*. 1980;30:912–919.

4. Heyer NJ, Franklin GM. Work-related traumatic brain injury in Washington State, 1988 through 1990. *Am J Public Health*. 1994;84(7):1106–1109.

5. Wrona RM. The use of state workers' compensation administrative data to identify injury scenarios and quantify costs of work-related traumatic brain injuries. *J Safety Res*. 2006;37(1):75–81.

6. Kristman VL, Côté P, Van Eerd D, et al. Prevalence of lost-time claims for mild traumatic brain injury in the working population: improving estimates using workers compensation databases. *Brain Inj*. 2008;22(1):51–59.

7. Wrona RM. Disability and return to work outcomes after traumatic brain injury: results from the Washington State Industrial Insurance Fund. *Disabil Rehabil*. 2010;32(8):650–655.

59

Developing a Life Care Plan

Roger O. Weed and Debra E. Berens

BACKGROUND

- Definition: "A life care plan is a dynamic document based upon published standards of practice, comprehensive assessment, data analysis and research, which provides an organized concise plan for current and future needs with associated costs, for individuals who have experienced catastrophic injury or have chronic health care needs" [1].
- Use: Identification of lifelong anticipated care for patients who will not fully recover (i.e., have a permanent disability).
- Historical relevance: The term "life care plan" was introduced into the legal literature in 1981 and came to be recognized as a valuable tool within the rehabilitation field that identifies and projects the impact of catastrophic injury on an individual's future [1–2].
- Includes expected short and long-term or lifelong needs and costs of medical care; residential placement (facility and in-home); transportation; home/architectural modifications; medical and nonmedical supplies, equipment, and adaptive devices; physical, occupational, speech, recreational, and other therapies; medications; and other needs as related to, or a result of, the traumatic brain injury (TBI).
- Routine healthcare needs/costs typically are not included, as the need or service would have occurred independent of the brain injury. Similarly, preexisting conditions typically are not included unless the brain injury exacerbated the condition or had another concomitant effect.

DIAGNOSIS: FOR WHOM IS A LIFE CARE PLAN APPROPRIATE?

- Life care plans for individuals with TBI may be generated for the following situations [2–8]:
  - Hospital or rehabilitation facility discharge planning

Portions of this chapter, reprinted with permission, appeared in the Demos publication: Weed R, Berens D. Life care planning after TBI: clinical and forensic issues. In: Zasler N, Katz D, Zafonte R, eds. *Neurorehabilitation of Traumatic Brain Injury*. New York: Demos Medical Publishing; 2006:1223–1240.

- Medical-legal cases (e.g., personal injury litigation, medical malpractice litigation)
- Adoption of special needs children
- Elder care planning
- Workers compensation claims
- Managed care health plans and reserve setting
- Trust-funded care for people with disabilities
- Medicare set-asides
- Vaccine injury fund cases
- Wounded warrior or veterans with injuries

MANAGEMENT: HOW IS A LIFE CARE PLAN GENERATED?

Elements of the Life Care Plan

These include the following:

- Projected evaluations: nonphysician or allied health evaluations that will occur on a periodic basis
- Projected therapeutic modalities: ongoing or episodic treatment
- Diagnostic testing/educational assessments, for example, neuropsychological, psychological, vocational evaluations, and, for children, developmental and/or psychoeducational testing
- Wheelchair needs, accessories, and maintenance: type and configuration of recommended wheelchairs, specialty cushions and covers, carry bags, gloves, and yearly maintenance/service requirements
- Aids for independent function (includes assistive technology and adapted devices)
- Orthotics and prosthetics
- Home furnishing and accessories
- Drug and supply needs: prescribed and over-the-counter drugs, and supplies including incontinence, feeding, tracheostomy, wound care, etc.
- Home care/facility care: living in the least restrictive setting is preferred. However, home care may not be the most cost effective alternative nor the most medically appropriate for the client depending on his/her needs and brain injury sequelae.
  - For clients recommended to live at home, the level of in-home care should be identified (e.g., skill level of providers, hours per day the providers are needed, shift care vs hourly care vs live-in care).
  - Facility care may be most appropriate for those who have no capability of living at home or whose needs exceed capabilities available in a home environment.
  - There also may be need for specialty programs such as yearly summer camps.

- Future medical care: typically provided by a physiatrist/physician with expertise in brain injury
- Transportation: adapted driving evaluation and training if client has potential to drive, vehicle modifications, wheelchair modifications, private driver, or public transportation
- Health and strength maintenance (aka recreation and leisure time activities): home exercise program, adapted sports or recreation activities, and gym or health club membership as an avenue for structured exercise and socialization or community integration
- Architectural renovations: typically included for clients who are to be cared for at home
    - For the military, the Veterans Administration has established certain allowances that are reevaluated each year. See http://www.homeloans.va.gov/sah.htm for current allowances.
- Potential complications: conditions for which the client with TBI is at higher risk to occur. Included for information only as no frequency or duration of complications are typically predictable. Costs of complications generally are not included unless they are "expected" and can be quantified
- Future medical care/surgical intervention or aggressive treatment
- Orthopedic equipment needs/durable medical equipment
- Vocational/educational plan

The Life Care Planning Team Members

These include the following:

- Client or evaluee (i.e., the person with the disability) [9]. Assuming that the client/evaluee is accessible (i.e., legally permitted) and capable of appropriate interaction, interview him or her. If not possible, one alternative is to have a videotaped "day in the life" of the client. It is recommended that the client interview take place in the client's residence (home or facility) for (1) client convenience, (2) the opportunity to assess potential home modification needs, and (3) to observe medications, equipment, and supplies.
- Family members/caregivers
- Physiatrist (or other physician with expertise in management of TBI):
    - Often designated the team leader
    - Can assist in establishing medical foundation for a life care plan [1,10,11]
    - The physician evaluation should include functional limitations, expected future medical treatment including referral to other specialties, review of medications, supplies, and/or durable medical equipment and related topics.

- Neuropsychologist: will establish cognitive, affective, behavioral, social, and functional capabilities as well as identify current and future needs, including aging-related needs
- Occupational therapist: addresses seating and positioning needs (may also be done by physical therapist), activities of daily living training, adaptive aids, safety in the residence, and other vocationally related issues
- Speech and language pathologist (may also be called communication disorders specialist): identifies speech and language abilities as well as augmentative communication needs for clients with severe communication disorders; cognitive remediation needs
- Physical therapist: reviews durable medical equipment needs including wheelchair design and specifications. If appropriate, may conduct a functional capacity evaluation (may also be performed by the occupational therapist).
- Educational consultant: identifies needed educational programs/services. Under the federal Individuals with Disabilities Education Act, the public school system is responsible for providing specialized services to *eligible* school-age children with disabilities up to the age of 22. Each state also offers early intervention programs for children with brain injury from birth to age 3.
- Case manager: coordinates care, equipment acquisition, and problem-solving support
- Vocational evaluator (if client has work potential): identifiies client's vocational capabilities [5]
- Rehabilitation counselor (aka vocational rehabilitation counselor): assists in coordinating a job and/or labor market analysis. Provides vocational guidance and counseling including job-seeking skills training, job development, selective job placement, supported employment, and/or postplacement services, and serves as a job coach and/or provides work adjustment training. A rehabilitation counselor with at least a Masters degree who holds the national CRC (certified rehabilitation counselor) credential is recommended.
- Economist: if litigation-related (forensic), calculates the cost of "damages" over the client's lifetime as related to the brain injury. The economist will rely on the base costs of the items and services recommended in the life care plan to project the cost of care throughout the client's life expectancy [12]. Table 59.1 shows an example entry from a life care plan that provides relevant information for the economist to make appropriate cost projections. In order for an economist to project the cost of care, certain details must be included in the life care plan, including the expected type and amount of treatment or service, date to start treatment, date to stop treatment, and base cost of treatment (in today's dollars; see Table 59.1). For products, such as durable medical equipment and supplies, include specifications, date to purchase, expected cost, and replacement schedules. It is strongly recommended

Table 59.1 Relevant Life Care Plan Information for Economist

Example Minimum Information Needed for an Economist to Project Costs
Psychiatric evaluation in 6/2010 at a cost of $750 (includes complete evaluation with report and recommendations).
Expect counseling to start in 7/2010, frequency one time per week, for 1 hour session each, for 26 weeks at a cost of $150 per hour from PhD level brain injury specialist.
Expect group counseling beginning 1/2011, frequency one time per week for 12 months then one time every 2 weeks for 12 months at a cost of $50 per session.
Expect medical follow-up four times per year until 1/2012 by psychiatrist at a cost of $75 each visit.
Expect medication as prescribed: Prozac, one 20 mg per day, from 7/2010 to 1/2012 at cost of $53.86 for 30 pills.

that the life care planner defer to an economist or other trained and qualified professional to determine the ultimate cost of the life care plan, unless (1) he/she has specific training in this specialized area or (2) he/she is in a position to apply special rules pertaining to economic projections (e.g., the Alaska Rule) that eliminate complex formulas.

General Life Care Planning Procedures/Additional Considerations

- Request and review all medical records and (if available) depositions of health care professionals regarding the client's brain injury [1]. May also be appropriate to request preinjury records and/or records regarding preexisting or comorbid conditions to determine the client's overall general health condition.
- Conduct an in-person interview with the client and/or reliable family member/caregiver. If client is unable to participate in interview, conduct observation of client.
- Begin identifying long-term care issues and options, including considerations for aging.
- Define the source of each recommendation, consistent with appropriate and reasonable care.
- Ensure familiarity with the client's particular situation and the literature with regard to probable needs as related to the TBI. Are the clinicians' recommendations reasonable and consistent with the accepted standard of care?
- Once an adequate foundation is established for the future care needs and recommendations, an initial life care plan is developed. The

process of developing a life care plan also includes an investigation into resources, availability of services, and cost research.

- The life care plan is then typically presented to, and reviewed by, the client/family (if clinically appropriate) and, at times, the treatment team. An alternative is to have the physician or health care provider(s) who participated in development of the plan review and sign off or endorse their medically based recommendations as being a reasonable plan of care for the client.

ADDITIONAL READING

Electronic References

American Association of Nurse Life Care Planners. http://www.aanlcp.org

The Internal Commission of Health Care Certification http://www.ichcc.org

International Academy of Life Care Planners has published peer-reviewed standards of practice which Academy members pledge to follow. http://www.rehabpro.org/sections/ialcp/focus/standards/ialcp-standards-of-practice

Weed RO, Berens DE. Private sector rehabilitation. In: Stone JH, Blouin M, eds. *International Encyclopedia of Rehabilitation* [online]. 2008. http://cirrie.buffalo.edu/encyclopedia/article.php?id=11&language=en

Textbooks/Chapters

Deutsch P, Sawyer H. *A Guide to Rehabilitation.* New York: Matthew Bender; 1985. (out of print.)

Riddick-Grisham S, ed. *Pediatric Life Care Planning and Case Management.* Boca Raton, FL: CRC Press; 2004.

Weed R, Berens D, eds. *Life Care Planning and Case Management Handbook.* 3rd ed. Boca Raton, FL: CRC Press; 2010. (Includes individual chapters for most of the topics discussed in this pocket guide.)

Weed R, Berens D. Life care planning after TBI: clinical and forensic issues. In: Zasler N, Katz D, Zafonte R, eds. *Neurorehabilitation of Traumatic Brain Injury.* New York: Demos Medical Publishing; 2006:1223–1240.

Journal Articles

Countiss R, Deutsch P. The life care planner, the judge and Mr. Daubert. *Journal of Life Care Planning,* 2002;1(1):35–43.

Weed R. Life care planning and earnings capacity analysis for brain injured clients involved in personal injury litigation utilizing the RAPEL method. *Journal of neurorehabilitation,* 1996;7(2):119–135.

REFERENCES

1. Weed R. Life care planning: past, present and future. In: Weed R, Berens D, eds. *Life Care Planning and Case Management Handbook.* 3rd ed. Boca Raton, FL: CRC Press; 2010:1–13.
2. Deutsch P, Sawyer H. *A Guide to Rehabilitation.* New York: Matthew Bender; 1985:2003. (Out of print.)

3. Weed R. Life care plans as a managed care tool. *Med Interface.* 1995;8(2):111–118.

4. Weed R. Life care planning: an overview. *Directions in Rehabilitation.* 1998;9(11):135–147.

5. Weed R, Field T. *The Rehabilitation Consultant's Handbook.* 3rd ed. Athens: E&F Vocational Services; 2001.

6. Weed R, Riddick S. Life care plans as a case management tool. *The Individual Case Manager Journal.* 1992;3(1):26–35.

7. Riddick S, Weed R. The life care planning process for managing catastrophically impaired patients. In: Bancett S, Flarey D, eds. *Case Studies in Nursing Case Management.* Gaithersburg, MD: Aspen; 1996:61–91.

8. Ripley D, Weed R. Life care planning for acquired brain injury. In: Weed R, Berens D, eds. *Life Care Planning and Case Management Handbook.* 3rd ed. Boca Raton, FL: CRC Press; 2010:349–381.

9. Weed R. Aging with a brain injury: the effects on life care plans and vocational opinions. *The Rehabilitation Professional.* 1998;6(5):30–34.

10. Bonfiglio R. The role of the physiatrist in life care planning. In: Weed R, Berens D, eds. *Life Care Planning and Case Management Handbook.* 3rd ed. Boca Raton, FL: CRC Press; 2010:17–25.

11. Zasler N. A physiatric perspective on life care planning. *Journal of Private Sector Rehabilitation.* 1994;9(2&3):57–61.

12. Dillman E. The role of the economist in life care planning. In: Weed R, Berens D, eds. *Life Care Planning and Case Management Handbook.* 3rd ed. Boca Raton, FL: CRC Press; 2010:303–317.

60

Medical–Legal Considerations in Traumatic Brain Injury

Robert E. Hanlon, Diana S. Goldstein, and Michael D. Carter

BASIC LEGAL CONCEPTS IN TBI LITIGATION

- Traumatic brain injury (TBI) lawsuits are generally based on a theory of negligence:
  - Defendant owed the plaintiff a legal duty of care
  - Defendant breached that duty of care
  - Breach caused the plaintiff's injury
  - Plaintiff suffered damages as a result of the breach
- Plaintiff must establish negligence based on the facts. Proof of negligence is required. A diagnosis of TBI is necessary
- Admissibility of evidence
  - Any point in contention may be proven by using a "more likely than not" standard. Proof beyond a reasonable doubt, proof by clear and convincing evidence, or strict scientific proof is not required
  - A witness allowed to offer testimony must have scientific, technical, or other specialized knowledge, which will assist the trier-of-fact to understand the evidence or determine a fact in issue.
  - The methodology employed to support conclusions and opinions must be reliable.
  - An expert witness may rely upon materials commonly relied upon by similar professionals, as well as his/her own experience, when forming opinions.

TYPES OF LAW SUITS INVOLVING TRAUMATICALLY BRAIN INJURED INDIVIDUALS

- Personal injury cases associated with motor vehicle collisions, motor vehicle versus pedestrian collisions, bicycle accidents, injuries sustained from being struck by a falling object, falls, playground accidents, sports-related injuries, physical abuse, and assaults

- Worker's compensation cases associated with falls, inadequate safety practices, equipment malfunction, supervisor and/or coworker negligence, workplace violence, and injuries sustained from being struck by a falling object
- Disability cases due to TBI
- Medical malpractice cases associated with medication mismanagement, inadequate supervision and/or protection of acutely confused patients, complications associated with surgical intervention, falls, and suicide
- Mental competency and guardianship cases
- Product liability cases

FACT WITNESS VERSUS EXPERT WITNESS

- Fact witnesses are healthcare providers involved in the examination and/or treatment of a patient who subsequently initiates litigation.
- Expert witnesses, specialized by training in the diagnosis and treatment of TBI, who may or may not actually examine the plaintiff, are commonly subpoenaed to testify with respect to opinions regarding the diagnosis of TBI, as well as the extent, severity, and permanence of damages.
- Ethical standards of numerous professional organizations discourage clinicians from assuming an expert witness role when a doctor-patient relationship exists. In general, treating clinicians are advocates for their patients and have concern for their welfare, whereas an expert witness is an advocate for the truth and guards against forming a therapeutic alliance. The two roles present obvious conflict.
- Lawyers are not required to know or follow the ethical guidelines or codes of conduct of a particular clinician; it is the sole responsibility of the clinician to ensure against transgressions by avoiding offering expert opinions if they are in a treating role.

ROLE OF THE TREATING CLINICIAN IN TBI LITIGATION

- Whether one actively seeks a forensic role as independent evaluator or is called upon to provide information to fact finders about a patient for purposes of litigation or another compensation-seeking context, clinicians are immediately subject to, and responsible for, following guidelines for forensic practitioners in their respective field. The American Academy of Neurology (AAN) adopted a Code of Professional Conduct in 1989 [1] to govern its members, and revised the "Qualifications and guidelines for the physician expert witness" in 2005 [2], making them comparable to those of the American Medical Association (AMA) and the American Association of Neurological Surgeons (AANS). Specialty guidelines for psychologists engaging in forensic work were similarly published in 1991 and revised in 2004 [3].

- The AMA has taken the position that forensic practice is the practice of medicine. Providing medical testimony is the practice of medicine by extension, a position upheld by a 7th Circuit Appeals Court when challenged [4].

- The AAN and AANS have assumed leadership roles regarding the integrity of expert medical testimony, and other associations are following [5]. Organizations have been created for the sole purpose of addressing expert medical testimony reform (e.g., Coalition and Center for Ethical Medical Testimony and Medical Justice) [6]. Clinicians must be knowledgeable about their ethical obligations when involved in forensic matters.

MODERATE TO SEVERE TBI

- Determination and documentation of severity

  - Glasgow Coma Scale is the most frequently recognized measure of severity of TBI by the court. Emergence from coma and regaining of consciousness are most reliably established by the consistent ability to follow commands [7].

  - Duration of posttraumatic amnesia (PTA) is also a commonly recognized measure of TBI severity by the court, and should be objectively assessed by an experienced examiner.

- Complications (e.g., posttraumatic epilepsy, hydrocephalus) may be expected to have a negative impact on functional outcome and, as a result, may be key factors in TBI litigation.

- Objective outcome measures

  - Results of serial neuropsychological evaluations are commonly used to objectively determine the functional capacity of TBI litigants and are frequently recognized by the court as key factors in making determinations regarding the extent and severity of damages.

  - The following schedule of serial neuropsychological evaluations is recommended [8,9] to objectively document neurocognitive recovery and neuropsychological outcome: (1) at resolution of PTA; (2) 3 months post injury; (3) 6 months post injury (4) 1 year post injury; and (5) 2 years post injury.

MILD TBI

- Diagnosis: Is there evidence of brain injury or not? [10–12]

  - A very small percentage of mild TBI (MTBI) patients report symptoms persisting beyond 3 months, and are diagnosed with postconcussion syndrome. Litigation status is increasingly recognized as a factor associated with protracted recovery.

- External incentives
  - Empirical data strongly support the association between involvement in litigation and persistent, worsening or more severe symptom complaints, deficits in cognitive test performance beyond the 3-month recovery period, and poor functional outcome such as prolonged delay or failure to return to work, and disability [13–16].
  - The 2004 World Health Organization Collaborating Centre Task Force on MTBI described litigation status or other compensation-seeking as one of the most reliable predictors of poor outcome [17].
- Objective outcome measures
  - Neuropsychological testing is sensitive to subtle dysfunction following MTBI and is commonly recognized by the court as a primary factor in making determinations regarding the extent and severity of damages. Optimal referral time for initial neuropsychological evaluation is 1 month post injury. Follow-up neuropsychological evaluation is typically conducted at 1 year [9].
  - Inclusion of measures to assess effort in neuropsychological evaluations of TBI litigants is critical to determining what impact, if any, motivational factors may have on clinical presentation.
  - Base rates of malingering of cognitive impairment vary across settings, but are significant [18,19].

ADDITIONAL READING

Electronic References

Regarding Custodial Care in TBI. http://www.nursingcenter.com/pdf.asp?AID=796406

Legal Services for Veterans. http://www.jmls.edu/veterans/

Textbooks/Chapters

Larrabee GJ. *Forensic Neuropsychology: A Scientific Approach.* New York: Oxford University Press; 2005.

Boone KB. *Assessment of Feigned Cognitive Impairment: A Neuropsychological Perspective.* New York: Guilford Press; 2007.

Journal Article

Williams MA, Mackin GA, Beresford HR, et al. American Academy of Neurology Qualifications and guidelines for the physician expert witness. *Neurology.* 2006;66(1):13–14.

REFERENCES

1. American Academy of Neurology Code of Professional Conduct. 1989;6.4.
2. www.aan.com/globals/axon/assets/7708.pdf. Accessed on July 18, 2010.
3. Specialty guidelines for forensic psychologists. *Law Hum Behav.* 2004;15(6):655–665.
4. Austin v. American Association of Neurological Surgeons, 253 F.3rd 967 (7th Cir. 2001).
5. Sagsveen MG. American Academy of Neurology policy on expert medical testimony. *Neurology.* 2004;63:1555–1556.
6. Shaw G. Dueling neurologists: as expert witness testimony increases, so do complaints. *Neurology Today.* 2004;12:14.
7. Giacino JT, Ashwal S, Childs N, et al. The minimally conscious state: definition and diagnostic criteria. *Neurology.* 2002;58:349–353.
8. Sherer M, Madison CF. Moderate and severe traumatic brain injury. In: GJ Larrabee, ed. *Forensic Neuropsychology: A Scientific Approach.* New York: Oxford University Press; 2005:237–270.
9. Sherer M, Novack T. Neuropsychological assessment after traumatic brain injury in adults. In: GP Prigatano, NH Pliskin, eds. *Clinical Neuropsychology and Cost Outcome Research.* New York: Psychology Press; 2003:39–60.
10. Iverson GL. Outcome from mild traumatic brain injury. *Curr Opin Psychiatry.* 2005;18:301–317.
11. Carroll LJ, Cassidy JD, Holm L, Kraus J, Coronado VG. Methodological issues and research recommendations for mild traumatic brain injury: the WHO Collaborating Centre Task Force on Mild Traumatic Brain Injury. *J Rehabil Med.* 2004(43 suppl):13–125.
12. McCrea MA. *Mild Traumatic Brain Injury and Postconcussion Syndrome.* Oxford: Oxford University Press, 2008.
13. Binder LM, Rohling ML. Money matters: a meta-analytic review of the effects of financial incentives on recovery after closed head injury. *Am J Psychiatry.* 1996;153:7–10.
14. Paniak C, Reynolds S, Toller-Lobe G, Melnyk A, Nagy J, Schmidt D. A longitudinal study of the relationship between financial compensation and symptoms after treated mild traumatic brain injury. *J Clin Exp Neuropsychol.* 2002;24:187–193.
15. Paniak C, Toller-Lobe G, Melnyk A, Nagy J. Prediction of vocational status three to four months after treated mild traumatic brain injury. *J Musculoske Pain.* 2000;8:193–200.
16. Belanger HG, Curtiss G, Demery JA, Lebowitz BK, Vanderploeg RD. Factors moderating neuropsychological outcomes following mild traumatic brain injury: a meta-analysis. *J Int Neuropsychol Soc.* 2005;11:215–227.
17. Carroll LJ, Cassidy JD, Peloso PM, et al. Prognosis for mild traumatic brain injury: results of the WHO Collaborating Centre Task Force on Mild Traumatic Brain Injury. *J Rehabil Med.* 2004:84–105.
18. Mittenberg W, Patton C, Canyock EM, Condit DC. Base rates of malingering and symptom exaggeration. *J Clin Exper Neuropsychol.* 2002;24(8):1094–1102.
19. Larabee GJ. Detection of malingering using atypical performance patterns on neuropsychological tests. *Clin Neuropsychol.* 2003;17:410–425.

61

Alcohol Misuse and Traumatic Brain Injury

John D. Corrigan

GENERAL PRINCIPLES

- Note that this chapter addresses alcohol but not illicit drugs or misuse of prescription drugs except as a complicating factor
- Definitions
  - Alcohol use disorders
    - Dependence (*International Statistical Classification of Diseases and Related Health Problems*. 10th Revision revision [ICD-10]) [1]: Three or more of the following occurring together for at least 1 month, or if less than 1 month, occurring together repeatedly within a 12-month period:
      - Need for significantly increased amounts of alcohol to achieve intoxication or desired effect, or markedly diminished effect with continued use of the same amount of alcohol
      - Physiological symptoms characteristic of the withdrawal syndrome for alcohol, or use of alcohol (or closely related substance) to relieve or avoid withdrawal symptoms
      - Difficulties controlling drinking (where, when, or amounts consumed)
      - Important alternative pleasures or interests given up or reduced to accommodate drinking or its effects
      - Persisting with drinking despite clear evidence and knowledge of harmful physical or psychological consequences
      - Strong desire or sense of compulsion to drink
    - Abuse/harmful use (ICD-10) [1]: Clear evidence that alcohol use contributed to physical or psychological harm, which may lead to disability/adverse consequences (pattern of use has persisted 1 month or occurred repeatedly over a 12-month period)
  - Alcohol misuse in the absence of alcohol use disorder [2]—recommended maximum consumption:
    - Men

- • ≤65 years old—no more than 4 drinks in a sitting or 14 drinks in a week
  - • >65 years old—no more than 3 drinks in a sitting or 7 drinks in a week
  - ▪ Women—no more than 3 drinks in a sitting or 7 drinks in a week
  - ▪ Less use may be considered misuse in the presence of medication interactions or contraindicated medical conditions.
  - ▪ There is no consensus in the field whether a traumatic brain injury (TBI) is a contraindicated medical condition; however, many clinicians have concluded that abstinence from alcohol is the only safe recommendation that can be made.
  - ▪ Low-risk use—use that does not meet criteria for misuse
  - ▪ Abstinence—no use of alcohol

- ▪ Epidemiology
  - ▪ Among those hospitalized due to TBI, approximately half will engage in binge drinking 1 year after injury [3].
  - ▪ Among those treated in acute rehabilitation, approximately 20% have problem alcohol or drug use 1 year post injury [4].
  - ▪ Substances most likely misused follow national trends, but alcohol is most available, most used, and most misused [5].

- ▪ Etiology
  - ▪ The greater one's intoxication at time of injury the more likely the injury will include a TBI [6].
  - ▪ Individuals with a history of substance use disorder prior to injury are as much as 10 times more likely to exhibit problematic substance use post injury, when compared to those without such history [7].
  - ▪ Large proportion of patients treated for TBI have prior histories of substance use disorder [8,9].
  - ▪ 5% to 10% of rehabilitation patients with no prior history develop problem use following injury [4].
  - ▪ Early childhood TBI may predispose to adolescent and early adulthood substance misuse [10].

TREATMENT

- ▪ Screening
  - ▪ Clinical interview
    - • Determine levels of use and consequences.
    - • To promote transparency, a supportive and nonjudgmental presentation is essential.
    - • Open-ended questions normally elicit more information than multiple, yes/no, or short response questions.

- Structured screening instruments (for brief descriptions, content, and cut-off scores see the American College of Surgeons Committee on Trauma Alcohol Screening and Brief Intervention Quick Guide. www.facs.org/trauma/publications/sbirtguide.pdf) [11]
  - AUDIT (Alcohol Use Disorders Identification Test): 10-items requiring 2 to 3 minutes administration; extensive validation; sensitive to entire spectrum of drinking problems [12]
  - CAGE + consumption: seven items, has extensive validation. Sensitive to alcohol use disorders [11,13]
  - CRAFFT: six items designed for screening in adolescents by asking about risky use situations but not actual questions about consumption [14]
  - Binge drinking question: single item inquiring when last time binged. If in last 3 months, considered positive. Allows conclusion that misuse or worse is present [15]
- Laboratory studies
  - Indices of impaired liver functioning are only sensitive to chronic use
  - Blood alcohol content at time of injury
    - Indicates intoxication at time of injury but not history of misuse
    - High values (e.g., 80 mg/dl exceeds the legal limit for operating a motor vehicle in all 50 states) a basis for assuming at least misuse
    - Very elevated values may suggest tolerance for alcohol associated with dependence.
    - If blood is not drawn for testing near the time of injury, add 15 mg/dl for each hour from injury to blood draw [11].
- Treatment in rehabilitation settings: In a rehabilitation setting, recommended interventions are education, screening, and brief intervention and referral for treatment, as indicated [16].
  - Education
    - Recommend all patients in rehabilitation for TBI receive education about the negative consequences of alcohol use [16,17]
      - Even if there was no premorbid misuse, patients should know that their acute recovery, if not lifetime health, will be more vulnerable to alcohol use than people who have not had a serious TBI [17].
      - Patient and family defensiveness can be minimized by emphasizing this is information that everyone who has had a TBI should know.
    - Content recommendations have been published (see Table 61.1) [17,18].
  - Brief intervention

Table 61.1 Eight Educational Messages Presented in a User's Manual for Faster, More Reliable Operation of a Brain After Injury

1.	People who use alcohol or other drugs after they have a brain injury don't recover as much.
2.	Brain injuries cause problems in balance, walking, or talking that get worse when a person uses alcohol or other drugs.
3.	People who have had a brain injury often say or do things without thinking first, a problem that is made worse by using alcohol and other drugs.
4.	Brain injuries cause problems with thinking, like concentration or memory, and using alcohol or other drugs makes these problems worse.
5.	After brain injury, alcohol and other drugs have a more powerful effect.
6.	People who have had a brain injury are more likely to have times during which they feel low or depressed, and drinking alcohol and getting high on other drugs makes this worse.
7.	After a brain injury, drinking alcohol or using other drugs can cause a seizure.
8.	People who drink alcohol or use other drugs after a brain injury are more likely to have another brain injury.

From Ref. [18].

- Standard structure (National Institute of Alcoholism and Alcohol Abuse Pocket Guide [see Web Sites])
- Screening:
  - Distinguish among abstainers, low-risk use, at-risk use, and substance use disorder.
- Intervention:
  - If low risk, advise not to increase.
  - If at risk, advise and assist depending on readiness to change.
  - If substance use disorder, advise, refer, and/or treat.
- "FRAMES" method [19]
  - FRAMES components:
    - Feedback—respectfully give specific information that concerns the patient
    - Responsibility—stress that the patient is responsible for any change
    - Advice—respectfully give advice to the patient
    - Menu—offer the patient choices
    - Empathy—listen and reflect

- Self-efficacy—reinforce that change is possible and will be beneficial
- Assess readiness to change:
  - If precontemplative, goal is to raise doubt.
  - If contemplative, goal is to increase ambivalence.
  - If ready to take action, goal is to elicit a commitment.
- Close on good terms
- Referral for treatment [17]
  - Locate appropriate referral source in the person's home community.
  - Discuss referral with the person and obtain release for referral and follow-up.
  - Contact referral source, verify cultural relevance, and make referral.
  - Facilitate patient's contact with the referral source to make an appointment.
  - Forward information including biographical data and plans for discharge.
  - Identify possible barriers to referral, such as transportation, scheduling or family compliance, and address prior to initial appointment.
  - Follow up with referral source after initial appointment to confirm attendance. If patient did not attend, determine how to facilitate participation.

ADDITIONAL READING

Electronic References

American College of Surgeons Committee on Trauma Alcohol Screening and Brief Intervention Quick Guide. www.facs.org/trauma/publications/sbirtguide.pdf

www.cdc.gov/InjuryResponse/alcohol-screening/resources.html

NIAAA Pocket Guide for Alcohol Screening and Brief Intervention. http://pubs.niaaa.nih.gov/publications/practitioner/PocketGuide/pocket.pdf

Textbook/Chapter

Corrigan JD. The treatment of substance abuse. In: Zasler N, Katz D, Zafonte R, eds. *Brain Injury Medicine: Principles and Practice.* New York: Demos Medical Publishing; 2007:1105–1115.

Journal Articles

Babor TF, McRee BG, Kassebaum PA, et al. Screening, brief intervention, and referral to treatment (SBIRT): toward a public health approach to the management of substance abuse. *Subst Abus.* 2007:28(3):7–30.

Corrigan JD. Substance abuse as a mediating factor in outcome from traumatic brain injury. *Arch Phys Med Rehabil.* 1995;76(4):302–309.

Hungerford DW, Pollock DA. *Alcohol Problems among Emergency Department Patients: Proceedings of a Research Conference on Identification and Intervention.* Atlanta, GA: National Center for Injury Prevention and Control, Centers for Disease Control and Prevention; 2002.

Ohio Valley Center for Brain Injury Prevention and Rehabilitation. *Substance Use and Abuse After Brain Injury: A Programmer's Guide.* Ohio State University; 2001. www.ohiovalley.org.

Ohio Valley Center for Brain Injury Prevention and Rehabilitation. *User's Manual for Faster More Reliable Operation of a Brain After Injury.* Ohio State University; 2004. www.ohiovalley.org.

REFERENCES

1. World Health Organization. *International Statistical Classification of Diseases and Related Health Problems.* 10th revision ed. Geneva, Switzerland: World Health Organization; 1993.

2. National Institute of Alcoholism and Alcohol Abuse. What is a Safe Level of Drinking? www.niaaa.nih.gov/FAQs. Accessed January 17, 2011.

3. Horner MD, Ferguson PL, Selassie AW, Labbate LA, Kniele K, Corrigan JD. Patterns of alcohol use 1 year after traumatic brain injury: a population-based, epidemiological study. *J Int Neuropsychol Soc.* 2005;11(3):322–330.

4. TBI Model Systems National Data and Statistical Center. Traumatic Brain Injury Model Systems National Database Syllabus. www.tbindsc.org/Syllabus.aspx. Updated 2010. Accessed January 17, 2011.

5. Substance Abuse and Mental Health Services Administration. *Results from the 2008 National Survey on Drug Use and Health: National Findings.* Rockville, MD: Office of Applied Studies, NSDUH Series H-36, HHS Publication No. SMA 09-4434; 2009.

6. Savola O, Niemela O, Hillbom M. Alcohol intake and the pattern of trauma in young adults and working aged people admitted after trauma. *Alcohol Alcohol.* 2005;40(4):269–273.

7. Bombardier CH, Temkin NR, Machamer J, Dikmen SS. The natural history of drinking and alcohol-related problems after traumatic brain injury. *Arch Phys Med Rehabil.* 2003;84(2):185–191.

8. Graham DP, Cardon AL. An update on substance use and treatment following traumatic brain injury. *Ann N Y Acad Sci.* 2008;1141:148–162.

9. Parry-Jones BL, Vaughan FL, Miles Cox W. Traumatic brain injury and substance misuse: a systematic review of prevalence and outcomes research (1994–2004). *Neuropsychol Rehabil.* 2006;16(5):537–560.

10. McKinlay A, Grace R, Horwood J, Fergusson D, MacFarlane M. Adolescent psychiatric symptoms following preschool childhood mild traumatic brain injury: evidence from a birth cohort. *Head Trauma Rehabil.* 2009;24(3):221–227.

11. Committee on Trauma. Screening and Brief Intervention Quick Guide. www.facs.org/trauma/publications/sbirtguide.pdf.

12. Babor TF, Higgins-Biddle JC, Saunders JB, Monteiro MG. *The Alcohol Use Disorders Identification Test: Guidelines for Use in Primary Care.* 2nd ed. Geneva, Switzerland: World Health Organization; 2001.

13. Ewing J. Detecting alcoholism, the CAGE questionnaire. *JAMA.* 1984;252(14):1905–1907.

14. Knight JR, Sherritt L, Shirier LA, Harris SK, Chang G. Validity of the CRAFFT substance abuse screening test among adolescent clinic patients. *Arch Pediatr Adolesc Med.* 2002;156(6):607–614.

15. Williams RH, Vinson DC. Validation of a single question screen for problem drinking. *J Fam Pract.* 2001;50(4):307–312.

16. Corrigan JD, Bogner JA, Lamb-Hart GL. Substance abuse and brain injury. In: Rosenthal M, Griffith ER, Miller JD, Kreutzer J, eds. *Rehabilitation of the Adult and Child with Traumatic Brain Injury.* 3rd ed. Philadelphia, PA: F.A. Davis Co; 1999:556–571.

17. Ohio Valley Center for Brain Injury Prevention and Rehabilitation. *Substance Use and Abuse After Brain Injury: A Programmer's Guide.* Columbus, OH: Ohio State University; 2001.

18. Ohio Valley Center for Brain Injury Prevention and Rehabilitation. *User's Manual for Faster More Reliable Operation of a Brain After Injury.* Columbus, OH: Ohio State University; 2004.

19. Gentilello LM, Riveara FP, Donovan DM, et al. Alcohol interventions in a trauma center as a means of reducing the risk of injury recurrence. *Ann Surg.* 1999;230(4):473–480.

62

Ethical Considerations

Debjani Mukherjee

DEFINITIONS AND KEY POINTS

- Ethics are a "set of moral principles; a theory or system of moral values" [1]
- Various theories and frameworks can be used to analyze ethical considerations, including a focus on principles, relationships, virtues, consequences, rules, or process
- Traumatic brain injury (TBI) can pose unprecedented ethical dilemmas and/or bring up age-old debates about what it means to live a good life. There are webs of lives affected by one injury [2]
- Core principles of biomedical ethics [3] include

  - Beneficence: providing benefit and balancing risks to bring forth the best results
  - Respect for autonomy: fostering self-determination and respecting individual differences
  - Nonmaleficence: doing no harm
  - Justice: upholding concepts of fairness and equity

- Clinical ethics involves analyzing and resolving practical ethical issues drawing on an analysis of medical indications, patient preferences, quality of life (QOL), and contextual factors [4]
- Ethical issues may arise when there are competing interests or values, or disagreements about the "right" or "wrong" way to approach a problem; terms such as moral dilemma, moral uncertainty, and moral distress describe the tension between the perceived course of right action and constraints [5]

PARTIAL LIST OF ETHICAL ISSUES IN TBI

- Decisions about withdrawal of life support
- Consideration of preinjury and postinjury interests and "selves"
- Communication of prognostic uncertainty
- The reverberating impact of the injury on the family system
- Assessment of decision-making capacity

- Decisional capacity versus performative capacity
- QOL judgments by persons other than the injured
- Identifying surrogate decision makers
- Assent versus consent in medical decision making
- Infantilization of adults with TBI
- Use of behavioral restraints
- Access to healthcare and social services
- Safe discharge options
- Allocation of resources
- Participation of vulnerable populations in research
- The role of spirituality in adjustment to TBI
- Addressing biases and stigma associated with cognitive disability

QUALITY OF LIFE

QOL is hard to define and measure [6]. Healthcare providers often rate QOL lower than people living with a disability [7]. Notions of a "good" life change over time and with new life experiences. The best interest standard is often used to discuss QOL, but factors such as the severity of the injury, access to services, premorbid personality characteristics, and social support can complicate the notion of what is in the patient's best interest. Family members and surrogate decision makers are dealing with their own emotional reactions and fears, and may not make decisions based on a "substituted judgment," or what the patients themselves would want. Understanding the values, preferences, hopes, and life satisfaction of persons with TBI is important in exploring ethical issues.

SENSE OF SELF AND PERSONHOOD

TBI raises dilemmas about a sense of self and personhood. Are individuals fundamentally changed if their personalities, memories, or functional capacities are altered? The definition of personhood is distinct from personality, and various legal, theological, and philosophical theories define the concept in specific ways [8]. Vegetative states, minimally conscious states, and other disorders of consciousness raise fundamental issues about how we define the self in relation to QOL, prognosis, and time post injury [9].

ISSUES TO CONSIDER BASED ON
BIOMEDICAL ETHICAL PRINCIPLES

1. Beneficence
   - Best interest of the patient
   - Who defines best interest?

- Benefits and burdens of each treatment
- Use of evidence-based guidelines in medical decision making
- Clear communication of information

2. Respect for patient autonomy/self-determination

- What is the patient's current decision-making capacity?
- Do they have an advance directive?
- Have they identified a surrogate decision maker?
- Has the patient made his/her preferences known? When?
- Has the TBI fundamentally changed the patient's sense of self?

3. Nonmaleficence

- Refers to harms of action as well as harms of nonaction
- If the patient does not fully understand what is being considered, is he/she being harmed?

4. Justice

- Discrimination because of diagnosis or some other category
- Allocation of resources: medical, social, and financial

OTHER FACTORS TO CONSIDER IN CLINICAL ETHICAL ANALYSES [4,10]

1. Identify the moral dilemma, moral uncertainty, or moral distress
2. Determine the facts of the case

- Medical: diagnosis, prognosis, symptoms, risks and benefits of treatment, and goals of treatment
- Social: family members, living situation, social support, occupation, and experiences with the healthcare system
- Spiritual and cultural: belief systems, values, and religious practices that may influence treatment decisions

3. List the stakeholders and the nature of their interests (e.g., patient, family, healthcare providers, facility, payers, community members, and others?)
4. Name the problem/dilemma(s):

- Values in conflict
- Communication difficulties
- Applicable laws and/or institutional policies
- Violations of codes of ethics

5. Gather additional information

- Are there any perspectives missing?
- Where are you getting your facts? Who is telling the story?

6. Consider the alternatives

- List arguments for and against each alternative

- Eliminate options that are "out of bounds" (illegal, against policy)
- Examine how each alternative may affect patients and other interested parties
- Are the choices consistent with the patient's moral, religious, or social beliefs? With the team members' beliefs? With your own beliefs?
- Examine the fairness of the action
- Will the action build goodwill?
- Who ultimately makes the decision/takes action?

7. Implementation and follow-up

- Identify next steps
- Determine the extent of agreement on a proper course of action
- Decide who should be informed
- Learn from the case
- What went right?
- What went wrong?
- What would you do differently in the future?

Ethical considerations range from withdrawal of life support decisions in severe TBI to the ability of a participant with a mild TBI to consent to a low-risk research project. There are numerous frameworks and philosophies that can be used to analyze ethical issues in TBI. The nature of the injury, striking at the core of the sense of self and personhood, can lead to philosophical and practical ethical considerations. The list of factors to consider is presented as a starting point to understanding the complexities involved.

ADDITIONAL READING

Electronic Reference
http://virtualmentor.ama-assn.org/2008/03/pdf/ccas1-0803.pdf

Textbooks/Chapters
Amundson R. Disability, ideology and quality of life: a bias in biomedical ethics. In: Wasserman D, Bickenbach J, Wachbroit R, eds. *Quality of Life and Human Difference.* Cambridge: Cambridge University Press; 2005:101–124.

Kothari S, Kirschner KL. Decision-making capacity after brain injury: clinical assessment and ethical implications. In: Zasler N, Zafonte R, Katz D, eds. *Neurorehabilitation of Traumatic Brain Injury.* New York: Demos Medical Publishing; 2007:1205–1222.

Journal Articles
Bernat JL. Ethical issues in the treatment of severe brain injury: the impact of new technologies. *Ann N Y Acad Sci.* 2009;1157:117–130.

Fins JJ. Lessons from the injured brain: a bioethicist in the vineyards of neuroscience. *Camb Q Healthc Ethics.* 2009;18(1):7–13.

Gill CJ. Disability, constructed vulnerability, and socially conscious palliative care. *J Palliat Care*. 2006;22(3):183–189.

Jennings B. Traumatic brain injury and the goals of care. The ordeal of reminding. *Hastings Cent Rep*. 2006;36(2):29–37.

Kirschner KL. When written advance directives are not enough. *Clin Geriatr Med*. 2005;21:193–209.

REFERENCES

1. Merriam-Webster's Online Dictionary. Ethics. http://www.merriam-webster.com/netdict/ethics. Accessed March 27, 2010.

2. Donnelley SD, Kirschner, KL. (Eds.) *Mapping the Moral Landscape: Families and Persons with Traumatic Brain Injury: The Hypothetical Case of Jeff.* Alexandria, VA: Brain Injury Association; 2003.

3. Beauchamp TL, Childress JF. *Principles of Biomedical Ethics*. 6th ed. New York: Oxford University Press; 2009.

4. Jonsen AR, Siegler M, Winslade WJ. *Clinical Ethics: A Practical Approach to Ethical Decisions in Clinical Medicine*. 6th ed. New York: McGraw-Hill; 2006.

5. Jameton A. *Nursing Practice: The Ethical Issues. Englewood Cliffs*. NJ: Prentice Hall; 1984.

6. Dunn DS, Brody C. Defining the good life following acquired physical disability. *Rehabil Psychol*. 2008;53(4):413–425.

7. Kothari S, Kirschner KL. Abandoning the golden rule: the problem with "putting ourselves in the patient's place". *Top Stroke Rehabil*. 2006;13(4):68–73.

8. Kirschner KL. Decision making in a case of personality change. Virtual Mentor. March 2008. http://virtualmentor.ama-assn.org/2008/03/ccas1–0803.html. Accessed January 11, 2011.

9. Fins JJ. The ethics of measuring and modulating consciousness: the imperative of minding time. *Prog Brain Res*. 2009;1773:371–382.

10. Kornblau B, Starling, S. *Ethics in Rehabilitation: A Clinical Approach*. Thorofare, NJ: Slack Incorporated; 2000.

63

Special Considerations for Military Personnel
Unique Aspects of Blast Injury

Shane D. McNamee, Gary Goldberg, and Ajit B. Pai

OVERVIEW

- Explosive ordinance in the form of improvised explosive devices (IEDs), mines, and rocket-propelled grenades are increasingly being deployed against military and civilian populations.

- In current armed conflicts, nearly half of all injured service members were injured by explosive devices and suffered neurotrauma [1]. As in the civilian population, mild traumatic brain injury (MTBI) is the most common severity of head injury in the combat population [2,3]. It is estimated that up to 20% of deployed service members have suffered an MTBI from blast injury [4]. Because of the ubiquity of IEDs, TBI is referred to as the "signature injury" of the current wars [2,5]. As the use of IEDs rises, civilians are also increasingly targeted and injured [6].

- Historically, blast exposures and subsequent impairments have been given a variety of labels such as "shell shock," "post combat neurosis," deployment-related psychological injury, and blast concussion. Posttraumatic stress disorder (PTSD) is also frequently encountered in those exposed to combat and can cause significant cognitive, physical, and emotional impairments that affect community re-entry and ultimately quality of life [7,8]. In evaluating those with blast exposures and persistent symptoms, psychological wellness must be evaluated, addressed, and prioritized to optimize recovery.

Authors' Note: The views expressed in this chapter are those of the authors and do not reflect the official policy of the Department of Army, Department of Defense, or U.S. Government.

DIFFERENCES FROM SPORTS CONCUSSION MODEL

- Combat sustained blast injuries occur in an emotionally and psychologically complex context. Service members operate at an elevated baseline of attentive hypervigilance for extended periods of time. In addition, combat exposure is associated with significant emotional trauma.

- Global bodily injury from blast dynamics are typically more complex and severe than focal brain injuries caused by sports concussion. It is currently unclear whether the severity and rate of persistent symptoms after concussion due to the blast mechanism itself differ from traditional concussion [9].

- Lessons learned from the study of sports concussion do translate to the combat theater. These include methods for early rapid assessment and consensus guidelines for return-to-duty decisions similar to those developed for return-to-play decisions in athletes following concussion. Also, cumulative effects of multiple blast exposures may be analogous to chronic traumatic encephalopathy in athletes.

- The tendency on the part of athletes to deny and mask postconcussive symptoms so that they can return to play is similar to the tendency of some soldiers to minimize postconcussion symptoms in order to return to action with their "battle buddies."

- There are significant differences in patterns of comorbid injuries and conditions that occur in military blast injuries from those seen in sports concussion. These include comorbid physical trauma such as burns, complex fractures, and limb loss, as well as comorbid psychological injury associated with combat exposure.

- Decisions about return to duty must be made with the recognition that residual cognitive impairment can significantly affect the response of the individual to demanding combat-related contingencies and thus may place other soldiers' lives at risk.

BLAST WAVE PHYSICS

Explosive blasts produce transient pressure waves, which can reach the speed of sound [10]. This is characterized by an initial high pressure wave followed by a protracted low pressure wave. This has been well studied and known to affect fluid- and air-filled structures (e.g., eyes, ears, lungs, and gastrointestinal tract). Blast waves also may include heat and electromagnetic waves, which can further disrupt metabolic process and injure tissue.

MECHANISMS OF BLAST-INDUCED TBI

Blast waves can cause TBI by several different commonly accepted mechanisms [1,11–21]. Primary, secondary, and quaternary mechanisms are generally considered unique to blast injury. The tertiary mechanism is akin to traditional closed head injuries.

- *Primary injury* represents the transduction of the blast wave itself, which can disrupt tissues. The direct effect upon the brain is still poorly understood and hotly debated. It is unclear if the direct effect of the blast wave differs from more traditional causes of TBI in pathophysiology, neurological damage, or upon recovery patterns [9]. The three prevailing theories developed from animal models include:
  - Transduction of blast wave through skull causing biochemical dysfunction
  - Vascular congestion from thorax injury causing transient pressure oscillations in the brain [22]
  - Retrograde cerebrospinal fluid pressure from compression in the spinal column causing increased pressure in the cranial cavity
- *Secondary injury* signifies the damage caused by objects traveling at high rates of speed and striking the victim. TBI can be caused by:
  - Penetrating head injury due to shrapnel or other foreign bodies
  - Traditional closed head injury patterns with focal contusions and diffuse axonal injury due to rapid acceleration and deceleration
- *Tertiary injuries* occur when the individual is thrown from high rates of speed and strike stationary objects. TBI is caused by traditional closed head injury mechanics such as rapid acceleration and deceleration in multiple planes.
- *Quaternary injuries* represent effects from thermal and inhalation injuries. Brain injury is thought to be caused by hypoxic or toxic effects upon cerebral tissue.

ACUTE MANAGEMENT OF BLAST-RELATED TBI IN FORWARD AND TACTICAL ENVIRONMENTS

- In-theater medical care is directly affected by the situation at hand:
  - Hostility within the tactical environment will dictate appropriateness and completeness of care. A complete history and assessment may be impossible because of the presence of heavy fire, chemical or biological agents, and the need for movement. Combat Medics are highly trained in the acute assessment and management of TBI.
  - In 2005, collaboration between the Defense and Veterans Brain Injury Center and the Brain Trauma Foundation produced Guidelines for the Field Management of Combat-Related Head Trauma [23].
- Blast-related management of moderate to severe and penetrating TBI is akin to traditional closed head injury. Stabilization of oxygenation, circulation with aggressive fluid resuscitation, secondary assessment,

and rapid evacuation are prioritized. Aggressive neurosurgical capabilities are available to allow rapid surgical management.

- Glasgow Coma Scale (GCS) determination is highly important, although difficult to obtain while in theater. Individuals with GCS < 13 are rapidly evacuated from the forward environment [23].

- Vasospasm can occur in up to 50% of individuals with blast-related TBI [24]. Vasospasm can occur up to 2 weeks post injury. Individuals with vasospasm incur a longer ICU stay and lower GCS scores upon discharge [25].

- Secondary blast injury can include penetrating injury from a variety of objects. Aggressive debridement and prophylaxis with broad-spectrum antibiotics is standard of care [26].

- Approximately 12% suffer early seizures after blast-related or penetrating brain injury [25]. Long-term risk of posttraumatic epilepsy is highest in those with penetrating head injuries; however, individuals with closed head injuries are still at significant risk. If cortical damage is seen on imaging, the risk is between 10% and 25%, but drops to 5% when there is no injury visualized on imaging [27].

- Secondary survey includes assessment for ocular injuries, otologic damage, respiratory injuries, colonic or ileocecal wall injuries, burns, and orthopedic damage.

COMORBIDITIES

Besides the combat-related psychological injury referenced earlier, blast injuries are associated with higher risk of significant physical comorbidities including impairment to visual and auditory sensory function.

- Dual sensory impairment with involvement of both visual and auditory function in association with an MTBI can occur due to both peripheral and central etiologies.

- More than 60% of veterans of Operation Iraqi Freedom with history of blast-related MTBI were found to have some degree of sensorineural hearing loss [28].

- The presence of central auditory processing impairments appears to be common in soldiers with blast exposure, although the underlying cause is unknown.

- Research on veterans with blast-related and other forms of TBI found that, in patients with moderate or severe TBI, 38.2% experienced an associated ocular injury. Reduced visual acuity was found in 16.7%, whereas 32.2% had visual field defects [29].

- Special expertise in auditory and visual rehabilitation is necessary for the complete rehabilitation approach to blast-injured military personnel [28].

CONCLUSION AND SUMMARY

- Individuals exposed to blasts are at a high risk for developing cognitive, emotional, and physical impairments that affect community reentry. Given the predilection for damage to the central nervous system, vulnerability of the sensory organs, and associated emotional trauma, an integrated diagnostic and therapeutic approach is a necessity.
- Understanding blast effects upon the central nervous system is an evolving science. Both the direct effects of the blast wave upon the brain and the possible sequelae of repeated exposure are currently debated and intensely investigated.

ADDITIONAL READING

Electronic References

http://www.dvbic.org/TBI---The-Military/Blast-Injuries.aspx
http://emedicine.medscape.com/article/822587-overview
http://www.pdhealth.mil/TBI.asp
http://www.army.mil/-news/2010/07/22/42650-new-policies-protect-troops-from-mild-traumatic-brain-injuries/
http://www.rand.org/multi/military/veterans/
http://www.apa.org/about/gr/issues/military/resources.aspx
http://www.mirecc.va.gov/visn19/VISN_19_Education.asp

Textbook/Chapter

Elsayed NM, Adkins JL. *Explosion and Blast-Related Injuries: Effects of Explosion and Blast from Military Operations and Acts of Terrorism.* London: Elsevier; 2008.

Journal Articles

Dennis AM, Kochanek PM. Pathobiology of blast injury. *Intensive Care Med.* 2007;21:1011–1022.

Hicks RR, Fertig SJ, Desrocher RE, Koroshetz WJ, Pancrazio JJ. Neurological effects of blast injury. *J Trauma.* 2010;68:1257–1263.

Ling G, Bandak F, Armonda R, Grant G, Ecklund J. Explosive blast neurotrauma. *J Neurotrauma.* 2009;26(6):815–825.

Moore DF, Jaffee MS. Special issue: military traumatic brain injury and blast. *Neurorehabilitation.* 2010;26:179–290.

Ritenour AE, Blackbourne LH, Kelly JF, et al. Incidence of primary blast injury in US military overseas contingency operations: a retrospective study. *Ann Surg.* 2010;251:1140–1144.

REFERENCES

1. Taber KH, Warden DL, Hurley RA. Blast-related traumatic brain injury: what is known? *J Neuropsychiatry Clin Neurosci.* 2006;18(2):141–145.
2. Warden D. Military TBI during the Iraq and Afghanistan wars. *J Head Trauma Rehabil.* 2006;21(5):398–402.

3. Gulf War and Health, Volume 7. *Long-term Consequences of Traumatic Brain Injury.* Washington, DC: Institute of Medicine; 2009.

4. Sayer NA, Cifu DX, McNamee S, et al. Rehabilitation needs of combat-injured service members admitted to the VA Polytrauma Rehabilitation Centers: the role of PM&R in the care of wounded warriors. *PM R.* 2009;1(1):23–28.

5. Martin EM, Lu WC, Helmick K, French L, Warden DL. Traumatic brain injuries sustained in the Afghanistan and Iraq wars. *Am J Nurs.* 2008;108(4):40–7; quiz 47.

6. Lucci EB. Civilian preparedness and counter-terrorism: conventional weapons. *Surg Clin North Am.* 2006;86(3):579–600.

7. Sundin J, Fear NT, Iversen A, Rona RJ, Wessely S. PTSD after deployment to Iraq: conflicting rates, conflicting claims. *Psychol Med.* 2010;40(3):367–382.

8. Carlson KF, Kehle SM, Meis LA, et al. Prevalence, Assessment, and Treatment of Mild Traumatic Brain Injury and Posttraumatic Stress Disorder: A Systematic Review of the Evidence. *J Head Trauma Rehabil.* 2010;[Epub ahead of print].

9. Wilk JE, Thomas JL, McGurk DM, Riviere LA, Castro CA, Hoge CW. Mild traumatic brain injury (concussion) during combat: lack of association of blast mechanism with persistent postconcussive symptoms. *J Head Trauma Rehabil.* 2010;25(1):9–14.

10. Cullis IG. Blast waves and how they interact with structures. *J R Army Med Corps.* 2001;147(1):16–26.

11. Belanger HG, Kretzmer T, Yoash-Gantz R, Pickett T, Tupler LA. Cognitive sequelae of blast-related versus other mechanisms of brain trauma. *J Int Neuropsychol Soc.* 2009;15(1):1–8.

12. Bochicchio GV, Lumpkins K, O'Connor J, et al. Blast injury in a civilian trauma setting is associated with a delay in diagnosis of traumatic brain injury. *Am Surg.* 2008;74(3):267–270.

13. Champion HR, Holcomb JB, Young LA. Injuries from explosions: physics, biophysics, pathology, and required research focus. *J Trauma.* 2009;66(5):1468–77; discussion 1477.

14. Cooper GJ, Maynard RL, Cross NL, Hill JF. Casualties from terrorist bombings. *J Trauma.* 1983;23(11):955–967.

15. Elder GA, Cristian A. Blast-related mild traumatic brain injury: mechanisms of injury and impact on clinical care. *Mt Sinai J Med.* 2009;76(2):111–118.

16. Finkel MF. The neurological consequences of explosives. *J Neurol Sci.* 2006;249(1):63–67.

17. Leibovici D, Gofrit ON, Stein M, et al. Blast injuries: bus versus open-air bombings–a comparative study of injuries in survivors of open-air versus confined-space explosions. *J Trauma.* 1996;41(6):1030–1035.

18. Ling G, Bandak F, Armonda R, Grant G, Ecklund J. Explosive blast neurotrauma. *J Neurotrauma.* 2009;26(6):815–825.

19. Moore DF, Jérusalem A, Nyein M, Noels L, Jaffee MS, Radovitzky RA. Computational biology—modeling of primary blast effects on the central nervous system. *Neuroimage.* 2009;47 suppl 2:T10–T20.

20. Taylor PA, Ford CC. Simulation of blast-induced early-time intracranial wave physics leading to traumatic brain injury. *J Biomech Eng.* 2009;131(6):061007.

21. Turégano-Fuentes F, Caba-Doussoux P, Jover-Navalón JM, et al. Injury patterns from major urban terrorist bombings in trains: the Madrid experience. *World J Surg.* 2008;32(6):1168–1175.

22. Cernak I, Savic J, Malicevic Z, et al. Involvement of the central nervous system in the general response to pulmonary blast injury. *J Trauma.* 1996;40(3 suppl):S100–S104.

23. Knuth TLP, Ling G, Moores LE, Rhee P, Tauber D, Trask A. *Guidelines for the Field Management of Combat-Related Head Trauma.* New York, NY: Brain Trauma Foundation; 2005:1–95.

24. Armonda RA, Bell RS, Vo AH, et al. Wartime traumatic cerebral vasospasm: recent review of combat casualties. *Neurosurgery.* 2006;59(6):1215–25; discussion 1225.

25. Bell RS, Vo AH, Neal CJ, et al. Military traumatic brain and spinal column injury: a 5-year study of the impact blast and other military grade weaponry on the central nervous system. *J Trauma.* 2009;66(4 suppl):S104–S111.

26. Antibiotic prophylaxis for penetrating brain injury. *J Trauma.* 2001;51(2 suppl):S34–S40.

27. Chen JW, Ruff RL, Eavey R, Wasterlain CG. Posttraumatic epilepsy and treatment. *J Rehabil Res Dev.* 2009;46(6):685–696.

28. Lew HL, Garvert DW, Pogoda TK, et al. Auditory and visual impairments in patients with blast-related traumatic brain injury: Effect of dual sensory impairment on Functional Independence Measure. *J Rehabil Res Dev.* 2009;46(6):819–826.

29. Brahm KD, Wilgenburg HM, Kirby J, Ingalla S, Chang CY, Goodrich GL. Visual impairment and dysfunction in combat-injured servicemembers with traumatic brain injury. *Optom Vis Sci.* 2009;86(7):817–825.

64

Treatment and Rehabilitation Services for Mild to Moderate Traumatic Brain Injury in the Military

Grant L. Iverson and Louis M. French

INTRODUCTION

- Traumatic brain injuries (TBIs) in the military can occur before, during, or after operational deployment. Although most are mild in degree, these injuries can result in serious short-term physical, emotional, and cognitive symptoms, and sometimes result in long-term changes in functioning.
- Many service members experience a combination of physical injuries, psychological trauma, and mild TBI. A mild TBI and traumatic stress reaction can occur as a result of the same event, or separate events. Service members who are wounded in combat are at an increased risk for chronic pain conditions [1], depression [2], and posttraumatic stress disorder (PTSD) [3].

SCOPE OF THE PROBLEM

- The United States Department of Defense (DoD) classification system for TBI is presented in Table 63.1. The estimated numbers of TBIs per year, based on DoD surveillance statistics and stratified by severity, are provided in Table 63.2.
- Postdeployment screening studies have yielded far greater estimates for mild TBI in military personnel returning from Iraq and Afghanistan (e.g., 11.2% to 22.8%) [4,5], although these estimates have methodological limitations that limit their accuracy [6]. It is essential to appreciate that screening positive for a mild TBI on a questionnaire is not definitive evidence that the injury actually occurred. Moreover, screening estimates do not yield data on the numbers of military personnel that suffer from residual symptoms or cognitive deficits that are directly

Table 64.1 US DoD Traumatic Brain Injury Classification System

Classification	Duration of Unconsciousness	AOC	Posttraumatic Amnesia
Mild	<30 minutes	A moment up to 24 hours	<24 hours
Moderate	30 minutes to 24 hours	If AOC > 24 hours, then severity based on other criteria	1–7 days
Severe	>24 hours		>7 days

AOC, alteration of consciousness

attributable to a brain injury [6]. Follow-up clinical evaluations are necessary to make such determinations.

COMORBIDITIES

- PTSD—A substantial minority of service members screen positive for PTSD on postdeployment questionnaires [3]. Screening positive for PTSD is associated with number of deployments [7], deployment-related stressors [8], greater combat exposure [9], getting wounded [10], sustaining a mild TBI [4], and greater general medical burden [11]. Careful diagnostic interviewing by a clinician results in more accurate identification of combat-related PTSD and reduces false-positive diagnoses [12,13]. Depression frequently co-occurs with PTSD in military personnel [4,13].

- Depression—In postdeployment surveys, 5.7% to 15.7% of service members screen positive for depression [14,15], although some surveys of those in the Veterans Administration (VA) care system have shown rates of 39% to 48% [16]. Similar to screening estimates for mild TBI and PTSD, these prevalence estimates decline when screening is followed by interviewing with a clinician [13]. Symptoms of depression are very similar to symptoms associated with postconcussion syndrome [17].

- Amputation—Between September 2001 and January 2009, there were 1,286 service members who underwent an amputation. These individuals often experienced other orthopedic injuries, internal organ injuries, and/or brain injuries. Some of these service members developed PTSD, depression, chronic pain, or a combination of these problems. Individuals undergoing amputations are at significant risk for depression, anxiety, and body image problems [18].

- Body image—Military personnel who suffer facial disfigurement, complex scars to their limbs or torso, spinal cord injuries, or amputations

Table 64.2 Traumatic Brain Injuries in the Military: 2000–2009

	2000	2001	2002	2003	2004	2005	2006	2007	2008	2009
Total	10,963	11,830	12,469	12,886	13,271	12,025	16,873	23,002	28,557	27,862
Mild	6,340	7,779	8,998	9,795	10,542	9,778	13,989	18,775	22,038	21,859
Moderate	4,141	3,536	3,058	2,618	2,240	1,803	2,328	3,456	2,999	3,059
Severe	174	186	149	167	145	151	186	194	226	258
Penetrating	271	290	223	270	310	234	299	349	420	404
Not classifiable	37	39	41	36	34	59	1	228	2874	2282

Source: Defense and Veterans Brain Injury Center, http://www.dvbic.org/TBI-Numbers.aspx Downloaded May 16, 2010. Numbers were extracted from tables.

frequently deal with psychological problems relating to their body image. Psychological adjustment issues and problems associated with body image can interfere with social and occupational functioning.

- Chronic pain—Pain lasting more than 6 months is defined as chronic. Chronic pain is a common problem in veterans [19], and it is frequently comorbid with TBI [20]. People who suffer from chronic pain often report subjectively experienced cognitive impairment [21], and they are likely to report postconcussion-like symptoms in the absence of a past mild TBI [22]. Those with chronic pain are also at risk for comorbid depression.

- Insomnia—Problems with sleep often occur during deployment [23], and they are commonly reported post deployment [24]. Persistent problems with falling asleep, staying asleep, or waking too early can occur as a primary insomnia condition or be associated with a comorbid condition (e.g., depression, PTSD, or chronic pain). Sleep problems can be associated with obesity [25] or tinnitus [26]. People with chronic sleep problems often report perceived cognitive problems [24].

- Substance misuse and dependence—Substance misuse and dependence can be a problem for service members and veterans. This problem can have an adverse effect on cognition, co-occur with mental health problems, and cause problems with social and occupational functioning.

- Life stress and community re-entry issues—Some service members struggle with resuming their home and work life and responsibilities following deployment [27]. These problems can be compounded by the stress of being deployed again after less than a year home. Repeated deployments can contribute to PTSD symptoms [7]. This life stress can contribute to substance misuse and mental health problems.

TREATMENT AND REHABILITATION SERVICES

- In-theatre management of mild TBI:
  - A clinical practice guideline sets out the procedures for managing an uncomplicated mild TBI during deployment (see Additional Reading: Web Sites).

- In-theatre management of moderate-to-severe TBI and military echelons of care:
  - Level I care is unit level care provided by medics at the point of injury. Level II care involves the Forward Surgical Team, where physicians can provide trauma life support and surgical stabilization. Level III care is the Combat Support Hospital, which provides intensive care unit and medical subspecialty care. This is also the point for medical evacuation as necessary to level IV care. Level IV care involves transport out of the war zone, usually en route

to the United States. In this conflict, level IV care is at Landstuhl Regional Medical Center in Germany. Level V care is represented by a Military Treatment Facility (MTF) in the United States. Current major MTFs include Walter Reed Army Medical Center, National Naval Medical Center, Brooke Army Medical Center, Madigan Army Medical Center, and Tripler Army Medical Center. In some cases, following stabilization and treatment, specialized rehabilitation is provided through the VA polytrauma care system [28].

- Guidelines for the in-theatre management of moderate to severe TBI were developed by the Defense and Veterans Brain Injury Center and the Brain Trauma Foundation in 2005. They can be found at: https://www.braintrauma.org/pdf/protected/btf_field_management_guidelines.pdf
- Recent military experience, especially as related to blast-related head trauma, has highlighted the importance of aggressive treatment of cerebral vasospasm [29], and the use of early decompressive craniectomy for penetrating and severe closed injuries [30]. A discussion of the evolution of the treatment of traumatic cerebrovascular injury during wartime can be found in Bell et al. [31].

- Service members who have experienced polytrauma may suffer from chronic pain, insomnia, depression, and/or PTSD [1,32]. It is important to aggressively treat chronic pain, and it is often helpful to focus treatment and rehabilitation services on the comorbidities of chronic pain and anxiety [33]. Depression frequently occurs following TBI, and when present it can be associated with both anxiety and aggressive behavior [34].
- General principles for providing treatment and rehabilitation services, from the VA/DoD Clinical Practice Guidelines [35], are reprinted in Table 63.3.
- For service members with complex comorbidities, treatment and rehabilitation services are often multimodal and interdisciplinary. Some components are listed in the following:
  - Medications (e.g., for sleep, headaches, bodily pain, and mental health)
  - Physical therapy [36], including treatment of vestibular problems and dizziness
  - Occupational therapy [37], including assessment and treatment of cognitive dysfunction and its effect on activities of daily living
  - Speech and language pathology—for the assessment of swallowing disorders after severe TBI or polytrauma, especially involving the face; and for the assessment and treatment of cognitive-communication disorders [38]
  - Physical conditioning and exercise—moderate-intensity aerobic exercise has been associated with positive effects on mood and

Table 64.3 General Principles for Providing Treatment and Rehabilitation Services

Treatment of somatic complaints (e.g., sleep, dizziness or coordination problems, vision, fatigue) should be based upon individual factors and symptom presentation
Headache is the single most common symptom and assessment and management of headaches in individuals should parallel those for other causes of headache
Medication for ameliorating the neurocognitive effects attributed to mild TBI is not recommended
Medications for headaches, musculoskeletal pain, or depression or anxiety should be carefully prescribed to avoid the sedating properties, which can have an impact upon a person's attention, cognition, and motor functioning
Treatment of psychiatric symptoms and problems should be based upon individual factors and the nature and severity of symptom presentation, and may include both psychotherapeutic and pharmacological treatment modalities
In patients with persistent postconcussive symptoms that have been refractory to treatment, consideration should be given to other factors including psychiatric, psychosocial support, and compensatory or litigation issues

Source: The Management of Concussion/mTBI Working Group. (2009). *VA/ DoD clinical practice guideline for management of concussion/mild traumatic brain injury (mTBI)*. Retrieved April 18, 2010, from http://www.healthquality. va.gov/mtbi/concussion_mtbi_full_1_0.pdf

self-esteem, and it promotes a general sense of well-being. In clinical populations, exercise has been shown to be a good adjunctive treatment for depression and anxiety, and there is some evidence that it is associated with reduced pain and disability in patients with chronic low back pain [39]. There is evidence that exercise promotes neurogenesis [40], and researchers are beginning to use exercise as a treatment modality for people who are slow to recover from a mild TBI [41].

- Psychological treatment—effective for reducing symptoms and improving functioning in patients with PTSD [42], and there is some evidence that psychological treatment can reduce symptoms in patients with comorbid mild TBI and anxiety problems [43]. Psychological and behavioral treatments can also be effective for improving sleep and reducing psychological distress in people with insomnia [24].

- The primary goal of treatment and rehabilitation in military personnel who have persistent symptoms and comorbidities is to reduce symptoms and improve functioning. Specific recommendations for treatment and rehabilitation can be found in the VA/DoD Clinical Practice Guideline listed under electronic references. Further information about treatment of specific TBI-related conditions and comorbidities is as described elsewhere throughout this text.

ADDITIONAL READING

Electronic Reference
The Management of Concussion/mTBI Working Group. *VA/DoD clinical practice guideline for management of concussion/mild traumatic brain injury (mTBI)*. 2009. http://www.healthquality.va.gov/mtbi/concussion_mtbi_full_1_0.pdf

Textbooks/Chapters
Committee on the Initial Assessment of Readjustment Needs of Military Personnel V, and Their Families, Populations BotHoS, Medicine Io. *Returning Home from Iraq and Afghanistan: Preliminary Assessment of Readjustment Needs of Veterans, Service Members, and Their Families*. Washington, DC: The National Academies Press; 2010.

Tanielian T, Jaycox LH, eds. *Invisible Wounds of War: Psychological and Cognitive Injuries, Their Consequences, and Services to Assist Recovery*. Santa Monica, CA: Rand Corporation; 2008.

Journal Articles
Belanger HG, Uomoto JM, Vanderploeg RD. The veterans health administration system of care for mild traumatic brain injury: costs, benefits, and controversies. *J Head Trauma Rehabil*. 2009;24(1):4–13.

McCrea M, Pliskin N, Barth J, et al. Official position of the military TBI task force on the role of neuropsychology and rehabilitation psychology in the evaluation, management, and research of military veterans with traumatic brain injury. *Clin Neuropsychol*. 2008;22(1):10–26.

Okie S. Traumatic brain injury in the war zone. *N Engl J Med*. 2005;352(20):2043–2047.

Rohling ML, Faust ME, Beverly B, Demakis G. Effectiveness of cognitive rehabilitation following acquired brain injury: a meta-analytic re-examination of Cicerone et al's (2000, 2005) systematic reviews. *Neuropsychology*. 2009;23(1):20–39.

REFERENCES

1. Dobscha SK, Clark ME, Morasco BJ, Freeman M, Campbell R, Helfand M. Systematic review of the literature on pain in patients with polytrauma including traumatic brain injury. *Pain Med*. 2009;10(7):1200–1217.

2. Grieger TA, Cozza SJ, Ursano RJ, et al. Posttraumatic stress disorder and depression in battle-injured soldiers. *Am J Psychiatry*. 2006;163(10):1777–83; quiz 1860.

3. Ramchand R, Schell TL, Karney BR, Osilla KC, Burns RM, Caldarone LB. Disparate prevalence estimates of PTSD among service members who served in Iraq and Afghanistan: possible explanations. *J Trauma Stress*. 2010;23(1):59–68.

4. Hoge CW, McGurk D, Thomas JL, Cox AL, Engel CC, Castro CA. Mild traumatic brain injury in U.S. soldiers returning from Iraq. *N Engl J Med.* 2008;358(5):453–463.

5. Terrio H, Brenner LA, Ivins BJ, et al. Traumatic brain injury screening: preliminary findings in a US Army Brigade Combat Team. *J Head Trauma Rehabil.* 2009;24(1):14–23.

6. Iverson GL, Langlois JA, McCrea MA, Kelly JP. Challenges associated with post-deployment screening for mild traumatic brain injury in military personnel. *Clin Neuropsychol.* 2009;23(8):1299–1314.

7. Reger MA, Gahm GA, Swanson RD, Duma SJ. Association between number of deployments to Iraq and mental health screening outcomes in US Army soldiers. *J Clin Psychiatry.* 2009;70(9):1266–1272.

8. Booth-Kewley S, Larson GE, Highfill-McRoy RM, Garland CF, Gaskin TA. Correlates of posttraumatic stress disorder symptoms in Marines back from war. *J Trauma Stress.* 2010;23(1):69–77.

9. Vasterling JJ, Proctor SP, Friedman MJ, et al. PTSD symptom increases in Iraq-deployed soldiers: comparison with nondeployed soldiers and associations with baseline symptoms, deployment experiences, and postdeployment stress. *J Trauma Stress.* 2010;23(1):41–51.

10. Koren D, Norman D, Cohen A, Berman J, Klein EM. Increased PTSD risk with combat-related injury: a matched comparison study of injured and uninjured soldiers experiencing the same combat events. *Am J Psychiatry.* 2005;162(2):276–282.

11. Hoge CW, Terhakopian A, Castro CA, Messer SC, Engel CC. Association of posttraumatic stress disorder with somatic symptoms, health care visits, and absenteeism among Iraq war veterans. *Am J Psychiatry.* 2007;164(1):150–153.

12. Hill JJ III, Mobo BH Jr, Cullen MR. Separating deployment-related traumatic brain injury and posttraumatic stress disorder in veterans: preliminary findings from the Veterans Affairs traumatic brain injury screening program. *Am J Phys Med Rehabil.* 2009;88(8):605–614.

13. Vasterling JJ, Schumm J, Proctor SP, Gentry E, King DW, King LA. Posttraumatic stress disorder and health functioning in a non-treatment-seeking sample of Iraq war veterans: a prospective analysis. *J Rehabil Res Dev.* 2008;45(3):347–358.

14. Hoge CW, Castro CA, Messer SC, McGurk D, Cotting DI, Koffman RL. Combat duty in Iraq and Afghanistan, mental health problems, and barriers to care. *N Engl J Med.* 2004;351(1):13–22.

15. Wells TS, LeardMann CA, Fortuna SO, et al.; Millennium Cohort Study Team. A prospective study of depression following combat deployment in support of the wars in Iraq and Afghanistan. *Am J Public Health.* 2010;100(1):90–99.

16. Haskell SG, Gordon KS, Mattocks K, et al. Gender differences in rates of depression, PTSD, pain, obesity, and military sexual trauma among Connecticut War Veterans of Iraq and Afghanistan. *J Womens Health (Larchmt).* 2010;19(2):267–271.

17. Iverson GL. Misdiagnosis of the persistent postconcussion syndrome in patients with depression. *Arch Clin Neuropsychol.* 2006;21(4):303–310.

18. Horgan O, MacLachlan M. Psychosocial adjustment to lower-limb amputation: a review. *Disabil Rehabil.* 2004;26(14–15):837–850.

19. Gironda RJ, Clark ME, Massengale JP, Walker RL. Pain among veterans of Operations Enduring Freedom and Iraqi Freedom. *Pain Med.* 2006;7(4):339–343.

20. Nampiaparampil DE. Prevalence of chronic pain after traumatic brain injury: a systematic review. *JAMA.* 2008;300(6):711–719.

21. Smith-Seemiller L, Fow NR, Kant R, Franzen MD. Presence of post-concussion syndrome symptoms in patients with chronic pain vs mild traumatic brain injury. *Brain Inj.* 2003;17(3):199–206.

22. Iverson GL, McCracken LM. 'Postconcussive' symptoms in persons with chronic pain. *Brain Inj.* 1997;11(11):783–790.

23. Peterson AL, Goodie JL, Satterfield WA, Brim WL. Sleep disturbance during military deployment. *Mil Med.* 2008;173(3):230–235.

24. Zeitzer JM, Hubbard J, Litsch S, Luzon A, Friedman L, O'Hara R. Sleep disorders in the context of traumatic brain injury. In: *State of the Art (SOTA).* Arlington, VA: Department of Veterans Affairs; 2008.

25. Kryger MH, Pouliot Z, Peters M, Neufeld H, Delaive K. Sleep disorders in a military population. *Mil Med.* 2003;168(1):7–10.

26. Alster J, Shemesh Z, Ornan M, Attias J. Sleep disturbance associated with chronic tinnitus. *Biol Psychiatry.* 1993;34(1–2):84–90.

27. Sayers SL, Farrow VA, Ross J, Oslin DW. Family problems among recently returned military veterans referred for a mental health evaluation. *J Clin Psychiatry.* 2009;70(2):163–170.

28. MacLennan D, Clausen S, Pagel N, et al. Developing a polytrauma rehabilitation center: a pioneer experience in building, staffing, and training. *Rehabil Nurs.* 2008;33(5):198–204, 213.

29. Armonda RA, Bell RS, Vo AH, et al. Wartime traumatic cerebral vasospasm: recent review of combat casualties. *Neurosurgery.* 2006;59(6):1215–25; discussion 1225.

30. Bell RS, Mossop CM, Dirks MS, et al. Early decompressive craniectomy for severe penetrating and closed head injury during wartime. *Neurosurg Focus.* 2010;28(5):E1.

31. Bell RS, Ecker RD, Severson MA 3rd, Wanebo JE, Crandall B, Armonda RA. The evolution of the treatment of traumatic cerebrovascular injury during wartime. *Neurosurg Focus.* 2010;28(5):E5.

32. Sayer NA, Chiros CE, Sigford B, et al. Characteristics and rehabilitation outcomes among patients with blast and other injuries sustained during the Global War on Terror. *Arch Phys Med Rehabil.* 2008;89(1):163–170.

33. Asmundson GJ, Katz J. Understanding the co-occurrence of anxiety disorders and chronic pain: state-of-the-art. *Depress Anxiety.* 2009;26(10):888–901.

34. Jorge RE, Robinson RG, Moser D, Tateno A, Crespo-Facorro B, Arndt S. Major depression following traumatic brain injury. *Arch Gen Psychiatry.* 2004;61(1):42–50.

35. The Management of Concussion/mTBI Working Group. VA/DoD clinical practice guideline for management of concussion/mild traumatic brain injury (mTBI). 2009. Accessed April 18, 2010 from http://www.healthquality.va.gov/mtbi/concussion_mtbi_full_1_0.pdf

36. Radomski MV, Davidson L, Voydetich D, Erickson MW. Occupational therapy for service members with mild traumatic brain injury. *Am J Occup Ther.* 2009;63(5):646–655.

37. Weightman MM, Bolgla R, McCulloch KL, Peterson MD. Physical therapy recommendations for service members with mild traumatic brain injury. *J Head Trauma Rehabil.* 2010;25(3):206–218.

38. American Speech-Language-Hearing Association. Roles of speech-language pathologists in the identification, diagnosis, and treatment of individuals with cognitive-communication disorders: Position statement; 2005. Accessed from www.asha.org/policy

39. Bell JA, Burnett A. Exercise for the primary, secondary and tertiary prevention of low back pain in the workplace: a systematic review. *J Occup Rehabil.* 2009;19(1):8–24.

40. van Praag H. Neurogenesis and exercise: past and future directions. *Neuromolecular Med.* 2008;10(2):128–140.

41. Leddy JJ, Kozlowski K, Donnelly JP, Pendergast DR, Epstein LH, Willer B. A preliminary study of subsymptom threshold exercise training for refractory post-concussion syndrome. *Clin J Sport Med.* 2010;20(1):21–27.

42. Bisson J, Andrew M. Psychological treatment of post-traumatic stress disorder (PTSD). *Cochrane Database Syst Rev.* 2007;3:CD003388.

43. Soo C, Tate R. Psychological treatment for anxiety in people with traumatic brain injury. *Cochrane Database Syst Rev.* 2007;(3):CD005239.

65

Management of Traumatic Brain Injury in the Older Adult

Sheital Bavishi and David Cifu

INTRODUCTION

This chapter will review the general aspects of traumatic brain injury (TBI) rehabilitation with a focus on the older adult (aged 65 and older).

DEMOGRAPHICS ON AGING

In the United States, the proportion of the population aged 65 years and older is projected to increase from 12.4% in 2000 to 19.6% in 2030. The number of persons aged 65 years and older is expected to increase from approximately 35 million in 2000 to an estimated 71 million in 2030, and the number of persons aged 80 years and older is expected to increase from 9.3 million in 2000 to 19.5 million in 2030 [1].

ETIOLOGY OF INJURY AND INJURY PREVENTION

Older adults (aged 65 and above) have the second highest rate of hospitalization for TBI. Falls are the leading cause of TBI for older adults (51%), followed by motor vehicle traffic crashes (9%) [2].

Risk Factors for falls may be stratified: (1) chronic (i.e., neurological disease, sensory impairment, dementia, general medical condition, or musculoskeletal disease, particularly affecting the lower extremities), (2) short-term (i.e., episodic postural hypotension, acute illness, alcohol use, or medication effects), (3) activity related (i.e., tripping while walking, descending stairs, climbing ladders), and (4) environmental (i.e., poor lighting, nonsecure throw rugs, or ill-fitting shoes). Slow reaction time and walking pace can also predispose older adults to motor vehicle accidents and pedestrian accidents, respectively [2,3].

MECHANISM OF INJURY

Falls, which are typically low velocity injuries, result in focal brain injuries, most commonly subdural hematomas (SDH) and/or focal cortical contusions [4]. Elders on anticoagulation have a higher likelihood of having intracerebral hemorrhages after a fall. Motor vehicle crashes may result in diffuse axonal injury (DAI), focal contusions, or SDHs [5]. Pedestrian-motor vehicle collisions frequently occur at crosswalks and in parking lots. These accidents result in DAI, SDH, or focal contusions but can also involve skeletal trauma and visceral injuries. Assaults and violent acts, although rare, are increasing among elderly people, and may result in focal contusions, skull fractures with SDH, epidural hematomas, and intracranial bone or bullet fragments.

When compared with younger individuals, older adults most often have an initial Glasgow Coma Scale score of 13 to 15 (i.e., mild TBI), with a time from onset of injury to following commands usually at 1 day or less. SDH is also more common in older adults than in younger individuals. Elderly individuals are particularly vulnerable to SDH because bridging veins become more susceptible to shearing forces as the brain naturally atrophies with advancing age. Because older adults more frequently experience TBI due to falls, often resulting in focal cortical injury (in contrast to high velocity events with more diffuse injuries), they spend less time in coma as compared to younger individuals [6].

MORBIDITY

TBI in the older adult often results in a higher morbidity because of concomitant medical problems. These medical problems can be the determining factors for acute discharge planning to an independent rehabilitation facility as compared to a skilled nursing facility. A brain injury physiatrist should be involved from the initial hospitalization to assist in minimizing the effects of prolonged bedrest (i.e., prevention of pressure sores, contractures, deep venous thromboembolism, cardiac deconditioning, aspiration precautions, bowel/bladder management), as well as comorbidities, such as cardiovascular disease, diabetes, neuromuscular disease, and dementia, which may have challenged function before injury.

COMMON COMORBID COMPLICATIONS

- Fractures—affect weight-bearing status and need for assistance
- Cardiopulmonary complications—low ejection fraction and vital capacity can affect ability to participate in rehabilitation and live independently

- Pain—can be preinjury neuropathic, musculoskeletal or vascular pain, or postinjury pain caused by trauma. Regardless of cause, pain must be assessed and treated appropriately
- Swallowing—may be compromised from injury or preexisting pathology (e.g., cerebrovascular accident), resulting in need for alternative feeding methods or modified diet
- Polypharmacy—specific to older adults who may be on multiple preinjury medications and may have difficulty managing medication administration instructions
- Deep venous thrombosis prophylaxis and treatment—need to consider both optimal timing of initiating prophylaxis as well as whether fall risk mitigates against starting therapeutic anticoagulation

REHABILITATION

The rehabilitation approach to an older adult with TBI requires an understanding of preinjury level of functional deficits, medical comorbidities, cognitive limitations, and behavioral issues. In addition to a thorough medical review of the older adult, a detailed review of the elder's social support network is critical. This is a key factor to help focus the rehabilitation program, to help develop needed goals to facilitate discharge planning.

Specific areas of focus in a rehabilitation program for the older adult are discussed in the following sections.

Medication Management

The majority of the population above 65 years of age takes at least one prescription medication daily, and over-the-counter medications are used commonly. Medications may change in the acute and chronic recovery periods. Therefore, medication education is important when transitioning a patient through the acute phase to rehabilitation and eventually to discharge from a hospital setting.

Substance Abuse

Alcoholism is one of the most common mental disorders among elderly men in the United States. Screening for substance abuse is vital in older adults. Current treatments for substance abuse are designed for the younger adult and are often held in group settings, which may not be the best setting for the older adult. An aggressive, tailored treatment program for substance abuse in the older adult is important. Family education is a key component of these programs.

Elder Abuse

Elder abuse has been increasing in prevalence, especially among those with poor social support. Not only physical abuse, but also emotional (e.g., neglect), financial, and emotional abuse are increasing. The importance of understanding a person's social support and family education cannot be emphasized enough in the rehabilitation program after a TBI [7].

Bladder and Bowel Continence

Normal aging may affect bladder function because of prostate hypertrophy (in men), pelvic relaxation (in women), decreased bladder capacity with urinary frequency, and decreased capability to suppress bladder contractions at low volumes resulting in urinary urgency [8]. TBI can result in urinary incontinence related to an inability to sense bladder fullness, an inability to suppress the pontine micturition center's automatic emptying at key volumes, or increased frequency caused by a urinary tract infection [9]. Assessment of preinjury voiding patterns is helpful in discerning underlying pathology, independent of the effects of TBI.

As with the bladder, bowel routines are typically disrupted during hospitalization. In the older adult, disruption of the bowel routine can become a preoccupation unless properly addressed. Assessing preinjury bowel routine is the first step in establishing goals. Continence should be a significant focus of rehabilitation efforts in older adults, because this can determine an individual's independence and level of caregiver burden.

Sensory Health

Vision

Normal aging is associated with changes in visual acuity and refractive power, decrements in extraocular motion, increases in intraocular pressure, decreased tear secretion, and decreased corneal and lens function. Finding easily correctable visual problems can aid in the rehabilitation process.

Hearing

Normal aging is associated with high frequency hearing loss and signal distortion at higher frequencies, difficulty localizing signals needed for binaural hearing, and difficulty understanding speech in unfavorable listening conditions. Traumatic injuries can result in disruption of the ossicular chain, or cranial nerve VIII can be selectively damaged. Preinjury hearing aids may be less effective, which can hinder the accurate communication needed to help older adults through the rehabilitation process.

Smell

The olfactory nerve is the most frequently injured cranial nerve in a TBI. Disruption of smell may affect an individual's appetite and the ability to detect burning objects. Home evaluation should include appropriate placement of smoke detectors.

Taste

Normal aging is accompanied by the loss of lingual papillae, decreased saliva volume, and relative decrement of taste acuity. Loss of smell caused by a TBI may further impair the sense of taste, which can result in poor oral intake.

Touch, Vibration, Joint Position Sense

Position sense diminishes with age, and this can be accelerated by the presence of peripheral neuropathy, which should be worked up and treated/managed. Compensation techniques and assistive devices may help an individual adapt to these impairments [10].

Behavior and Cognition

Dementia affects 3% to 11% of community-dwelling adults above the age of 65, and 20% to 50% of adults above the age of 85. Preinjury cognition and behavior as needs to be assessed in order to set appropriate rehabilitation goals. Neurostimulants, typically used to address arousal and attention in patients with TBI, should be used with caution in those with a history of arrhythmia [11].

Sleep Disturbance

Normalizing the sleep-wake cycle is important after a TBI. Behavioral and environmental modifications are usually the first line for improving sleep. In considering medication management, note the following considering specific to older adults: (1) diphenhydramine should not be used owing to the risk for urinary retention and cognitive worsening; (2) benzodiazepines should be avoided due to paradoxical reactions in the elderly people; and (3) tricyclic antidepressants can cause postural hypotension and urinary retention and are poorly tolerated.

Sexuality

Sexuality is commonly ignored in older adults, but at any age sexuality can give someone a sense of self, capacity to show love and affection, and maintain relationships. Normal aging can result in physiologic changes to the vaginal mucosa, erectile and orgasmic performance. Sexual desire may change (increase or decrease) after TBI; therefore, it is important to screen for sexual and relationship concerns in older adults. Sildenafil, tadalafil, and vardenafil are usually contraindicated in older adults because of cardiac conditions, such as coronary artery disease and hypertension [12].

Safety

Home evaluations are important to assess safety risks in the home to prevent future injury secondary to falls or wandering.

AGING WITH TBI

After a TBI, there can be an earlier onset of Alzheimer's dementia in a sub-population of those already susceptible to it [13]. In addition, repeated TBIs appear to predispose to accelerated degeneration of the brain, most classically seen in chronic traumatic encephalopathy [14]. Neuropsychological impairments after a TBI in the older adult often parallel the changes with normal aging, with diminished ability to attend, concentrate, and recall, although long-term recall is more often affected with aging.

OUTCOME

Data from the National Institute on Disability and Rehabilitation Research (NIDRR) TBI Model systems from 1995 to 2002 revealed that when compared with individuals aged 50 years or younger, individuals aged 55 years and older had only a 5-day longer rehabilitation length of stay and marginally higher costs but demonstrated greater disability as measured on the Disability Rating Scale (DRS) and Functional Independence Measure (FIM), and a decreased percentage of return to a private residence at discharge. On the Supervision Rating Scale (SRS), individuals aged 65 and above have demonstrated the need for a higher degree of supervision for their day-to-day care 1 year post injury [15].

COMMUNITY REINTEGRATION

Mobility can often be impaired after a TBI. Rehabilitation programs should focus on route finding, negotiating different terrains, and appropriate use of public transportation. This can help with an individual's ability to resume leisure activities and minimize feelings of isolation.

ADDITIONAL READING

Electronic Reference
http://biaoregon.org/seniors.htm

Textbook/Chapter

Englander J, Cifu DX, Tran TT. The older adult. In: Zasler N, Katz D, Zafonte R, eds. *Brain Injury Medicine: Principles and Practice.* New York, NY: Demos Medical Publishing; 2007:315–332.

Journal Articles

Bodenheimer C, Roig R, Worsowicz G, Cifu DX. Geriatric rehabilitation. 5. The societal aspects of disability in the older adult. *Arch Phys Med Rehabil.* 2004;85(7):23–26.

Duong TT, EnglanderJ, Wright J, Cifu DX, Greenwald BD, Brown AW. Relationship between strength, balance, and swallowing deficits to outcome after traumatic brain injury: a multicenter analysis. *Arch Phys Med Rehabil.* 2004;85:1291–1297.

Foxx-Orenstein A, Kolakowsky-Hayner S, Marwitz J, et al. Incidence, risk factors, and outcomes of fecal incontinence after acute brain injury: findings from the Traumatic Brain Injury Model Systems National Database. *Arch Phys Med Rehabil.* 2003;84:231–237.

Frankel J, Marwitz J, Cifu DX, Kreutzer JS, Englander J, Rosenthal M. A follow-up study of older adults with traumatic brain injury: taking into account decreasing length of stay. *Arch Phys Med Rehabil.* 2006;87:57–62.

Kreutzer JS, Kolakowsky-Hayner SA, Ripley D, et al. Charges and lengths of stay for acute and inpatient rehabilitation treatment of traumatic brain injury 1990–1996. *Brain Injury.* 2001;15(9):763–774.

Phillips E, Bodenheimer C, Roig R, Cifu DX. Geriatric rehabilitation 4. Physical medicine and rehabilitation interventions for age-related physiologic changes. *Arch Phys Med Rehabil.* 2004;85(7):18–22.

REFERENCES

1. U.S. Census Bureau. International database. Table 094. Midyear population, by age and sex. Available at http://www.census.gov/population/www/projections/natdet-D1A.html

2. Thompson HJ, McCormick WC, Kagan SH. Traumatic brain injury in older adults: epidemiology, outcomes, and future implications. *J Am Geriatr Soc.* 2006;54(10):1590–1595.

3. Tinetti ME, Speechley M. Prevention of falls among the elderly. *N Engl J Med.* 1989;320(16):1055–1059.

4. Rakier A, Guilburd JN, Soustiel JF, Zaaroor M, Feinsod M. Head injuries in the elderly. *Brain Inj.* 1995;9(2):187–193.

5. Katz DI, Alexander MP. Traumatic brain injury. Predicting course of recovery and outcome for patients admitted to rehabilitation. *Arch Neurol.* 1994;51(7):661–670.

6. TBI Model Systems National Data Center. TBI Model Systems Database. http://www.tbindsc.org/

7. Dyer CB, Picken S, Burnett J. When it is no longer safe to live alone. *JAMA.* 2007;298:1448–1450.

8. Chutka DS, Fleming KC, Evans MP, Evans JM, Andrews KL. Urinary incontinence in the elderly population. *Mayo Clin Proc.* 1996;71(1):93–101.

9. Opitz JL, Thornsteinsson G, Schutt AH, et al. Neurogenic bladder and bowel. In: *Rehabilitation Medicine: Principles and Practice*. 3rd ed. Philadelphia, PA: JB Lippincott; 1993:441–459.

10. Kane RL, Ouslander JG, Abrass IB. *Essentials of Clinical Geriatrics*. 4th ed. New York, NY: McGraw-Hill; 1999:256–291.

11. Flanagan SR, Hibbard MR, Riordan B, Gordon WA. Traumatic brain injury in the elderly: diagnostic and treatment challenges. *Clin Geriatr Med*. 2006;22(2):449–68; x.

12. Herstein GA, Griffith ER. Sexuality and sexual dysfunction. In: Rosenthal M, Griffith ER, Kreutzer JS, Pentland B, eds. *Rehabilitation of the Adult and Child with Traumatic Injury*. 3rd ed. Philadelphia, PA: FA Davis; 1999:470–502.

13. Koponen S, Taiminen T, Kairisto V, et al. APOE-epsilon4 predicts dementia but not other psychiatric disorders after traumatic brain injury. *Neurology*. 2004;63(4):749–750.

14. McKee AC, Cantu RC, Nowinski CJ, et al. Chronic traumatic encephalopathy in athletes: progressive tauopathy after repetitive head injury. *J Neuropathol Exp Neurol*. 2009;68(7):709–735.

15. Frankel JE, Marwitz JH, Cifu DX, Kreutzer JS, Englander J, Rosenthal M. A follow-up study of older adults with traumatic brain injury: taking into account decreasing length of stay. *Arch Phys Med Rehabil*. 2006;87(1):57–62.

66

Complementary and Alternative Medicine in Traumatic Brain Injury

Felise S. Zollman

BACKGROUND

Definitions

- Complementary and alternative medicine (CAM)—a group of diverse medical and healthcare systems, practices, and products that are not generally considered to be part of conventional medicine [1].
- Conventional medicine—current accepted Western medical practice.
- Complementary medicine—modalities that complement—but don't replace—conventional medical interventions.
- Alternative medicine—modalities used in lieu of conventional medical interventions.

Partial Listing of CAM Practices

Homeopathy/naturopathy; herbal medicine; aromatherapy; relaxation techniques (meditation, hypnosis, music or humor therapy, guided imagery); biofeedback; energy-based therapies (healing touch, reflexology, Reiki, massage); craniosacral manipulation; electromagnetic therapy (transcranial magnetic stimulation, crystals); movement therapies (Alexander, Feldenkrais, Qi Gong, Tai Qi, Yoga); hyperbaric oxygen; Chinese medicine/acupuncture. This chapter will focus on those areas for which there is published data addressing use in those with TBI.

Published Data in TBI Exists for the Following

Meditation (Mindfulness)
Basic principles:

- Mindfulness is a form of meditation, which involves attending to relevant aspects of one's experience in a nonjudgmental manner. The goal of mindfulness is to maintain awareness moment by moment, disengaging oneself from strong attachment to beliefs, thoughts, or emotions, thereby developing a greater sense of emotional balance and well-being [2].

Mindfulness in traumatic brain injury (TBI):

- Trisha Meili (the "Central Park Jogger") describes learning to "live inside again." In contrast to prevailing medical views, Meili sees lack of memory and insight as an opportunity to develop the ability to focus on the present ("Here it is.... This is my situation"), not as an impairment to be overcome [3].
- In a pilot intervention study, 10 subjects attended 12 weekly group sessions consisting of meditation, breathing exercises, guided visualization, and group discussion. Outcome: SF-36 (a widely recognized life satisfaction scale in which higher numbers indicate greater satisfaction) increased from 37 to 52 [4]

Tai Qi/Qi Gong (Also Known as Tai Chi, Chi Gong, Qi Quong)

- Basic principles: Tai Qi, literally meaning "great energy," is both a healing art and martial arts discipline. Qi Gong literally means "energy work." Qi Gong generally involves slower movements, and is considered easier to perform; there is a specific focus on mindfulness and physical health.
- Tai Qi in TBI: while the literature is scant, two case series and one case/control study showed beneficial effects with respect to motor function [5], mood [6,7], and/or self-esteem [7].

Acupuncture

Basic principles:

- From a Chinese medicine perspective, the human body is viewed as a microcosmic reflection of the universe. The physician's role is to aid in maintenance of harmonious balance, both internally and in relation to the external environment.
- Vital energy, known as "Qi," flows through channels, or meridians, creating an interwoven network of circulation.
- Meridians are a multilayered, interconnecting network of channels or energy pathways that establish an interface between an individual's internal and external environments. These energy pathways are named for organs whose realms of influence are expanded from their conventional biomedical physiology to include functional, energetic, and metaphorical qualities. Pathology involves disharmony/disruption of energy flow [8]. The relationship between these organs and their broader spheres of influence is often represented via a Table of Correspondences:

Table 66.1 Table of Correspondences

Element	Water	Wood	Fire	Earth	Metal
Season	Winter	Spring	Summer	Late summer	Fall
Associated pathogen	Cold	Wind	Heat	Damp	Dryness
Yin organ	Kidney	Liver	Heart and SNS[a]	Spleen	Lung
Yang organ	Bladder	Gallbladder	Small intestine and PNS[b]	Stomach	Large intestine
Primary sense organ	Ears	Eyes	Tongue	Mouth	Nose
Body tissue	Bone	Ligaments and tendons	Blood	Muscles	Skin
Emotion	Fear	Anger	Joy/Mania	Worry	Grief
Taste	Salty	Sour	Bitter	Sweet	Spicy
Color	Blue	Green	Red	Yellow	White

[a] Sympathetic nervous system (also known as pericardium or master of the heart).
[b] Parasympathetic nervous system (also known as triple heater or triple burner).

Source: Adapted from Beinfield H, Korngold, E. *Between Heaven and Earth: A Guide to Chinese Medicine.* New York: Ballantine Books; 1992.

- The five-phases approach to diagnosis: The dynamic energy balance among pathways/organs can be viewed diagrammatically by arranging five elements, and the organs with which they are associated, as follows (Figure 66.1, on facing page).
- Any of the correspondences (e.g., emotions, organs) from Table 66.1 can be overlaid onto this construct to understand the relative influence of one to the other. For example, the emotion of *water* is fear, the emotion of *wood* is anger or irritability, and the emotion of *fire* is joy/mania. The five-phases relationship tells us that fear nourishes anger and controls (or mitigates) joy/mania.

Use of acupuncture in TBI:

- TBI from a Chinese medicine perspective: Two syndromes are typically recognized: *Qibi* (or blockage of Qi)—presents with an agitated, hyperadrenergic state; *Qituo* (or exhaustion of Qi)—presents with

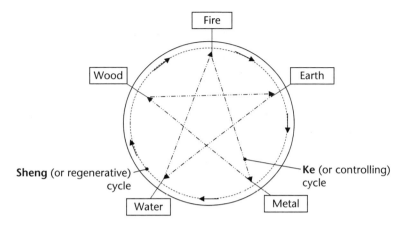

Figure 66.1 5-phases relationships.

unresponsiveness. Additional factors may include Kidney Yin deficiency and Liver Yin deficiency/Liver Yang excess (capitalized organ names represent both associated characteristic energetic qualities and meridian pathway labels).

- Though the data is again scant, acupuncture has been reported to be of benefit in TBI, both with respect to improvement in level of consciousness, as well as outcomes [9,10]. One study in particular, an interventional controlled study of subjects in coma, compared 17 subjects to 15 historical controls. Diagnoses included TBI and ruptured internal carotid artery. Subjects within 1 week of injury underwent four acupuncture treatments at 12-hour intervals: "A significantly greater number of patients in the acupuncture group (59%) had a >50% neurological recovery, than the patients in the no acupuncture group (20%) (P = .025)." Study conclusion: Early acupuncture intervention may be a reasonable adjunctive treatment for brain-injured patients [10]. Acupuncture has also been shown to be of benefit in treating insomnia Post-TBI [11].

ASSESSMENT

- Determine candidacy for a particular intervention.
  - For meditation/mindfulness: Is the individual able to attend to the mindfulness exercise? Is trying to develop focused attention more likely to increase the patient's frustration level, or is it valuable to him/her to hone this skill?
  - For Tai Qi/Qi Gong: Probably most appropriate for addressing balance/motor deficits, though there is a component of mindfulness about movement that might (theoretically) aid attention as well.

- Acupuncture: (1) Will the patient tolerate needle placement? For a Rancho Level IV patient in particular, this may be a challenge. (2) What is the goal of treatment? It's important to identify specific impairments or functional gains which are to be the focus of treatment and monitor progress accordingly.

- Ensure that appropriately trained/qualified providers are available to provide the service being considered. For example, acupuncturists may be (1) physicians trained in medical acupuncture, (2) licensed acupuncturists (typically trained as Oriental Medical Doctors), and occasionally (3) chiropractors. Physician acupuncturists may be located via the Academy of Medical Acupuncture website [see Electronic References]. Consider the medical complexity of the situation in identifying an appropriate provider: patients who have significant medical comorbidities (such as someone with a moderate to severe TBI) may be better served by seeing a physician acupuncturist, while someone with residual sequelae of a mild TBI (e.g., headaches, fatigue) may be just as well served by seeing a licensed acupuncturist.

TREATMENT

Meditation/mindfulness:

- Fundamental principle involves attending to the present and to awareness of self. This process is undertaken in a nonjudgmental fashion, observing our natural tendency for our mind to stray, then returning to self-awareness [2].
- This process can be facilitated via breathing exercises, guided imagery, and use of external cues (e.g., meditative object).

Tai Qi/Qi Gong:

- Both disciplines incorporate smooth, balanced movement with mindfulness.
- Specific "forms" are intended to promote the smooth flow of Qi along certain meridians and/or (particularly with respect to Qi Gong) for the purpose of nourishing certain organs or organ qualities.

Acupuncture:

- The technique involves penetrating the skin with thin, solid, metallic needles that are manipulated by the hands, using a heat source, or by electrical stimulation [12].
- Acupuncture treatment is designed to restore the smooth balanced flow of Qi through meridian channels and their associated organs. This is accomplished through the manipulation of acupuncture points, primarily via the use of needles.
- Acupuncture needles have unique bioelectrical characteristics:
- They are typically bimetallic (e.g., stainless steel shaft, copper/silver/bronze alloy handle) and therefore effectively create a battery.

One needle inserted causes local agitation. Two or more needles cause a directional current flow. Current flow can be enhanced with the use of heat and electricity.

- Once needles are placed, they may be manipulated in one of the following ways: (a) no manipulation/neutral/dispersion; (b) manual tonification (manipulation); (c) heat; or (d) electrical stimulation, which facilitates the directed flow of Qi (electrons) (Figures 66.2–66.4). Low frequency electrical stimulation results in an endorphin-mediated generalized effect. High frequency stimulation results in a monoamine-mediated, more rapid onset, segmental response [8].

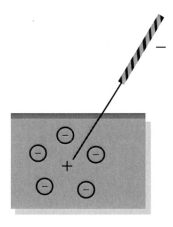

Figure 66.2 Dispersion. *Source*: From Ref. [8].

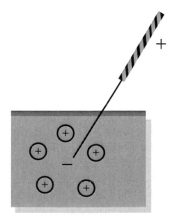

Figure 66.3 Tonification. *Source*: From Ref. [8].

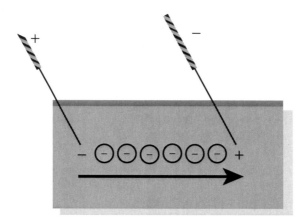

Figure 66.4 Directed flow of Qi facilitated with electrical stimulation. *Source*: From Ref. [8].

- Risks/side-effects include bleeding/bruising, infection, needle shock/fainting, nerve irritation, and puncture of an organ/vital structure (very rare).
- In general, acupuncture is a very safe and well-tolerated procedure.

ADDITIONAL READING

Electronic References

American Academy of Medical Acupuncture. www.medicalacupuncture.org/
NIH National Center for Complementary and Alternative Medicine (NCCAM). http://nccam.nih.gov/

Textbooks/Chapters

Beinfield H, Korngold E. *Between Heaven and Earth: A Guide to Chinese Medicine*. New York: Ballantine Books; 1992.
Helms JM. *Acupuncture Energetics: A Clinical Approach for Physicians*. 1st ed. Berkeley, CA: Medical Acupuncture Publishers; 1995.

Journal Articles

Acupuncture. *NIH Consensus Statement*. 1997;15(5):1–34.
Cheshire A, Powell L, Barlow J. Use of complementary and alternative medicine for children with brain injury in the United Kingdom. *J Altern Complement Med*. 2007;13(7):703–704.
Ludwig DS, Kabat-Zinn J. Mindfulness in medicine. *JAMA*. 2008;300(11):1350–1352.

REFERENCES

1. NCCAM website. http://nccam.nih.gov/
2. Ludwig DS, Kabat-Zinn J. Mindfulness in medicine. *JAMA.* 2008;300(11):1350–1352.
3. Meili T, Kabat-Zinn J, The power of the human heart: a story of trauma and recovery and its implications for rehabilitation and healing. *Adv Mind Body Med.* 2004;20(1):6–16.
4. Bedard M, Felteau M, Mazmnian D. Pilot evaluation of a mindfulness-based intervention to improve quality of life among individuals who sustained traumatic brain injury. *Disabil Rehabil.* 2003;25(13):722–731.
5. Shapira MY, Chelouche M, Yanai R. Tai Qi Chuan practice as a tool for rehabilitation of severe head trauma. *Arch PM&R.* 2001;82(9):1283–1285.
6. Gemmell C, Jeathem JM. A study investigating the effects of Tai Qi Chuan: individuals with traumatic brain injury compared to controls. *Brain Inj.* 2006;20(2):151–156.
7. Blake H, Batson M. Exercise intervention in brain injury: a pilot randomized study of Tai Qi Qigong. *Clin Rehabil.* 2009;23(7):589–598. Epub Feb 23.
8. Helms JM. *Acupuncture Energetics: A Clinical Approach for Physicians.* 1st ed. Berkeley, CA: Medical Acupuncture Publishers; 1995.
9. Wang XM, Yang SL. The effect of acupuncture in 90 cases of sequelae of brain concussion. *Journal of Traditional Chinese Medicine,* 1988;8(2):127–128.
10. Frost E. Acupuncture for the comatose patient. *Am J Acupunct.* 1976;4(1):45–48.
11. Zollman FS, Larson EB, Wasek-Throm LK, Cybroski CM, Bode RK. Acupuncture for treatment of insomnia in patients with traumatic brain injury: a pilot intervention study. *J Head Trauma Rehab.* Epub ahead of Print, Jan 2011.
12. NCCAM Publication No. D003; Date Revised: December 2004.

67

Return to Work Following Traumatic Brain Injury

Paul Wehman, Matthew Goodwin, Shane D. McNamee, and Pamela Sherron Targett

BACKGROUND

Importance

Traumatic brain injury (TBI) results in cognitive, physical, and psychosocial impairments that present barriers to return to work (RTW) [1]. The importance of successful RTW after a TBI cannot be overstated. Survivors who RTW report an improved sense of well-being and identity, better health status, greater community involvement, less usage of healthcare services, decreased social isolation, and better quality of life [2]. With supportive legislation in place and the improvement of medical and rehabilitation interventions, increasing numbers of TBI survivors have had the opportunity to RTW [1].

Incidence

It has been estimated that among patients who were employed prior to injury, 40.4% RTW at 1 year, and 40.8% at 2 years, with a range reported from 0% to 84% across studies [3]. Several factors contribute to the wide range of RTW rates, including varied classification of severity of TBI, differing definitions of RTW, financial incentives that promote or discourage RTW in different countries, and availability of vocational rehabilitation services [4].

Durability

Review of US TBI model systems data revealed that 34% of survivors were stably employed (i.e., employed at 1-, 2-, *and* 3- or 4-year follow-up), 27% were unstably employed (employed at one or two of the three follow-up visits), and 39% were unemployed at all three follow-ups [5].

Rehabilitation Continuum of Care

The full spectrum of TBI rehabilitative services includes acute inpatient rehabilitation, postacute rehabilitation, and community reentry and RTW with assistance as indicated. Vocational assistance may range from instruction on gaining employment to intensive on-the-job training, and outpatient follow-up to help adapt to new challenges and access community resources [4,6].

Primary Treatment Models

These include comprehensive/holistic programs that feature work readiness training and work trials [7], case coordination [8,9] and supported employment [10–12]. All treatments are "individualized" to some degree; more research is needed to determine unique effects of different treatment approaches on long-term outcomes [6].

Effectiveness

Supported employment can improve outcomes for individuals with severe TBI [12,13]. Those who go to work also seem to improve in nonvocational areas. Work has therapeutic benefits including social interaction, providing structure and purpose in life, enhancing perception of quality life and positively impacting self-concept.

Funding Sources for Vocational Interventions

These may include

- State vocational rehabilitation agency
- Insurance carrier
- Out of pocket

ASSESSMENT

Factors

A systematic review of the literature (1992–2008) for prognostic and nonprognostic factors impacting RTW in nontraumatic and TBI indicates the following: greater injury severity (Glasgow Coma Scale) and presence of depression or anxiety are negatively associated with RTW; longer inpatient stay, residual physical impairments, number/extent of injuries, and limitations in activities of daily living performance also appear to correlate with a reduced chance of RTW (Table 67.1) [3].

Table 67.1 Some of the Risk Factors Associated With Unsuccessful RTW for TBI

Age more than 40 years at time of injury	Lack of awareness of available work incentives
Unemployment pre injury	Lack of job placement assistance
Low preinjury education level	Inability to return to preinjury job or employer
Unskilled manual laborer pre injury	Lack of self-awareness
Greater number of neuropsychological deficits	Poor social support network
Length of inpatient rehabilitation stay	Psychiatric history and prior drug or EtOH use
Length of coma	Greater level of physical disability

From Refs. [1,4].

Note that RTW involves a complex interaction between premorbid characteristics, injury factors, postinjury impairments, and personal and environmental factors, making predicting outcomes only moderately accurate [4].

Physical Examination

A thorough physical examination and diagnostic workup including neuroimaging and neuropsychological testing is necessary for accurate diagnosis of the physical, cognitive, behavioral, and emotional sequelae of TBI. If returning to previous work, some type of release to return to duty may be required. Having a member of the team conduct a thorough job analysis can be very helpful.

Vocational Assessment

- Traditional vocational assessment, that is, a "place once and done" approach, has not been effective for individuals with more significant support needs [1,12].
- Functional vocational assessment: This assessment is designed to determine RTW options and support needs. It may involve examining the individual's ability to return to preinjury employment; a new job that capitalizes on use of the person's residual skills either with pre injury or new employer; or different type of job with new employer [1]. Assessment includes interviewing the individual and/or caregivers as well as a vocational situational assessment in a real (not simulated) work setting.

VOCATIONAL REHABILITATION INTERVENTION

Team Approach

This may include physiatry, vocational rehabilitation (including job coach if severe disability), social work, physical therapy, occupational therapy, vision therapy, speech therapy, and neuropsychology. Each discipline can offer unique insight that can be integrated into the survivor's RTW plan. It is also important to get solicit input from the family and patient.

Client Instruction and Advisement

Client instruction and advisement involves providing the client with information and instruction to assist with conducting a job search and, once employed, use of compensatory strategies at work. Many individuals with TBI will not be able to profit from this office-based intervention because of cognitive impairments.

Selective Placement

This involves job placement assistance followed by minimal interaction and intervention. This approach assumes that neither intensive on-the-job assistance nor ongoing support is necessary. Ongoing contact with the individual may be maintained more closely than with the employer.

Supported Employment

Supported employment is effective in increasing employment among those with TBI [12], with a job retention rate of more than 70% [14]. This approach is characterized by individualized employment support, provided and/or facilitated by a vocational rehabilitation specialist sometimes referred to as a job coach [1]. These services are specifically tailored to assist an individual with severe TBI with gaining and maintaining competitive employment. This approach begins with a functional vocational assessment, followed by an immediate job search (in place of prolonged preemployment training or treatment) that is aligned with the information gathered during client assessment and review of the employer's business needs. Once the job seeker is hired, the job coach facilitates on and off job-site supports. On-the-job training is often provided, including assisting the new hire with developing and learning to use various supports like compensatory memory strategies. The job coach gauges how the new hire is progressing toward meeting the employer's standards and expectations and adjusts instructional strategies accordingly. Ongoing long-term follow-up or job retention services are also provided throughout the individual's tenure. This could include assisting the employee with resolving novel challenges as they arise or new skills training if indicated [1,3,4,12,13].

Workplace Supports

Some common physical, cognitive, and emotional impairments and possible workplace supports are described in the following:

- Physical impairments (e.g., seizures, heterotopic ossification, spasticity) [15]: Some ways to help circumvent difficulties arising from physical sequelae of TBI include [16]
  - Developing a job that will utilize residual strengths versus merely avoiding points of weakness
  - Selecting or modifying the work environment to ensure safety in the event of the recurrence of a seizure or in the setting of balance dysfunction and dizziness; teaching the client to recognize symptoms and take steps to "be safe"; educating the employer on reaction to occurrence if appropriate
  - Rearranging the workspace to help accommodate decreased range of motion and strength
  - Considering ergonomic modifications
  - Considering how pattern or sequencing of activities impacts speed and accuracy, endurance and fatigue; making modifications where feasible
  - Utilizing assistive technology and/or adaptive equipment if necessary
- Cognitive and emotional impairments (e.g., memory impairment, impaired attention/concentration, lack of self-awareness, disinhibited behaviors). Some ways to help ameliorate cognitive, emotional, and behavioral dysfunction at work include
  - Cognitive rehabilitation [4]
  - Cognitive behavioral therapy that focuses on developing mechanisms for emotional and behavioral self-regulation and for developing self-awareness [4]
  - Employment supports [16]
  - Assistive technology
  - Procedural modifications or process reorganization (e.g., changing sequence of tasks)
  - Compensatory strategies: for example, creating associations and utilizing verbal rehearsing, check lists, flow charts, reference manuals, etc
  - Identifying/avoiding factors associated with triggering behaviors
  - Modeling positive interactions

- Providing counseling on emotional distress and difficulty adjusting to effects of injury

Additional Considerations

With the advent of supported employment, virtually no one should be considered too disabled to work. Workshop settings, a place where individuals with disabilities congregate together to perform contract work or to receive training, are not acceptable, nor are group models sometimes referred to as enclaves or mobile work crews. Even individuals with very severe injuries have been assisted to RTW through a supported approach [1,2,4,12–14]. Awareness of the distinctions among these vocational rehabilitation approaches is key, as TBI providers may need to take a leadership role in ensuring that the survivor is directed toward services that will lead to real work for real pay/competitive employment in every appropriate circumstance.

ADDITIONAL READING

Electronic Reference
Virginia Commonwealth University's Rehabilitation Research and Training Center on Workplace Supports and Job Retention. www.worksupport.com

Textbook/Chapter
Targett P, Yasuda S, Wehman P. Applications for Youth with TBI. In: Wehman P, ed. *Life Beyond the Classroom: Transition strategies for young people with disabilities* (pp. 601–624). Baltimore, MD: Paul H. Brookes Publishing; 2006.

Journal Articles
Shames J, Treger I, Ring H, Giaquinto S. Return to work following traumatic brain injury: trends and challenges. *Disabil Rehabil.* 2007;29;1387–1395.

Wehman P, Targett P, West M, Kregel J. Production work and employment for persons with traumatic brain injury: what have we learned? *J Head Trauma Rehabil.* 2005;20(2):115–127.

REFERENCES

1. West M, Targett P, Yasuda S, Wehman P. Return to work following TBI. In: Zasler ND, Katz DI, Zafonte RD, eds. *Brain Injury Medicine.* New York: Demos; 2007.

2. van Velzen JM, van Bennekom CA, Edelaar MJ, Sluiter JK, Frings-Dresen MH. How many people return to work after acquired brain injury?: a systematic review. *Brain Inj.* 2009;23(6):473–488.

3. Fadyl JK, McPherson KM. Approaches to vocational rehabilitation after traumatic brain injury: a review of the evidence. *J Head Trauma Rehabil.* 2009;24(3):195–212.

4. Shames J, Treger I, Ring H, Giaquinto S. Return to work following traumatic brain injury: trends and challenges. *Disabil Rehabil.* 2007;29(17):1387–1395.

5. Kreutzer JS, Marwitz JH, Walker W, et al. Moderating factors in return to work and job stability after traumatic brain injury. *J Head Trauma Rehabil.* 2003;18(2):128–138.

6. Hart T, Dijkers M, Whyte J, et al. Vocational interventions and supports following job placement for persons with traumatic brain injury. *Journal of Vocational Rehabilitation.* 2010;32(3):135–150.

7. Ben-Yishay Y, Rattok J, Lakin P, et al. Neuropsychological rehabilitation: quest for a holistic approach. *Seminars in Neurology.* 1985;5:252–259.

8. Malec JF, Buffington AL, Moessner AM, Degiorgio L. A medical/vocational case coordination system for persons with brain injury: an evaluation of employment outcomes. *Arch Phys Med Rehabil.* 2000;81(8):1007–1015.

9. Malec JF. Impact of comprehensive day treatment on societal participation for persons with acquired brain injury. *Arch Phys Med Rehabil.* 2001;82(7):885–895.

10. Wehman PH, Kreutzer JS, West MD, et al. Return to work for persons with traumatic brain injury: a supported employment approach. *Arch Phys Med Rehabil.* 1990;71(13):1047–1052.

11. Wehman P, Kregel J, Keyser-Marcus L, et al. Supported employment for persons with traumatic brain injury: a preliminary investigation of long-term follow-up costs and program efficiency. *Arch Phys Med Rehabil.* 2003;84(2):192–196.

12. Wehman P, Targett P, West M, Kregel J. Productive work and employment for persons with traumatic brain injury: what have we learned after 20 years? *J Head Trauma Rehabil.* 2005;20(2):115–127.

13. Chesnut RM, Carney N, Maynard H, Mann NC, Patterson P, Helfand M. Summary report: evidence for the effectiveness of rehabilitation for persons with traumatic brain injury. *J Head Trauma Rehabil.* 1999;14(2):176–188.

14. Wehman P, Sherron P, Kregel J, Kreutzer J, Tran S, Cifu D. Return to work for persons following severe TBI: supported employment outcomes after 5 years. *Am J Phys Med Rehabil.* 1993;72:355–363.

15. McNamee S, Walker W, Cifu DX, Wehman PH. Minimizing the effect of TBI-related physical sequelae on vocational return. *J Rehabil Res Dev.* 2009;46(6):893–908.

16. Wehman P, Bricout J, Targett P. Supported employment for people with traumatic brain injury. In: Fraser R, Clemmons D, eds. Traumatic brain injury rehabilitation practical vocational, neuropsychological and psychotherapy interventions (pp. 201–239). Boca Raton, FL: CRC Press; 2000.

68

Resources for Traumatic Brain Injury Survivors and Caregivers

Donna Zahara

BACKGROUND

Need for Transitional Support

Many brain injury survivors and their families will require significant support as they transition from hospital or rehabilitation to home and community. While many will need support throughout their lifetime, the type and amount of support needed is likely to change over time [1]. Because the residual effects of each brain injury will have a unique impact on the existing family unit, individualized transitional planning is important for successful community reintegration [2], an important aspect of quality of life [3]. As transitional plans are developed, it is useful to consider the general domains of living: (1) activities of daily living, (2) vocational/school reentry, and (3) leisure/social/wellness. Consideration also needs to be given to available community resources. Although it is widely acknowledged that many traumatic brain injury (TBI) survivors and their families need transitional support services following hospitalization, many do not receive services due to the lack of availability [1] or because barriers exist to accessing those services.

Barriers to Resource Access

Lack of Knowledgeable Providers
When developing a community support network for the survivor and the family, it is important to find reputable, experienced, and knowledgeable service providers. Most community programs simply do not employ staff educated in brain injury. Medical professionals, psychologists, and even rehabilitation professionals may not have had experience with the TBI population or their needs. However, knowledgeable staff can be found, and an effort should be made to identify them. For example, many large park districts have programming for those with

special needs; community mental health programs may have individuals who have worked with the TBI population, and some counties may have special community case management services available. In addition, advocacy groups often have experience working with TBI survivors and their families.

Financial/Funding Considerations

TBI affects not just the financial status of the survivor, but of the entire family [4]. Lost wages are a consideration for the survivor, but may affect the spouse or parent as well. Parents or spouses may become primary caretakers of the TBI survivor, impacting their employment status and the family's financial well-being. The cost to provide in-home care, outpatient rehabilitation, day care, and transportation services can be quite high [6]. Equipment and medications can be costly as well. Since these or other services may be required over a lifetime, the costs can become significant. Historically, community services for TBI survivors and their families have not been well funded in the public sector. However, financial support opportunities for eligible families are available. See, for example, http://www.traumaticbraininjury.com/content/fundingresources/tbi-funding-resources.html

Limited Local or Regional Resource Availability

The specific state or area in which the survivor/family reside may hinder service access. Some rural areas do not have the resources of larger urban centers. Also, states vary widely in the financial support made available to survivors/families or to the providers who offer services to persons with traumatic brain injuries.

RESOURCES

Although most resources for the TBI survivor and the family are accessed at a local level, they are usually first identified through national information sources. This resource list will therefore focus on general categories of support needs and national resources, which can, in turn, lead to local resource information.

TBI Education

The following organizations and centers provide Web-based access to TBI educational materials of value to both consumers and professionals:

- Brain Injury Association of America (BIAA). http://www.biausa.org
- Brain Injury Resource Center. http://www.headinjury.com

- Centers for Disease Control and Prevention. http://www.cdc.gov/ (Search: Traumatic Brain Injury)
- Disabilities Resources, Inc. http://www.disabilityresources.org

Medical

Ongoing medical management is important for most brain injury survivors. Physicians who specialize in TBI may be identified through selected professional organizations:

- American Academy of Physical Medicine and Rehabilitation. http://www.e-aapmr.org/imis/imisonline/findphys/find.cfm
- American Academy of Neurology. http://patients.aan.com/finda-neurologist
- Local academic medical centers may be able to assist in identifying physicians who have speciality expertise in managing TBI.
- There are currently 16 TBI Model System Centers located throughout the United States (see http://www.tbindsc.org/Centers.aspx). These centers are recognized providers of expert care for TBI.

Neuropsychological/Psychological

Neuropsychological assessments should be conducted and interpreted by those who have experience working with individuals with TBI. Neuropsychologists can significantly enhance understanding of the effects of the brain injury. In addition, psychologists who understand the effects of sudden loss or change on family systems can also be helpful to survivors and families trying to cope with the effects of brain injury. See:

- The American Psychological Association. http://www.apa.org (Search by city/state—does not provide information by subspecialty)
- BIAA. http://www.biausa.org (Local offices often maintain lists of psychologists/neuropsychologists with TBI experience.)

Neurorehabilitation

The ongoing rehabilitation needs of each survivor will vary according to the residual effects of the brain injury. Home health services, long term care/skilled nursing/subacute programs, day treatment and outpatient programs are the usual categories of programs that may be recommended for a survivor. One means of locating services available in your area is through your state Brain Injury Association chapter.

Caregiver Support/Resources

Caregiver burden is widely discussed in the literature. The burden experienced by a caregiver of a TBI survivor—generally a family member—may be particularly difficult given the lengthy recovery process and the altered abilities and personality of the survivor [5]. Often, the caregiver's wellness is sacrificed when their need for support is not understood and prioritized. Wellness, respite, and spiritual and social networking can be important components of a caregiver support plan. Support groups for the caregiver, as well as for the survivor, can be found throughout most states and are often important sources of caregiver wellness information. Your state BIAA chapter/affiliate is one helpful resource for locating these groups. The following are also useful caregiver resources:

- Family Caregiver Alliance. http://www.caregiver.org/caregiver/jsp/home.jsp
- The Rehabilitation Institute of Chicago—Life Center. http://lifecenter.ric.org (click "Patient and Family Resource Guide Handouts")

Advocacy/Legal

In seeking out and obtaining needed services, advocacy is often necessary at some juncture. The advocacy role is generally played by the spouse, parent, or caregiver.

- Every state and territory in the United States has a Protection and Advocacy Agency. All of these agencies are part of a network known as The National Disability Rights Network. A state-specific search for your local agency can be initiated via http://www.napas.org/aboutus/PA_CAP.htm
- For assistance with independent living, consider contacting Centers for Independent Living, http://www.virtualcil.net/cils, which provides links to independent living centers throughout the country.
- For legal information/resources see http://www.ada.gov/cguide.htm

Vocational

Supported employment interventions improve job placement and retention for TBI survivors [6]. Vocational counselors and job coaches experienced in working with TBI survivors can be an invaluable resource, advocating with employers, recommending job modifications, and providing individualized retraining. Every state has a Department or Division of Rehabilitation Services that may help with vocational support. The following Web site may also be helpful: http://www.headinjury.com/jobs.htm.

Leisure/Social Networking for Survivors

Leisure and social relationships are often adversely affected by a TBI [6]. Support groups, special "clubhouses" for survivors, and local park districts can become core aspects of community reentry and social interaction. In additional to undertaking a Web site search under "Special Recreation Associations TBI" or "Parks & Recreation TBI," the following resources can provide assistance:

- International Brain Injury Clubhouse Alliance. http://www.braininjuryclubhouses.net/. (choose "Find a Clubhouse Near You")
- BIAA. http://www.biausa.org

Research

- Several "model systems" across the nation have been funded by the National Institute on Disability and Rehabilitation Research to conduct ongoing TBI research. Their studies can be accessed at http://msktc. washington.edu/tbi
- To locate current clinical trials, http://clinicaltrials.gov (search TBI)

SPECIALIZED NEEDS

Military

Those who have served in the military and their families have access to support through:

- DBVIC (Defense and Veterans Brain Injury Center). http://www.dvbic. org/
- Department of Veterans Affairs. http://www.va.gov/
- Polytrauma Rehabilitation Family Education Manual. http://www. hsrd.minneapolis.med.va.gov/FCM/PDF/FamilyEdMan.pdf
- Military healthcare (Tricare) benefit information. http://www.military. com/benefits/tricare

Pediatrics/Adolescents

For children and adolescents, the major focus of community reentry will be return to school. Issues related to Pediatric TBI and education have been widely discussed [7,8]. Individualized supports and accommodations may be in place via federal and local laws. Families/caregivers should seek support to assure that an appropriate *Individualized Education Plan* (IEP) is in place and reviewed regularly as required by local law. Western Oregon University supports the Center on Brain Injury Research & Training which contains information on IEPS (http://www.cbirt.org/tbieducation/formalized-support/iep-and-program-development-tbi/). Neuropsychologists with expertise in pediatric neuropsychological testing are good resources to assure appropriate placement and support, especially for those children with cognitive issues.

Mild TBI

Because mild TBI (MTBI) deficits are often subtle, individuals with MTBI may not be easily identified and may be misunderstood by community agency personnel. The following resources may be of use:

- Centers for Disease Control and Prevention. http://www.cdc.gov/ncipc/tbi
- Physicians Tool kit. http://www.cdc.gov/concussion/HeadUp/physicians_tool_kit.html

REFERENCES

1. Kolakowsky-Hayner SA, Miner KD, Kreutzer JS. Long-term life quality and family needs after traumatic brain injury. *J Head Trauma Rehabil.* 2001;16(4):374–385.
2. Sander AM, Clark A, Pappadis MR. What is community integration anyway? Defining meaning following traumatic brain injury. *J Head Trauma Rehabil.* 2010;25(2):121–127.
3. Kalpakjian CZ, Lam CS, Toussaint LL, Merbitz NK. Describing quality of life and psychosocial outcomes after traumatic brain injury. *Am J Phys Med Rehabil.* 2004;83(4):255–265.
4. Vangel SJ Jr, Rapport LJ, Hanks RA, Black KL. Long-term medical care utilization and costs among traumatic brain injury survivors. *Am J Phys Med Rehabil.* 2005;84(3):153–160.
5. Kreutzer JS, Gervasio AH, Camplair PS. Primary caregivers' psychological status and family functioning after traumatic brain injury. *Brain Inj.* 1994;8(3):197–210.
6. McCabe P, Lippert C, Weiser M, Hilditch M, Hartridge C, Villamere J; Erabi Group. Community reintegration following acquired brain injury. *Brain Inj.* 2007;21(2):231–257.
7. Ylvisaker M, Todis B, Glang A, et al. Educating students with TBI: themes and recommendations. *J Head Trauma Rehabil.* 2001;16(1):76–93.
8. Savage RC, DePompei R, Tyler J, Lash M. Paediatric traumatic brain injury: a review of pertinent issues. *Pediatr Rehabil.* 2005;8(2):92–103.

69

Living With Traumatic Brain Injury
From a Survivor's Perspective

Jennifer Field

I was 17 years old. From the age of 6, I had been a competitive rider on the show circuit and was now at the Grand Prix level of show jumping. I was champion in the Junior Jumpers at the Washington International Horse Show in Landover, Maryland, and fresh off a third place win at the Maclay Equitation Finals at the Madison Square Garden horse show. My plan was to graduate early from high school and compete in Europe with an eye to the Olympics.

But on a snowy Friday in November, I wasn't thinking about any of that. The year had ended in the competitive show world, and I could finally take time for myself. My mother was leaving for the weekend and my boyfriend Matt was coming up from Connecticut College; we had schemed this secret rendezvous since our last time together at the Garden.

I skipped my last class to go home, change clothes, and make it back to school to meet Matt. I couldn't be late. Queen's *Under Pressure* blasted through my Black Saab 900 as I sped 55 mph down a winding country road. A severe, early-winter storm was predicted and it was just beginning to snow. I had lived in New Hampshire long enough to know that these conditions were the deadliest—but I was not deterred. I could only think of Matt.

Without warning, I hit black ice, skidded uncontrollably into the other lane and collided with a tractor-trailer barreling toward me. The bumper of the truck, towering above me, smashed the passenger-side rear window. The impact was so severe, my seat collapsed and my head ricocheted back through the driver side rear window. Glass was embedded in my skull. My neck was twisted, the airway was blocked, and I had stopped breathing.

In that moment, life as I had known it was over. From then on, I would become consumed with the search for a complete healing. At first, I wanted the old me, to regain my old life. Now, 18 years later, I realize on that day I was reborn. The intense training to become a champion rider would serve me well in this new journey, not only through the many, often tedious and certainly challenging, years of traditional and alternative medicine, therapies, spiritual healers, and physical training, but also in my creation and development of a one-woman show, called "A Distant Memory," which traces my life before and after this life-defining accident.

I'm not sure how long I lay there, unconscious, unable to breathe, but a volunteer firefighter was already in the area and arrived on the scene after hearing about the accident on his CB radio. He knew from the position of my head that I wasn't breathing, and although a fire crew was trying frantically to get me out of the car, the volunteer firefighter found the strength to open the door and reposition my head so that I could breathe again. The ambulance took me to the local community hospital where the emergency team quickly assessed the severity of my injury and made arrangements for me to be transported to a regional hospital.

> I picked up the phone and a voice said, "This is the Monadnock Community Hospital calling. Your daughter has been in an accident." So I asked how Jennifer was and the woman on the phone said, "I should really get the doctor," and I just went nuts. I just screamed and screamed and I guess the doctor came on and I asked "Is she alive?" and he said, "Yes." And then I don't think I could talk anymore.
>
> *Joanne Field—Jennifer's mom*

The doctors at the regional hospital had little hope for my survival. Tubes were coming out of my body, wires were attached to monitors, and I had a pressure gauge in my head. A renowned neurosurgeon from Chicago had been flown to New Hampshire to see if there was something more that could be done. After reading my CAT scan, he concluded that I could not be moved, that I would survive, but I might never speak again.

I lay in a coma for 3 weeks; I was on a respirator, my left arm and leg pumped continuously, of their own volition, and because of severe tone, my right arm curled inward and remained frozen for months. My vitals had begun to stabilize and the pressure gauge measuring swelling had been removed from my head.

Coma patients are evaluated on the Rancho Los Amigos scale, indicating the severity of the condition and the likelihood that the patient would respond to, and benefit from, treatment. Using this one-to-ten scale, I was ranked a "three." Given that a "one" indicates a vegetative state, I wasn't doing very well.

I was being fed through a tube, and was nonresponsive, so doctors suggested to my mom that she decorate my room with personal effects to stimulate a response. My mom brought photos, a saddle, some of my horse's mane, and even some manure. None of it created the response everyone was hoping for.

> One morning, nurses were washing her face and I saw Jennifer's left eye open. Stunned, I told the nurse her eye had opened, but the nurse said "Oh, Joanne, I know how badly you want this to happen..." and

just at that moment, "bing!" her eye opened again. I went tearing down the hallway of the hospital and told everyone in the waiting room—and this hoard of family and friends came thundering down the ICU, which was completely against the rules. Of course, both eyes were closed by the time we arrived in her room and remained closed for three days. And then, Jen opened her left eye and this time, it remained opened.

Joanne Field

My first awareness of being awake was my "coming to" on the floor of a blue padded room with Matt and my best friend, Kirstin, looking down at me, and I had absolutely no idea who Matt was. Someone had to tell me that he was my boyfriend.

I was put in that padded room as a safety precaution because as you come out of a coma you can get really violent and either hurt yourself, or someone else. It can be difficult for family members to watch a loved one coming out of a coma, and I'm sure that it's difficult, too, for families to muster patience in the face of just how slow recovery can be: weeks, months, even, as in my case, years.

I had sustained a diffuse, closed-head injury. Although the truck hit the right side of my head, the whiplash was so severe that the left side of my brain received the brunt of the trauma. The human body works in diagonals. The left part of the brain controls the right side of the body; the right controls the left. So when I eventually awoke, the right side of my body was completely paralyzed. I couldn't walk, talk, or use my right arm. And my right eye was completely closed.

During this time, I wasn't troubled by the severity of my condition. I remember being calm and tranquil. My moment-by-moment experiences were all I knew: My whole world was a blue padded room.

The rehabilitation schedule that followed my coming out of the coma was a series of good and bad days, each one including numerous doctors, specialists, therapists, exercises, tests, and evaluations. The good days were filled with small hard-won victories and the bad days were filled with insurmountable, soul-destroying and energy-sapping impossibilities. Some of the tests were so simple, such as clipping clothes pegs to an upright ruler, and yet I found this almost impossible to do. When I achieved that task with my right arm, which had been a cement block of severe tone, it was a tremendous victory.

Early in my rehabilitation, my mother went to Toys-R-Us and purchased puzzles, word games, and cards, anything that would stimulate my brain. She explained that although it might seem childish to me, my brain had been damaged and we had to work together to reconnect neural pathways by performing activities that had contributed to my development years earlier. Somehow I innately understood that I needed to heal my brain and challenge my neurological system. So, I was starting my life over again as a toddler, joined at the hip to my mother. I was learning how to wipe my face, dress and feed myself, brush my hair, and blow my nose, from the same woman who had taught me those basic skills the first time around.

Meanwhile my speech was hardly audible: My voice was whispery and my words were slurred and halting because of the cognitive challenge of trying to track what I had just said at the same time as I was trying to recall the word that meant what I hoped to say next. Suffice it to say, it wasn't easy for others to understand me.

At the culmination of long months of intensive rehabilitation, doctors told my mother, "Your daughter will make all her improvements in the first year and very few after that," and, "Don't you realize the severity of your daughter's injury? She will never get any better, this is it." On the verge of tears, my mother said nothing, but inside she thought, "No, this can't be it."

Back home in Peterborough, New Hampshire, as my mother lay in bed one night, a voice came into her head with the message, "Go downstairs and get your alternative medicine books, and search for another way."

This began a 2-year odyssey across the United States, to Mexico, Canada, and Europe in search of therapies that could address the cognitive and physical constraints that my mom and I were determined I would overcome. Standard medical rehabilitation techniques had helped me to regain a measure of function, but I was far from achieving even a semblance of physical independence. During this next period of my journey, I regained significant functionality from a combination of alternative therapies, including craniosacral therapy, soft-tissue manipulation, osteopathy, acupuncture, neuro-optometric rehabilitation, Neuropathways EEG Imaging, nutrition, hyperbaric oxygen, various healers, and Continuum Movement.

Experimenting with these modalities, and adjusting the degree of emphasis on each practice in my rehabilitation regimen, I began to increase my physical capacity and confidence—in my balance, in my ability to move and walk, in my capability to coordinate different functions, in my reasoning and thought process, and, finally, in my speech.

Finding, practicing, and testing the many therapies became a full-time job for my mom and me. It wasn't easy, it wasn't always fun, and it was often tiring for both of us, even with significant support from family and friends. Fortunately for me, diligence and unwavering determination were qualities that my mom had in abundance.

Years later, I would overhear her saying to her friends, "When I look back on my life, what gives me the most pride is Jennifer's recovery."

After 2 years of pursuing alternative therapies, I wanted more out of life. I wanted to go to college, to be "normal." I applied to Wheaton College, was accepted, and began my freshman classes in 1995. It required long hours of dedicated study on my part, extra help from others, and unlimited time on exams, but the result was an important personal victory: I graduated Magna Cum Laude in Art History in 2000. I was ready for my next challenge.

I left New England and moved to my own apartment in Santa Monica, California, in order to immerse myself in Continuum Movement practices, which I have found to be a vital tool for me to experience the fullness of what it means to be alive. At this time, my speech was still slow and halting—and word retrieval remained difficult. New people I encountered often thought I was drunk, or high, when I spoke.

Not all of the therapies I had engaged in were centered around my physical recovery. Some were about finding ways to express my "inner experience" of dealing with the day-to-day grind and how long my recovery was taking. Sometimes I became very frustrated with myself. When you lose your physical independence and have to start relying on other people for everything, you can feel helpless, "locked out," and forgotten. So, while searching for ways to express what was going on inside, I began to write and paint.

I had never considered taking up a creative practice. I had absolutely no idea if I were even capable of producing anything worth looking at or reading, but I did it anyway and it was a tremendous help. The first writing I did took the form of poetry, then my writing became more autobiographical. The colors I used in my paintings were expressive. Given my struggle with impaired speech, engaging in creative expression was a welcome change of pace.

From 2003 to 2006, I complemented writing, painting, and Continuum Movement work with acting classes, studying the Meisner Technique with The Ruskin Group Theatre Company. Acting was difficult for me at first, because of the need to memorize my lines. But the Meisner Technique's emphasis on "living truthfully under imaginary circumstances" gave me an additional outlet to express myself and deal with my head injury. When a friend suggested, "Why don't you turn what you're writing into a one-woman play about your life?" I just laughed, but that's exactly what I did.

I have performed my one-woman show, "A Distant Memory," in theaters and at colleges, high schools, hospitals, rehab centers, and conferences since 2006. The act of performing and repeating my story has strengthened my verbal skills, which continue to improve to this day. And it has helped me to build my confidence. Coming offstage after my very first performance of the show, I remember saying to John Ruskin, the director of the theater, "I have found the feeling I had when entering the ring on my horse to compete."

As John Lennon wrote, "Life is what happens while you're busy making other plans." I had my goal of riding and show jumping, but during my years of recovery, I started to realize that in my pursuit to become "normal," to get back to my "old self" and the life I had before the accident, I was actually living my life. As I grew to appreciate the meaning of this, it became easier to welcome new challenges and improve upon the life I was building. And I think that is the basis of a pretty "normal" and satisfying life.

When it first happened, everyone thought of my accident as "the horrific tragedy" that I would never really recover from. Well, I have recovered, and the more time passes, the more I find it difficult to use the words "accident" and "tragedy" to describe what happened to me. I have come to believe that in rising to overcome difficulties, our lives become enriched and we grow.

I think angels come into our lives in many different forms. Even in the forms of "tragedies" and "accidents." Not to punish, but to teach us. Maybe hitting that truck was a harsh and dramatic way to learn a lesson. I can't know what my life would have been like, or what kind of person I would be, if I had never had this challenge to overcome, but I am completely certain that this experience has helped me to develop a rich spiritual and emotional life. I doubt I would have achieved this on the course I was originally headed.

Years after the accident, I believe that a key to my healing was a conviction that both my mother and I developed: There is always an alternative. It may not be immediately apparent. You may have to search for it. But it's there.

You see, my own road to recovery began after someone else, who had been in this same situation, reached out to help me. My mother received a phone call 2 days after my accident from a woman whose daughter had suffered a similar brain injury in a fall from a horse. This daughter's mother said to my mother, "Don't listen to everything the doctors say. Stay with your daughter. DO NOT leave her. She will get better."

That woman was right. No one with a traumatic brain injury should ever have to accept someone saying, "You can't," "That's not going to be possible," "That's all that is available to you," or "That's all that can be done, you must learn to live with it."

My position, borne of experience, persistence, and hard work, is that you don't have to "just live with" the devastation of traumatic brain injury. There are always options. There is always hope. There is always possibility.

To learn more about Jennifer Field and the JField Foundation, visit jfield-foundation.org.

Index

Note: Page references followed by "*f*" and "*t*" denote figures and tables, respectively.

the Durotriges. Their name occurs in the *Geography* of Ptolemy, a Greek writing in Alexandria about 150 AD. And there are two stones found on Hadrian's Wall which name Durotrigian work parties employed on reconstruction.

In *Camulodunum* (Colchester) the Catuvellauni were already in contact with the Roman world by trade long before the conquest. As a result they began to use the Latin alphabet to write down their names. Thus we find coins with the name of their capital abbreviated to CAMU, and on the other side the name of their king – CUNO,

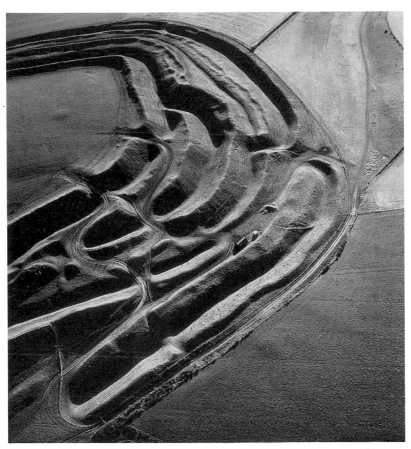

An aerial photograph of part of Maiden Castle, clearly showing the extraordinary complications of the western entrance.

standing for Cunobelinus (Shakespeare's Cymbeline).

The Durotriges of Dorset were using coins too, and the find spots of these coins give us our best idea of the extent of Durotrigian territory. In the place on their coins where you might expect to find a name there is sometimes a row of squiggles which are not real letters. As far as we know, they were illiterate.

Durotrigian territory extended from Hengistbury Head (south of Christchurch harbour) in the east, to the River Axe in the west. In the north Ilchester was a Durotrigian town in Roman times, and South Cadbury Castle was certainly included. Some scholars think they even had an outlet to the Bristol Channel.

The Durotriges were the major hillfort builders of Britain. Hillforts exist almost everywhere, but nowhere in such numbers and size as in their territory. Maiden Castle, Hod Hill, Hambledon, Eggardon, Badbury Rings and many others. No one has attempted to calculate the amount of earth shifted, but it was enormous. The Roman historian Suetonius, describing the attack on south-west Britain by the future emperor Vespasian, says he captured twenty towns, and he means the hillforts of the Durotriges.

The question of what was inside the hillforts depends partly on excavations, and partly on surface evidence from those which have not been ploughed. A small hillfort which is unploughed is Abbotsbury Castle. Here you can still see the ring of eleven circular huts which housed the inhabitants. There is a vast amount of empty space. One idea is that in times of trouble other farmers from the

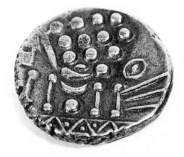 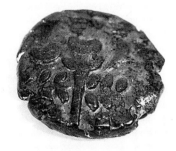

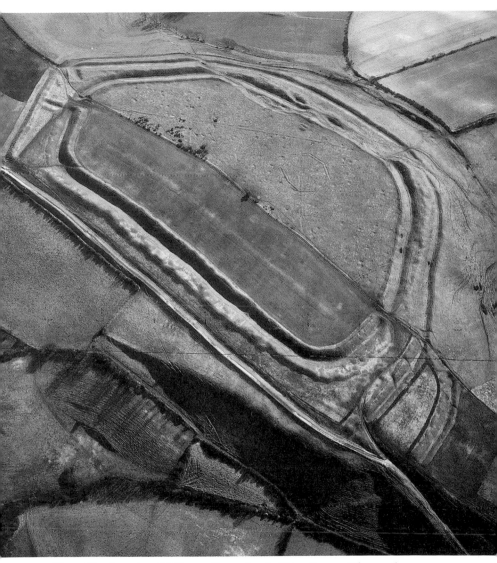

Above The Iron Age Hillfort at Eggardon in West Dorset. The northern
half has been ploughed, but the southern half shows clear traces
of its Iron Age and later occupation.
Opposite page Coins of the Durotriges, the Iron Age tribe
which inhabited Dorset.

surrounding countryside would take refuge in the hillfort, bringing their livestock with them.

Among the large hillforts, Hod Hill, north of Blandford, offers important evidence. Most of this site has now been ploughed at one time or another, but a famous aerial photograph taken in 1924 before most of the ploughing, shows that this major hillfort was closely covered with round huts, with streets showing clearly between them.

Excavation at Maiden Castle suggests a similar intensive occupation. In fact these hillforts were in the process of developing into towns. Among the more advanced tribes of south-east England such towns were already in existence, such as that at Prae Wood in Hertfordshire, which wasn't even situated on a hilltop.

At Danebury near Stockbridge in Hampshire, excavation has shown that by the time of the Roman conquest, the hillfort had been abandoned for more comfortable places to live.

It is not yet clear whether this was true of Dorset. The hillforts were clearly defended against the Romans. But were they still the great centres of political activity that they had been? There were extensive and crowded settlements on the land between Maiden Castle and Dorchester, but it is not yet clear whether these settlements appeared before or after the Roman conquest. It has recently been suggested that a major settlement already existed on the site of Dorchester itself before the construction of the Roman town *Durnovaria*. This is a very interesting hypothesis, but at present there is insufficient evidence to decide.

LIFE IN THE IRON AGE

The Iron Age chieftains lived a life surrounded by luxurious artefacts and what can only be described as works of art, many imported from the continent. There were two artistic styles, known to us as Hallstatt and La Tène, after sites in Austria and Switzerland respectively, where such objects were first recognised. La Tène follows Hallstatt somewhere about 500 BC. The La Tène style is the most spectacular. The patterns are abstract geometric designs involving swooping reverse curves and circles. The most spectacular piece found in

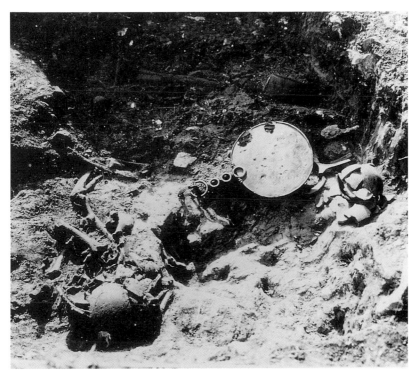

The burial of a wealthy Iron Age woman at Portesham, showing her mirror.

Dorset is the bronze mirror from Portesham near Abbotsbury, which can now be seen in Dorset County Museum. Although buried shortly after the Roman conquest, it represented the height of fashion in the late Iron Age. On its back was a beautiful pattern of La Tène curves and circles. The other side was, of course, polished to act as a mirror. It was a high status object. In the grave with it and the bones of a mature lady were pots, brooches, a Roman toilet set and a Roman strainer.

In terms of quality this grave parallels the male burial at Whitcombe, south-east of Dorchester, known as 'warrior burial', also on display in the Museum. He had his sword with its baldrick, a spear, a hammer and file and a spindle whorl.

One of the most successful industries of the Durotriges was the manufacture of pottery. Ball clay is still dug today in Purbeck for

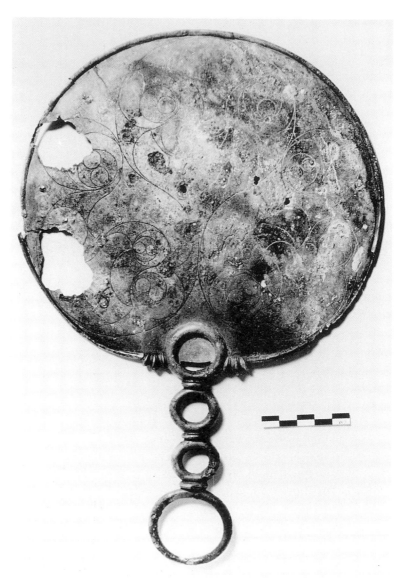

Above The bronze mirror from a grave near Portesham. The photograph shows the intricately decorated back in La Tène style. The other side was polished to form the reflecting surface.
Opposite The 'Whitcombe Warrior'. Found at Whitcombe near Dorchester, this Iron Age Warrior was buried with his great slashing sword beside him.

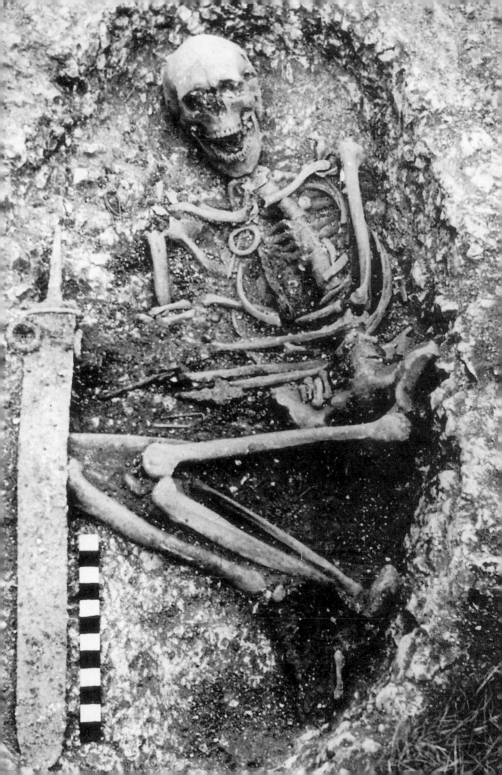

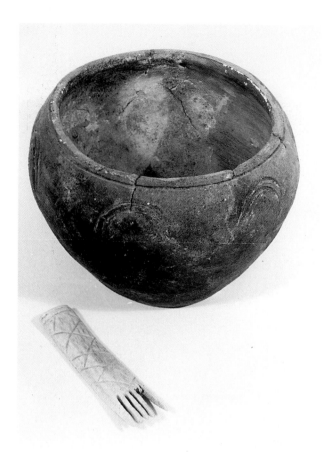

An Iron Age cooking pot and a comb from Maiden Castle.

pottery and other industries, and in Iron Age Dorset an even larger industry flourished. 'Durotrigian' pottery is found throughout Durotrigian territory and sometimes beyond. Distinctive bowls, cups and jars were made in reducing fires (kilns were not used) and the resulting dark grey or black ware finished by burnishing. Along with their coins this is one of the ways of distinguishing Durotrigian territory. So successful was the industry that it survived the Roman conquest and obtained lucrative contracts with the Roman army, which it continued to supply with a more Romanised product, even as far afield as Hadrian's Wall.

Between 100 BC and 50 BC the Durotriges were engaged in intensive trade with the continent through their harbour at Hengistbury Head. Excavations here have shown that large quantities of continental imports came into Britain at this point. Armorican coins are found. The Durotriges probably helped Armorica in their revolt against the Romans in 56 BC, and this may have brought an end to the trade through Hengistbury.

This may give a clue as to the origins of the Durotrigian people. Perhaps they started as groups of traders from Armorica, who later settled and intermarried with the native population, who were of course themselves already a mixture of peoples.

The Iron Age, at least in Dorset, was not generally a period of spectacular burials. Beyond the lady at Portesham and the warrior at Whitcombe, both of whom were undoubtedly members of the Durotrigian 'nobility', we have only the cemeteries such as that at Maiden Castle, where the dead were buried curled up on their sides, sometimes with pots of food. This is the only indication we have of their belief in an after life.

Temples are known elsewhere in Iron Age Britain, but few in Durotrigian territory beyond a small rectangular one in South Cadbury Castle, and a possible circular predecessor to the later Roman temple in Maiden Castle. It is possible, but not certain by any means, that the magnificent Cerne Giant represents one of the gods of the Durotriges, standing as he does in a busy Iron Age landscape of fields and farms. There are parallels in other parts of Britain to show that Iron Age people found deities in natural places like rivers, lakes and forests. There is little evidence in Dorset, but one of the most famous is the bog at Llyn Cerrig Bach in Anglesey. In this had been deposited as a votive offering a large hoard of La Tène items, including swords, spears, shields, chariot fittings, slave chains, a bronze trumpet and currency bars.

To the Romans, the main priests among the Iron Age people were the Druids. They were regarded as unspeakable because of their practice of sacrificing humans for the good of the community. This was probably true. The Romans went to enormous lengths to wipe them and their influence out completely, but there is no evidence for their activity in Dorset.

THE ROMAN CONQUEST

It is interesting to speculate how the Durotriges and the other Iron Age tribes of Britain might have developed their own civilization had they been left to their own devices. But it was not to be.

Julius Caesar had already invaded Britain in 55 and 54 BC as part of his campaigns in Gaul. He was only too aware of the close connections between the continental tribes and those of southern Britain. But although he defeated the tribes of the south-east in battle, other problems ensured that Britain was not permanently occupied by Rome at that time.

In the years that followed Britain became more closely linked to Rome through trade and ideas. We have already seen that the Durotrigian lady buried at Portesham with her splendid mirror also possessed a Roman toilet set and a Roman strainer. Contact was still closer in the south-east. Native kings at St. Albans, Winchester, Colchester and elsewhere were buried surrounded by imported luxury Roman articles. Rows of amphorae show they had acquired the taste for Roman wine, and Roman metalwork and pottery abound. The Roman business world must have seen Britain as a lucrative market.

But it was the political problems of the Emperor Claudius that eventually brought about the incorporation of Britain into the Roman empire. Claudius was an unexpected choice for emperor. He was a historian by instinct, and undertook the military and political task with reluctance. The power and security of Roman emperors depended on their popularity with the legions. They were unlikely to secure this without military experience and preferably a spectacular triumph.

Claudius consulted his advisors as to where he might achieve such a reputation, and the answer was Britain. Perhaps commercial interests encouraged this, and there had been the abortive adventure of Caesar which could be regarded as unfinished business. But the main reason can be seen in Claudius's triumphal arch in Rome which records the conquest of Britain as his main achievement. He even arranged for a fictitious set-back to occur during the crossing of the Thames by his general Aulus Plautius, so that Claudius could hurry to Britain in person and lead his troops in triumph into the Catuvellaunian capital at *Camulodunum* (Colchester).

This happened in 43 AD. The Durotriges were far from the centre of power in southern Britain, and we can only speculate on how soon the news reached them. However, they had trading connections with Armorica on the continent, and perhaps they heard soon enough.

It was the Second Legion Augusta which was given responsibility for the south-west. For political reasons the Atrebates in Hampshire welcomed the Roman presence, and the Second Legion built a secure base in friendly territory at Chichester. Their fortress lies under the modern city. By chance we know the name of their commander. Vespasian became emperor himself in 69 AD, and his biographer Suetonius gives us a tantalisingly small glimpse of his British command. 'He went to Britain, where he fought thirty battles, conquered two warlike tribes, and captured more then twenty towns, besides the whole of the Isle of Wight.' The Durotriges must have been one of two tribes, and their hillforts were the twenty towns.

Because of our Roman heritage, it is all too easy to see this event from the point of view of the Romans. But for the Durotriges it was a frightening and disastrous happening. There is dramatic evidence for what happened. Their hillforts were no match for the sophisticated Roman army. At Hod Hill archaeologists have found some of the hail of ballista bolts which rained down, fired from the legion's artillery. In the corner of the hillfort the Romans built a small short lived fort of their own. These earthworks are well preserved, and provide dramatic evidence of the conquest. At Maiden Castle one of the skeletons in the tribal cemetery still had the head of a Roman ballista bolt embedded in its spine.

The Durotriges seem to have defended their territory hillfort by hillfort. But in the end either each surrendered separately, or if there was an overall king, he eventually signed a treaty of surrender with Vespasian.

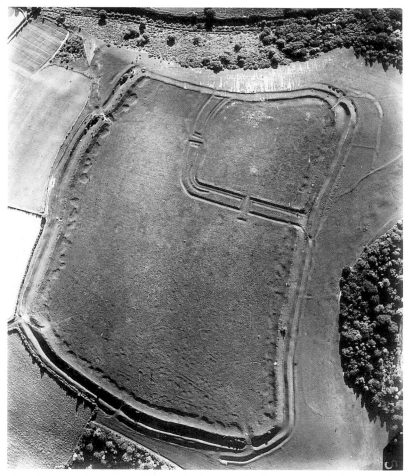

The Iron Age Hillfort at Hod Hill, showing the Roman Army's fort built in the north-west corner.

A half-legionary fortress was built by the Stour at Lake Farm near Wimborne, and a harbour was established at Hamworthy. A large donkey mill which probably belonged to the legion was found in the mud here, which must have fallen from a supply ship and not been recovered.

Hod Hill lay in advance of this position to protect it from interference. The legion's trunk road from Silchester led to Badbury Rings and from there to Hamworthy harbour via the Lake Farm fortress. Later the road was extended to a supply point at Weymouth harbour, and a fort was established at Dorchester. This position was protected by a fort on a hilltop at Waddon near Beaminster. Finally, when the conquest of the Durotriges was complete, the road was again extended to Seaton and eventually Exeter, where the legion moved its fortress in about 55 A D.

It's impossible to say with any certainty how long the conquest of the Durotriges took. The building of forts and harbours and roads takes time, and finds of pottery and coins cannot be dated with great precision. It certainly was not over in one summer, and the later stages must have been completed by an unknown general who took over from Vespasian.

For a while the Durotriges lived under the direct rule of the local Roman military commanders. But Roman policy was to romanise the native tribes, to encourage them to adopt the Roman way of life, and to contribute to their own prosperity and that of the Roman empire at large. The Roman authorities had done this frequently and were good at it. So we can imagine the Durotrigian leaders being taken to see the benefits of the Roman style of life in the commandant's house in the legionary fortress, being wined and dined on a lavish scale, and being treated to steam baths.

Since the Durotriges had put up a strong resistance and many had been killed, the process must have taken a longer time than in some other parts of Britain. But Roman Dorchester itself (*Durnovaria*) is evidence that in the end the Durotriges fully accepted their part in the Roman empire. Look at the baths excavated in Dorchester in 1977, or at the great walls that enclosed Roman Dorchester. Look at the complex aqueduct that brought the supply of running water, or the sophisticated country villas which the native leaders built for themselves.

When the Roman government relinquished its hold over Britain in 410 A D, the Durotrigian authorities in Dorchester will have seen this news as a disaster, depriving them of their place in the Roman world, rather than as a release from serfdom.

FINDING OUT ABOUT THE PAST

The days are long gone when wealthy amateurs amused themselves by digging up ancient sites, keeping only those objects which might prove attractive decoration for their mantelpiece or talking points with their friends. Modern excavation is a complex process and is normally professionally directed. This does not mean that amateurs wishing to learn for themselves the skills and thrills of archaeological research cannot do so. Volunteers are often wanted on expertly conducted digs, and courses abound in universities and elsewhere.

For Dorset, the Dorset Natural History and Archaeological Society publishes a list every spring of digs happening during the year. Their address is Dorset County Museum, High West Street, Dorchester, Dorset DT1 1XA, telephone 01305 262735.

Nationally, the Council for British Archaeology offers advice and details of archaeological opportunities. Write to the CBA, 111 Walmgate, York YO1 2UA, telephone 01904 671417.

Even the professional archaeological units which carry out the usually urgent digging in advance of development and new roads, sometimes avail themselves of the help of volunteers. Contact Wessex Archaeology, Portway House, Old Sarum, Salisbury SP4 6EB, telephone 01722 326867.

Courses in almost every aspect of archaeology can be found in various branches of adult education. Contact the Public Programmes Office of Bristol University (0117 928 7172) or the School of Conservation Sciences at Bournemouth University (01202 595178).

SCIENCE AND ARCHAEOLOGY

The archaeologists of today frequently have scientific training. The story of early Dorset told in this book would not be possible without the use of scientific techniques developed in recent years.

AERIAL PHOTOGRAPHY This powerful archaeological tool has developed since the First World War, when flyers with historical interests found that the view of sites from above gave an enormously valuable perspective on the past. Not only could a grasp of a site as a whole be obtained, but new features could be discovered by way of crop marks, shadow marks and soil marks.

There are two types of aerial photograph. First the high level vertical photographs taken by the RAF or commercial firms for mapping purposes. These may or may not contain archaeological information, depending on the weather or the time of year.

Secondly there are low level, usually oblique, potographs, taken by professionals or amateurs for archaeological purposes. These will have been taken because it is felt that archaeological sites are visible in them.

Aerial photographs can be found in County and District Council Planning offices, or in Museums and Record Offices, and it may be possible to arrange to copy them. Major collections of photographs can be found at the Department of Aerial Photography at the University of Cambridge, and at the National Monuments Record at Swindon. Photographs can be inspected at both locations by personal visits, but they will also answer questions about the availability of photographs of particular sites, and sell you copies.

What lies hidden in your photographs? There are several factors at work to reveal archaeological features to the aerial camera. Shadow marks on photographs are most useful for the exploration of low banks, walls and ditches remaining from former villages, field systems etc. This is particularly effective when the sun was low in the sky at the time of the photograph.

An equally important cause of revealing marks is the effect produced by the growth and ripening of crops (cropmarks). There is better growth over buried ditches and pits, and worse growth over buried walls, roads and stony areas. It is even possible for the soil itself to reveal the marks of buried features through its colour.

ANALYSING STONE TOOLS AND POTTERY If you look at neolithic axes in many of our museums, you will see a mark where a slice of stone has been removed by a diamond saw and the resulting slot filled with plaster. While it is undesirable to harm ancient

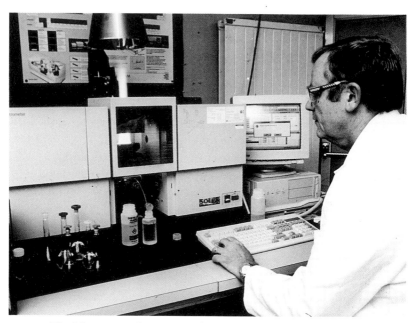

The laboratory: the Atomic Absorption Spectrometer analyses
the chemical composition of metals.

artefacts in this way, the results sometimes justify the damage. The
thin slice removed is polished to a thickness of only a fraction of a
millimetre. It can then be illuminated from behind in a microscope,
the constituent minerals identified and their relative quantities noted.

The results are compared with known samples taken by geologists
from a wide range of stone types in Britain and abroad, and thus
in many cases a firm opinion can be given as to their place of
origin. The most startling results from this have been in the Neolithic
period, where we now know that many fine axe types were sold far
away from where they were manufactured by travelling traders, presumably in return for food or other tradable commodities.

The same thing can be done with pottery, and here thin slicing has
shown from the minerals involved the likely area of the potters'
workshops.

ARCHAEOMAGNETISM It has long been known to geographers that the magnetic poles of the earth vary in position and intensity. When maps indicate the magnetic north pole, they have to include the date, without which the information is meaningless.

Where fired clay structures such as kilns and ovens are still in situ on an archaeological site, the position and the intensity of the poles is fossilised within the clay. It is the magnetic oxides haematite and magnetite that adopt the pattern of the earth's magnetism when they are heated, and keep it in their structure when they cool.

Obviously the samples have to be carefully marked with their position and orientation before they are moved to the laboratory for the magnetic pattern to be read. The results have then to be compared with the known pattern of movement of the poles in relation to Britain that has been built up over years of study, back for over two millennia.

DENDROCHRONOLOGY This is the dating of wood by the pattern of tree rings, and was the first of the absolute dating methods to be established for archaeology in the 1920s. A core sample of timber is taken from the wood, whether in excavation or from standing buildings.

This shows the annual growth rings produced by the tree. These rings vary in size year by year, according to the climate. Within limits the rings of trees from the same region will show similar patterns over the same period. By comparison with a master chart for your area the date after which the tree must have been cut down can be established.

EXCAVATION Excavation was once for the most part an amateur affair conducted mainly at weekends and in the university summer holidays. Nowadays it is mainly professional, though the amateur still has a part to play. Major excavations are done by archaeological units such as Wessex Archaeology. Small excavations may be done by local museums or societies, but are usually directed by professionals.

Excavation is a complex scientific process, not digging for treasure as it is commonly represented. After much preliminary research into the site, the ground is cut open in a way similar to a surgical operation, paying attention to the structure of the soil and how the various layers relate to one another. A careful record is made of everything, by writing, drawing and photography. Once the dig is over this will be the only record of what was there.

Excavation is always regarded as the last resort – after all it does destroy the site in the process. Nowadays every effort is made to preserve sites, if possible without excavation.

FIELDWORK Much time is spent by archaeologists studying and recording the landscape by methods other than excavation. If there are the fields of an Iron Age village still visible on the surface, it is a valuable but time consuming task to survey them in detail while they are still visible. Information about them will come from this survey – excavation might add little.

The positions, sizes and characteristics of a group of round barrows might similarly be studied with profit, especially comparing their condition with that of several years ago. This sort of archaeological research can be done without harm to the monuments themselves.

GEOPHYSICAL PROSPECTING Increasingly it is becoming possible to make some examination of what is buried under the ground without digging holes at all. There are three major types of instrument, each of which works well in some conditions but less well in others.

The resistivity meter is driven into the soil surface at regular intervals and reads the electrical resistance between its probes. This gives an indication of the presence of buried walls, ditches etc. Faster in use is the magnetometer which reads, disturbances to the earth's magnetic field caused by buried features. Finally there is the new technology of ground radar which alone can 'see' features several metres below the surface, for instance in a town site with many metres of archaeological deposits. This is however expensive and still under development.

There is now a guide to these prospecting methods, *Seeing beneath the soil*, by Anthony Clark (1990).

POLLEN ANALYSIS All flowering plants produce pollen as part of their reproductive processes. This pollen mostly ends up in the ground close by. Each grain of pollen is identifiable under the microscope by its shape. In suitable soils, mainly the acid ones, pollen survives and thus it can provide proof of the plants growing in the area of, say, a

[70]

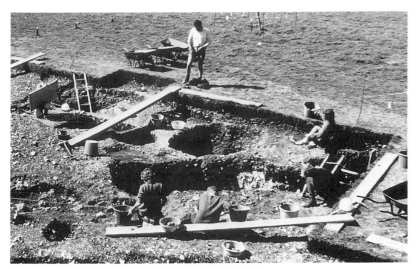

Large scale excavation at Maiden Castle in 1986.

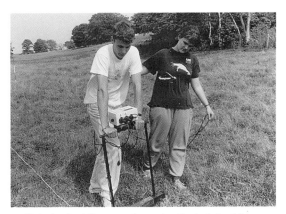

Geophysical Prospection: the Resistivity Meter
searches for archaeological features underground.

burial mound, just before its construction sealed the soil beneath it.

Essentially this provides information about the landscape, and particularly about cereal and other crops which might have been grown at that time. It will not provide a date, unless the changing pattern of vegetation is already known over a long period for the area, and the sample can be fitted into this pattern.

RADIO-CARBON DATING This was the greatest discovery of them all, one of the more useful by-products of atomic research in the Second World War. It has made possible absolute dating in remote periods where previously we could only guess. It is not surprising that the development of the technique has been called the radio-carbon revolution.

The radioactive isotope of carbon, C-14, is constantly produced in the atmosphere by radiation from the sun. All living matter, plant and animal, takes up C-14 during its life from the atmosphere, but ceases to do so on its death. After death the C-14 in the plant or animal decays at a known rate (it reduces by half every 5730 years). It follows that by measuring the C-14 present in an archaeological sample of bone or wood and calculating back, it is possible to determine at what date the sample would have been at the normal atmospheric level, and thus its absolute date.

As a result of the use of this process, the date of the construction of Stonehenge, the date of the arrival of farmers in Britain, are no longer vague guesses, but well-researched facts.

A full guide to radio-carbon and other dating methods is available; *Science based dating in archaeology*, by M. J. Aitken (1990).

THERMOLUMINESCENCE This is a remarkable method of dating pottery which is independent of the traditional methods of shape and pattern and fabric.

There are tiny quantities of radioactive matter in clay, emissions from which disturb electrons in quartz crystals. If the fired clay is reheated in a special chamber the electrons return and give off light in the process. The measurement of this light (and thus the amount of radioactive matter remaining) gives the date at which the original firing took place.

This is an important process when new cultures are discovered and there is no obvious point of comparison with known neighbours. Combined with, say, radio-carbon dating, a firm date range for the culture can be established.

PLACES TO VISIT

ABBOTSBURY CASTLE. Small Iron Age hillfort near Abbotsbury. Privately owned, but free access at all times. The interior has never been ploughed, and it is possible to see the huts in which the inhabitants lived. Turn off the B3157 Abbotsbury-Bridport road soon after the steep climb from the village. SY 556866

BADBURY RINGS. Iron Age hillfort near Wimborne, used as a point of alignment by several Roman roads. National Trust, but free access at all times. No dogs allowed. Car park off the B3082 Wimborne-Blandford road part way along the Kingston Lacy avenue of beeches. The hillfort has never been excavated. ST 964030

BOKERLEY DYKE. Bank and ditch forming the prehistoric boundary of Dorset on the north-east. Privately owned, but access free at all times from adjacent car park and footpaths. On the Blandford-Salisbury road (A354) just beyond Woodyates. SU 033199

CAME WOOD. Bronze Age barrow cemetery on either side of Culliford crossroads on the minor road from the Ridgeway (A354) to Broadmayne, near the turning to Preston and Sutton Poyntz. The barrows, including an excellent pond barrow, lie partly in the open field by the cross roads (no access) and partly in Came Wood. There are footpaths through the wood. The barrows are aligned with a bank barrow of probable Neolithic date which lies at the eastern end of the alignment. Park in the lay-by near the crossroads. SY 699853

DORSET COUNTY MUSEUM. In High West Street, Dorchester. Admission charge, free to members of the Dorset Natural History and Archaeological Society. Telephone 01305 262735. Substantial collections of artefacts from prehistoric (and later) sites in Dorset. Aerial photographs and interpretative displays.

EGGARDON. Iron Age hillfort in dramatic location at the western end of the chalk uplands of Dorset, overlooking the Marshwood Vale. In some parts of the interior it is still possible to see hollows caused by the sinking of Iron Age grain storage pits. Privately owned, but free access at all times. Park by the roadside and follow footpath. 10 miles west of Dorchester along the old Roman road. SY 542946

GRIMSTONE. Iron Age (later Roman) village and its fields, unploughed since Roman times. Privately owned. A footpath passes through the site, but permission is needed to walk over the full extent of the ancient fields. Park in Grimstone on the A37 Dorchester-Yeovil road, then through the railway arch and up the hill via the dairy. SY 646956

HAMBLEDON HILL. Spectacular Iron Age hillfort and Neolithic causewayed camp near Child Okeford. Interior unploughed – the sites of huts can be seen. Free access. Footpaths from north, east and west sides. About a mile further on from Hod Hill (see below). ST 845124

HELL STONE. Partially reconstructed Neolithic stone tomb from which the earth mound has weathered away. Privately owned, but footpaths from Portesham (B3157) or from the top of Portesham Hill. SY 605867

HENGISTBURY HEAD. Iron Age harbour in what is now Christchurch harbour. Double ramparts defend the hilltop dating to the first century BC when it was a port. Large car park outside the ramparts, Long walk, or use the 'land trains'. Signposted from the B3059 at Southbourne. SZ 175907

HOD HILL. Iron Age hillfort containing a smaller Roman fort, built at the time of the Roman conquest. National Trust. Free access at all times. Steep climb. Small car park off the minor road to Child

Okeford from the A350 Blandford-Shaftesbury, just north of Stour-paine. ST 855108

KINGSTON RUSSELL STONE CIRCLE. Small, much damaged stone circle of late Neolithic or early Bronze Age date. On private land, but free access at all times. Take footpath from the minor road from Hardye's Monument to Abbotsbury. SY 578878

KNOWLTON. The second late Neolithic religious centre after Dorchester. The middle sized henge monument survives intact, largely because of the derelict church inside it. The other henges are not easily visible. English Heritage site, free access at all times. Follow the B3078 north from Wimborne for 7 miles. SU 025103

MAIDEN CASTLE. The great hillfort of the Iron Age people of Dorset, the Durotriges. English Heritage site, but free access at all times. Turning marked off the Dorchester-Weymouth road (A354) in the outskirts of Dorchester. Car park. SY 667885

MAUMBURY RINGS. The visible monument is a Roman amphitheatre, but it contains buried within it the remains of a small Neolithic henge monument, which was converted by the Romans. Free access at all times. On the southern outskirts of Dorchester, just beyond the brewery. Park in the market car park. SY 690899

NEW BARN. Reconstructed Iron Age village in Bradford Peverell, three miles north-west of Dorchester on the A37. Open to the public. Entry charge. SY 656924.

NINE STONES. Small stone circle of late Neolithic or early Bronze Age date adjacent to the A35 Dorchester-Bridport road just west of Winterbourne Abbas. English Heritage site, but free access at all times. No car park. Stop near farm entrance towards the village, and cross the road carefully. SY 611903

OAKLEY DOWN. Best known of the Bronze Age round barrow cemeteries in Dorset. Privately owned. A good view of the barrows can be obtained from the road, but permission is needed to walk in the field. A footpath runs along the Roman road at the back of the field. There are several spectacular examples of the disc barrow, where a small mound lies within a large circular ditch and bank. Just north-east of the Sixpenny Handley roundabout on the A354 Blandford-Salisbury Road. SU 018173

PILSDEN PEN. Iron Age hillfort on steep hill close to the Birdsmoorgate-Broadwindsor road (B3164). Privately owned, but free access at all times. The low mounds in the interior are artificial rabbit warrens built much later than the hillfort. ST 413013

POOR LOT. Bronze Age barrow group on the A35 two miles west of Winterbourne Abbas. Parking difficult, but possible with care on the side road to the north. English Heritage site with free access at all times. SY 587908

RAWLESBURY. Small Iron Age hillfort with superb views. West of Bulbarrow. Privately owned, but access via footpaths. Near the minor road from Higher Ansty to Hazlebury Bryan. ST 767058

THICKTHORN DOWN. Southern terminal of the seven mile long Dorset Cursus, adjacent to a Neolithic long barrow. The monuments are on private property, but can be seen well from the road. They lie a short distance from the A354 Blandford-Salisbury road. Take the turning to Gussage St Michael. ST 970124

TURNWORTH. Iron Age (later Roman) farm with fields preserved from ploughing. Car park at Okeford Hill picnic site, then footpath to Ringmoor. Off minor road 5 miles north of Winterborne Whitchurch which is on the A354. National Trust, but free access at all times. ST 807087.

FURTHER READING

BOOKS ABOUT PREHISTORIC BRITAIN

Bahn, Paul G., *Prehistoric Art* (Cambridge Illustrated History) 1998
Barton, Nicholas, *Stone Age Britain* (English Heritage) 1997
Bowen, H.C., *Ancient Fields* 1970
Bradley, Richard, *The Prehistoric Settlement of Britain* 1978
Burl, Aubrey, *Prehistoric Astronomy and Ritual* (Shire Book) 1983
Burl, Aubrey, *Prehistoric Stone Circles* (Shire) 2nd ed 1983
Cavendish, Richard, *Prehistoric England* 1983
Cunliffe, Barry, *Danebury, Anatomy of an Iron Age Hillfort* 1983
Cunliffe, Barry, *Iron Age Britain* (English Heritage) 1995
Cunliffe, Barry, *Iron Age Communities in Britain* 1974
Cunliffe, Barry, *The Ancient Celts* 1997
Cunliffe, Barry, *The Oxford Illustrated Prehistory of Europe* 1994
Daniel, Glyn & Bahn, Paul, *Ancient Places, the Prehistoric and Celtic sites of Britain* 1987
Darvill, Timothy, *Prehistoric Britain* 1987
Darvill, Timothy, *Prehistoric Britain from the Air* 1996
Delaney, Frank, *Legends of the Celts* 1989
Dyer, James, *Ancient Britain* 1990
Green, Miranda Jane, *Celtic Myths* (British Museum) 1994
Jersey, Philip de, *Celtic Coinage in Britain* (Shire) 1996
Lawson, Andrew J., *Cave Art* (Shire) 1991
Manley, John, *Atlas of Prehistoric Britain* 1989
Pearson, Michael Parker, *Bronze Age Britain* (English Heritage) 1990
Reynolds, Peter J., *Butser, Ancient Farm* 1980
Ritchie, W.F. and J.N.G., *Celtic Warriors* (Shire Book) 1985
Spindler, Konrad, *The Man in the Ice* 1994
Stead, I.M., *Celtic Art* (British Museum) 1985
Thom, A., *Megalithic Sites in Britain* 1967
Thomas, Charles, *Celtic Britain* 1986
Timms, Peter, *Flint Implements of the Old Stone Age* (Shire) 1980
Wainwright, Geoffrey, *The Henge Monuments, Ceremony and Society in Prehistoric Britain* 1989
Wood, John Edwin, *Sun, Moon and Standing Stones* 1978
Wymer, John, *The Palaeolithic Age* 1982

Alcock, Leslie, *By South Cadbury is that Camelot* 1972

Castleden, Rodney, *The Cerne Giant* 1996

Cunliffe, Barry, *Hengistbury Head, Dorset,* Vol 1 1987

Grinsell, L.V., *Dorset Barrows* 1959

Mercer, Roger, *Hambledon Hill, A Neolithic Landscape* 1980

Penny, A. and Wood, J.E., *The Dorset Cursus Complex* (Arch Journal 130 for 1973) 1973

Putnam, Bill, *Roman Dorset* 1984

RCHME (Royal Commission for Historical Monuments for England) *An Inventory of the Historical Monuments in the County of Dorset* 1970

Sharples, N.M., *Maiden Castle, Excavations and Field Survey 1985-6* 1991

Sharples, Niall M., *Maiden Castle* (English Heritage) 1991

Smith, Roland J.C. *et al Excavations along the Route of the Dorchester By-pass, Dorset 1986-8* 1997

Wainwright, Geoffrey, *Mount Pleasant, Dorset: Excavations 1970-71* 1979

Wheeler, R.E.M. *Maiden Castle, Dorset* 19473

JOURNALS

Many articles about prehistoric Dorset appear annually in *The Proceedings of the Dorset Natural History and Archaeological Society.* More general articles about prehistoric Britain in general appear in *The Proceedings of the Prehistoric Society.* Up to date news on recent excavations appears in *Current Archaeology.*

ACKNOWLEDGEMENTS

I would like to thank Maureen Putnam for her help in the preparation of this book. I would also like to thank the following for allowing the inclusion of illustrations in their possession or for which they hold the copyright. Bournemouth University: pages 68, 71 (bottom): Cambridge University: page 50: Dorset County Museum: frontispiece, pages 14, 17, 19, 23, 28, 35, 41 (both), 54, 58, 59, 60: New Barn Field Centre, Bradford Peverell: page 48: Francesca Radcliffe: pages 25, 31, 37, 39, 47 (both), 49: Royal Commission Historical Monuments (England), © Crown Copyright: pages 6, 42, 52, 53, 64: Wessex Archaeology: the illustration on the front cover by Jane Brayne, pages 57, 71 (top).

The

DISCOVER DORSET

Series of Books

A series of paperback books providing informative illustrated
introductions to Dorset's history, culture and way of life.
The following titles have so far been published.

BRIDGES *David McFetrich and Jo Parsons*

CASTLES AND FORTS *Colin Pomeroy*

CRANBORNE CHASE *Desmond Hawkins*

GEOLOGY *Paul Ensom*

THE GEORGIANS *Jo Draper*

THE INDUSTRIAL PAST *Peter Stanier*

ISLE OF PURBECK *Paul Hyland*

LEGENDS *Jeremy Harte*

PORTLAND *Stuart Morris*

POTTERY *Penny Copland-Griffiths*

THE PREHISTORIC AGE *Bill Putnam*

SAXONS AND VIKINGS *David Hinton*

SHIPWRECKS *Maureen Attwooll*

STONE QUARRYING *Jo Thomas*

THE VICTORIANS *Jude James*

All the books about Dorset published by The Dovecote Press
are available in bookshops throughout the county,
or in case of difficulty direct from the publishers.
The Dovecote Press Ltd, Stanbridge,
Wimborne, Dorset BH21 4JD
Tel: 01258 840549.